Biomaterials for Bone Tissue Engineering

Biomaterials for Bone Tissue Engineering

Special Issue Editor
José A. Sanz-Herrera

MDPI • Basel • Beijing • Wuhan • Barcelona • Belgrade • Manchester • Tokyo • Cluj • Tianjin

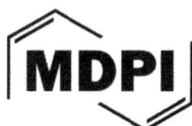

Special Issue Editor
José A. Sanz-Herrera
University of Sevilla
Spain

Editorial Office
MDPI
St. Alban-Anlage 66
4052 Basel, Switzerland

This is a reprint of articles from the Special Issue published online in the open access journal *Applied Sciences* (ISSN 2076-3417) (available at: https://www.mdpi.com/journal/applsci/special_issues/Bone_Tissue_Engineering).

For citation purposes, cite each article independently as indicated on the article page online and as indicated below:

LastName, A.A.; LastName, B.B.; LastName, C.C. Article Title. *Journal Name* **Year**, *Article Number*, Page Range.

ISBN 978-3-03928-965-3 (Hbk)
ISBN 978-3-03928-966-0 (PDF)

© 2020 by the authors. Articles in this book are Open Access and distributed under the Creative Commons Attribution (CC BY) license, which allows users to download, copy and build upon published articles, as long as the author and publisher are properly credited, which ensures maximum dissemination and a wider impact of our publications.

The book as a whole is distributed by MDPI under the terms and conditions of the Creative Commons license CC BY-NC-ND.

Contents

About the Special Issue Editor vii

José A. Sanz-Herrera
Special Issue on "Biomaterials for Bone Tissue Engineering"
Reprinted from: *Appl. Sci.* **2020**, *10*, 2660, doi:10.3390/app10082660 1

Thanh Danh Nguyen, Olufemi E. Kadri, Vassilios I. Sikavitsas and Roman S. Voronov
Scaffolds with a High Surface Area-to-Volume Ratio and Cultured Under Fast Flow Perfusion Result in Optimal O_2 Delivery to the Cells in Artificial Bone Tissues
Reprinted from: *Appl. Sci.* **2019**, *9*, 2381, doi:10.3390/app9112381 5

Ramin Rahmani, Maksim Antonov, Lauri Kollo, Yaroslav Holovenko and Konda Gokuldoss Prashanth
Mechanical Behavior of Ti6Al4V Scaffolds Filled with $CaSiO_3$ for Implant Applications
Reprinted from: *Appl. Sci.* **2019**, *9*, 3844, doi:10.3390/app9183844 19

Sheila Lascano, Cristina Arévalo, Isabel Montealegre-Melendez, Sergio Muñoz, José A. Rodriguez-Ortiz, Paloma Trueba and Yadir Torres
Porous Titanium for Biomedical Applications: Evaluation of the Conventional Powder Metallurgy Frontier and Space-Holder Technique
Reprinted from: *Appl. Sci.* **2019**, *9*, 982, doi:10.3390/app9050982 31

Yu-Che Cheng, Chien-Hsun Chen, Hong-Wei Kuo, Ting-Ling Yen, Ya-Yuan Mao and Wei-Wen Hu
Electrical Stimulation through Conductive Substrate to Enhance Osteo-Differentiation of Human Dental Pulp-Derived Stem Cells
Reprinted from: *Appl. Sci.* **2019**, *9*, 3938, doi:10.3390/app9183938 45

Masami Kanawa, Akira Igarashi, Katsumi Fujimoto, Veronica Sainik Ronald, Yukihito Higashi, Hidemi Kurihara, Yukio Kato and Takeshi Kawamoto
Potential Marker Genes for Predicting Adipogenic Differentiation of Mesenchymal Stromal Cells
Reprinted from: *Appl. Sci.* **2019**, *9*, 2942, doi:/10.3390/app9142942 61

Carlo F. Grottoli, Riccardo Ferracini, Mara Compagno, Alessandro Tombolesi, Osvaldo Rampado, Lucrezia Pilone, Alessandro Bistolfi, Alda Borrè, Alberto Cingolani and Giuseppe Perale
A Radiological Approach to Evaluate Bone Graft Integration in Reconstructive Surgeries
Reprinted from: *Appl. Sci.* **2019**, *9*, 1469, doi:10.3390/app9071469 71

Antonio Nappo, Carlo Rengo, Giuseppe Pantaleo, Gianrico Spagnuolo and Marco Ferrari
Influence of Implant Dimensions and Position on Implant Stability: A Prospective Clinical Study in Maxilla Using Resonance Frequency Analysis
Reprinted from: *Appl. Sci.* **2019**, *9*, 860, doi:10.3390/app9050860 85

Mantas Vaitiekūnas, Darius Jegelevičius, Andrius Sakalauskas and Simonas Grybauskasme
Automatic Method for Bone Segmentation in Cone Beam Computed Tomography Data Set
Reprinted from: *Appl. Sci.* **2020**, *10*, 236, doi:10.3390/app10010236 93

Hendrikje Raben, Peer W. Kämmerer, Rainer Bader, and Ursula van Rienen
Establishment of a Numerical Model to Design an Electro-Stimulating System for a Porcine Mandibular Critical Size Defect
Reprinted from: *Appl. Sci.* **2019**, *9*, 2160, doi:0.3390/app9102160 107

Jacobo Baldonedo, José R. Fernández, José A. López-Campos and AbrahamSegade
Analysis of Damage Models for Cortical Bone
Reprinted from: *Appl. Sci.* **2019**, *9*, 2710, doi:10.3390/app9132710 125

José A. Sanz-Herrera, Juan Mora-Macías, Esther Reina-Romo, Jaime Domínguez and Manuel Doblaré
Multiscale Characterisation of Cortical Bone Tissue
Reprinted from: *Appl. Sci.* **2019**, *9*, 5228, doi:10.3390/app9235228 137

Yong-Gon Koh, Jin-Ah Lee, Hwa-Yong Lee, Hyo-Jeong Kim and Kyoung-Tak Kang
Biomechanical Evaluation of the Effect of Mesenchymal Stem Cells on Cartilage Regeneration in Knee Joint Osteoarthritis
Reprinted from: *Appl. Sci.* **2019**, *9*, 1868, doi:10.3390/app9091868 155

Dae Woo Park, Aekyeong Lim, Jong Woong Park, Kwon Mook Lim and Hyun Guy Kang
Biomechanical Evaluation of a New Fixation Type in 3D-Printed Periacetabular Implants using a Finite Element Simulation
Reprinted from: *Appl. Sci.* **2019**, *9*, 820, doi:10.3390/app9050820 167

Algirdas Maknickas, Vidmantas Alekna, Oleg Ardatov, Olga Chabarova, Darius Zabulionis, Marija Tamulaitienė and Rimantas Kačianauskas
FEM-Based Compression Fracture Risk Assessment in Osteoporotic Lumbar Vertebra L1
Reprinted from: *Appl. Sci.* **2019**, *9*, 3013, doi:10.3390/app9153013 177

Dan T. Zaharie and Andrew T.M. Phillips
A Comparative Study of Continuum and Structural Modelling Approaches to Simulate Bone Adaptation in the Pelvic Construct
Reprinted from: *Appl. Sci.* **2019**, *9*, 3320, doi:10.3390/app9163320 199

Jose A. Sanz-Herrera and Esther Reina-Romo
Continuum Modeling and Simulation in Bone Tissue Engineering
Reprinted from: *Appl. Sci.* **2019**, *9*, 3674, doi:10.3390/app9183674 217

About the Special Issue Editor

José A. Sanz-Herrera is an Associate Professor at the School of Engineering of the University of Sevilla, Sevilla, Spain. He completed his Ph.D. degree in biomedical engineering at the University of Zaragoza, Zaragoza, Spain, and has held several visiting research positions at École Polytechnique, France; Massachusetts Institute of Technology, USA; Imperial College, UK; University of Colorado at Boulder, USA; and KU Leuven, Belgium. His research includes different aspects of computational biomechanics, biomaterials modelling, and tissue engineering, with a focus in the recent years on the modelling and simulation of cell-biomaterial interaction and cellular mechanics. He has more than 50 publications in these topics including peer-reviewed journals, book chapters, and conference proceedings.

Editorial

Special Issue on "Biomaterials for Bone Tissue Engineering"

José A. Sanz-Herrera

Escuela Técnica Superior de Ingeniería, Universidad de Sevilla, 41092 Sevilla, Spain; jsanz@us.es; Tel.: +34-95-448-7293

Received: 2 April 2020; Accepted: 10 April 2020; Published: 12 April 2020

---

1. Preface

The present Special Issue covers recent advances in the field of tissue engineering applied to bone tissue. Bone tissue engineering is a wide research topic, so different works from different transversal areas of research are shown. This Special Issue is a good example of a multidisciplinary collaboration in this research field. Authors from different disciplines, such as medical scientists, biomedical engineers, biologists, biomaterial researchers, clinicians, and mechanical engineers, are included from different laboratories and universities across the world. I specially thank the work and time of the reviewers, listed in Table A1 (in Appendix A), for their time and efforts in reviewing the papers compiled in this Special Issue.

2. Contents

The bone tissue engineering (BTE) field aims at the development of artificial bone substitutes that restore (partially or totally) the natural regeneration capability of bone tissue lost under the circumstances of injury, significant defects, or diseases, such as osteoporosis. BTE is a multidisciplinary area of research which includes the synthesis, fabrication, characterization, and experimentation of biomaterials. The modeling and simulation of biomaterials, bone tissue, and bone tissue interactions are also important methodologies in BTE. As a result, in this Special Issue, the 16 published papers can be classified within these general subfields.

Regarding the synthesis, characterization, and experimentation of biomaterials in BTE, Nguyen et al. [1] synthesized a class of scaffolds with a high surface area-to-volume ratio, which optimizes O_2 delivery to the scaffold interior. This topic is one of the most important challenges to grow artificial tissues of clinically relevant sizes. In order to evaluate the performance of different scaffold designs, the authors used high-resolution 3D X-ray images of two common scaffold types, namely lattice Boltzmann fluid dynamics and reactive Lagrangian scalar tracking mass transfer solvers. The mechanical performance of scaffolds is of utmost importance in BTE for two main reasons: (i) the scaffold should present an overall stiffness similar to the natural bone tissue [2], and (ii) the mechanical stimuli at the bone–biomaterial surface have been evidenced as an important design parameter in BTE scaffolds [3]. In this context, Rahmani et al. [4] evaluated in silico the mechanical performance of additively manufactured BTE scaffolds. Moreover, the scaffolds were experimentally characterized by means of compressive tests. The experimental results showed a good agreement versus the finite element simulations. Similarly, Lascano et al. [5] evaluated the industrial implementation and potential technology transfer of different powder metallurgy techniques to obtain porous titanium scaffolds for BTE. The microstructural and mechanical properties were obtained, and further assessed by finite element models. The authors discussed the feasibility of synthesizing BTE titanium scaffolds from powder metallurgy techniques.

Several works have been published in this Special Issue regarding the experimentation of the different techniques in BTE to enhance bone growth and regeneration processes. Cheng et al. [6]

applied an electrical stimulation on human dental pulp-derived stem cells to promote bone healing. The results presented in this work are promising, and reveal an enhancement in calcium deposition at different days of the tests. Specifically, increasing levels of bone morphogenetic proteins were found using electrical stimulation in the early stage of osteodifferentiation. On the other hand, Kanawa et al. [7] studied adipogenic differentiation of mesenchymal stromal cells (MSCs), i.e., the formation of adipocytes (fat cells) from MSCs. Adipogenesis is a key process when MSCs are used in tissue engineering and regenerative medicine. The authors identified three genes involved in this process. Grottoli et al. [8] investigated a non-invasive methodology to assess and quantify bone growth and regeneration. Specifically, the authors developed a novel radiological approach, in substitution of invasive histology, for evaluating the level of osteointegration and osteogenesis in orthopedics to oral and maxillofacial bone grafts. The authors concluded that the newly established radiological protocol allowed the tracking of the bone grafts, and showed effective integration and bone regeneration. Finally, Nappo et al. [9] evaluated the dimensions and positions of dental implants regarding their stability. This issue is relevant for the correct osteointegration and long-term success of dental implant treatments. The authors evidenced that the implant length, diameter, and the maxillary regions have an influence on primary stability.

Modeling and simulation of BTE and related bone tissue processes are an active field of research with increasing importance, as demonstrated in this Special Issue. A total of nine papers were published in this area. First, Vaitiekūnas et al. [10] presented an automatic method for bone segmentation for the clinical practice of endodontics, orthodontics, and oral and maxillofacial surgery. The automatic method showed clinically acceptable accuracy results versus an experienced oral and maxillofacial surgeon. This method allows one to efficiently reconstruct 3D bone geometries to be applied in oral and maxillofacial surgery for the performance of a 3D virtual surgical plan (VSP) or for postoperative follow-ups, as well as for their use as an input in in silico models. Raben et al. [11] modeled the electrical stimulation as a therapeutic approach for the regeneration of large bone defects. Electrically stimulated implants for critical size defects in the lower jaw were modeled using segmentation and finite element software. Electric field maps were shown along the bone geometry. The authors concluded that the parameters used in the numerical studies shall be applied in future in in vivo validation studies. Baldonedo et al. [12] compared the different mathematical models which included the mechanical evolution of bone tissue damage. The models were numerically implemented, using the finite element method, and compared in 1D and 2D geometries. Moreover, Sanz-Herrera et al. [13] presented a multiscale approach of the cortical bone tissue. The results were assessed by experimental data, and they showed both macro- and microstructural stress and strain patterns, highlighting their differences and emphasizing the importance of multiscale techniques for the characterization of bone tissue. On the other hand, Koh et al. [14] developed a biomechanical model which allows to study cartilage defect regeneration in the knee joint. The model considered a biphasic poroelastic formulation, which was implemented in a finite element framework. The results were shown in a knee joint model including cell and tissue distributions in the cartilage defect. The model was able to predict interesting applications, such as the benefits of the gait cycle loading with flexion versus the use of simple weight-bearing loading.

In silico biomechanical simulations for biomaterials and implants have also been included in this Special Issue. In particular, Park et al. [15] studied 3D periacetabular implants using finite element simulations. Different implant models were generated from computed tomographies and medical images. The outcome of the simulations established the biomechanical performances of different implant designs. This methodology can be used in the design phase of different orthopedic products before implantation. Biomechanical analyses are also useful to predict important conclusions in orthopedics. For example, Maknickas et al. [16] analyzed the risk of fracture in the osteoporotic lumbar vertebra L1. The risk of fracture was evaluated by means of Monte Carlo finite element simulations. The paper includes some validation from 3D printed vertebra models. The conclusions establish that the risk of fracture is substantially higher for low levels of apparent density. Zaharie and Phillips [17] compared different finite element models of the pelvis using different continuum and structural modeling approaches. On one hand, continuum isotropic, continuum orthotropic, hybrid isotropic, and hybrid orthotropic models were developed. On the other hand, a structural model previously developed by the authors was considered. The results show interesting conclusions and knowledge when compared with a computed tomography-derived model of the pelvis.

Finally, the Special Issue ends with a review of the state-of-the-art numerical modeling and simulation of BTE [18]. This paper emphasizes the importance of in silico simulations in two main contexts: First, to optimize and reduce in vitro and in vivo tests (and hence to reduce time and cost) to evaluate the performance of biomaterials in BTE processes. Second, an in silico methodology can be used as a powerful design tool for biomaterials in BTE. The conclusions highlight the importance of the experimental validation of the numerical models, and hence the multidisciplinary collaboration of the involved scientific fields.

3. Conclusions

BTE is a mature field of research. It is also an active and hot topic of research. However, its clinical practice is not as evident as the scientific results. Therefore, the transfer of methods and technology from scientific research to clinical practice is the fundamental keystone of the methodology. It requires the multidisciplinary and transversal collaboration of biomaterial scientists, modelers, biologists, and clinicians. Moreover, in silico simulations of BTE processes may be helpful to accomplish this task. This Special Issue covered the different state-of-the-art techniques and methods of BTE, including many successful examples of multidisciplinary collaboration in this area. Therefore, the scientific advances and accomplishments shown in this Special Issue may add some light to make BTE a clinical viable reality.

Funding: This research was funded by the Ministerio de Economía y Competitividad del Gobierno de España, grant number PGC2018-097257-B-C31; and Consejería de Economía, Conocimiento, Empresas y Universidad Junta de Andalucía, grant number US-1261691.

Acknowledgments: We would like to sincerely thank our assistant editor, Marin Ma (marin.ma@mdpi.com), for all the efforts during the different steps in the edition of this Special Issue.

Conflicts of Interest: The authors declare no conflict of interest.

Appendix A

Table A1. Special Issue reviewer list.

J. Teo	A. Dehghan	J. Lee	H. Almeida
E. Onal	H. Yuan	F. Alifui-Segbaya	P. Gentile
K. Tappa	I. Polozov	H.S. Moghaddam	M.A. Bonifacio
E. Pegg	A. Ballini	L.-C. Zhang	M. Schulze
Gaetano Isola	Seunghee Cha	Charles J. Malemud	G. Milcovich
D. Tomasz	A. Saboori	M. Klontzas	A. Celentano
Z. Khurshid	C. Rossa	M. Padial-Molina	J. Żmudzki
K.-T. Lim	P. Palma	S. A. Danesh-Sani	M. Ratajczak
J. Hu	F. Bernardello	A. Scherberich	B. Wildemann

References

1. Nguyen, T.; Kadri, O.; Sikavitsas, V.; Voronov, R. Scaffolds with a High Surface Area-to-Volume Ratio and Cultured Under Fast Flow Perfusion Result in Optimal O2 Delivery to the Cells in Artificial Bone Tissues. *Appl. Sci.* **2019**, *9*, 2381. [CrossRef]
2. Hutmacher, D.W. Scaffolds in tissue engineering bone and cartilage. *Biomaterials* **2000**, *21*, 2529–2543. [CrossRef]

3. Sanz-Herrera, J.A.; García-Aznar, J.M.; Doblaré, M. Scaffold microarchitecture determines internal bone directional growth structure: A numerical study. *J. Biomech.* **2010**, *43*, 2480–2486. [CrossRef] [PubMed]
4. Rahmani, R.; Antonov, M.; Kollo, L.; Holovenko, Y.; Prashanth, K. Mechanical Behavior of Ti6Al4V Scaffolds Filled with CaSiO3 for Implant Applications. *Appl. Sci.* **2019**, *9*, 3844. [CrossRef]
5. Lascano, S.; Arévalo, C.; Montealegre-Melendez, I.; Muñoz, S.; Rodriguez-Ortiz, J.; Trueba, P.; Torres, Y. Porous Titanium for Biomedical Applications: Evaluation of the Conventional Powder Metallurgy Frontier and Space-Holder Technique. *Appl. Sci.* **2019**, *9*, 982. [CrossRef]
6. Cheng, Y.; Chen, C.; Kuo, H.; Yen, T.; Mao, Y.; Hu, W. Electrical Stimulation through Conductive Substrate to Enhance Osteo-Differentiation of Human Dental Pulp-Derived Stem Cells. *Appl. Sci.* **2019**, *9*, 3938. [CrossRef]
7. Kanawa, M.; Igarashi, A.; Fujimoto, K.; Ronald, V.; Higashi, Y.; Kurihara, H.; Kato, Y.; Kawamoto, T. Potential Marker Genes for Predicting Adipogenic Differentiation of Mesenchymal Stromal Cells. *Appl. Sci.* **2019**, *9*, 2942. [CrossRef]
8. Grottoli, C.; Ferracini, R.; Compagno, M.; Tombolesi, A.; Rampado, O.; Pilone, L.; Bistolfi, A.; Borrè, A.; Cingolani, A.; Perale, G. A Radiological Approach to Evaluate Bone Graft Integration in Reconstructive Surgeries. *Appl. Sci.* **2019**, *9*, 1469. [CrossRef]
9. Nappo, A.; Rengo, C.; Pantaleo, G.; Spagnuolo, G.; Ferrari, M. Influence of Implant Dimensions and Position on Implant Stability: A Prospective Clinical Study in Maxilla Using Resonance Frequency Analysis. *Appl. Sci.* **2019**, *9*, 860. [CrossRef]
10. Vaitiekūnas, M.; Jegelevičius, D.; Sakalauskas, A.; Grybauskas, S. Automatic Method for Bone Segmentation in Cone Beam Computed Tomography Data Set. *Appl. Sci.* **2020**, *10*, 236. [CrossRef]
11. Raben, H.; Kämmerer, P.; Bader, R.; van Rienen, U. Establishment of a Numerical Model to Design an Electro-Stimulating System for a Porcine Mandibular Critical Size Defect. *Appl. Sci.* **2019**, *9*, 2160. [CrossRef]
12. Baldonedo, J.; Fernández, J.; López-Campos, J.; Segade, A. Analysis of Damage Models for Cortical Bone. *Appl. Sci.* **2019**, *9*, 2710. [CrossRef]
13. Sanz-Herrera, J.; Mora-Macías, J.; Reina-Romo, E.; Domínguez, J.; Doblaré, M. Multiscale Characterisation of Cortical Bone Tissue. *Appl. Sci.* **2019**, *9*, 5228. [CrossRef]
14. Koh, Y.; Lee, J.; Lee, H.; Kim, H.; Kang, K. Biomechanical Evaluation of the Effect of Mesenchymal Stem Cells on Cartilage Regeneration in Knee Joint Osteoarthritis. *Appl. Sci.* **2019**, *9*, 1868. [CrossRef]
15. Park, D.; Lim, A.; Park, J.; Lim, K.; Kang, H. Biomechanical Evaluation of a New Fixation Type in 3D-Printed Periacetabular Implants using a Finite Element Simulation. *Appl. Sci.* **2019**, *9*, 820. [CrossRef]
16. Maknickas, A.; Alekna, V.; Ardatov, O.; Chabarova, O.; Zabulionis, D.; Tamulaitienė, M.; Kačianauskas, R. FEM-Based Compression Fracture Risk Assessment in Osteoporotic Lumbar Vertebra L1. *Appl. Sci.* **2019**, *9*, 3013. [CrossRef]
17. Zaharie, D.; Phillips, A. A Comparative Study of Continuum and Structural Modelling Approaches to Simulate Bone Adaptation in the Pelvic Construct. *Appl. Sci.* **2019**, *9*, 3320. [CrossRef]
18. Sanz-Herrera, J.; Reina-Romo, E. Continuum Modeling and Simulation in Bone Tissue Engineering. *Appl. Sci.* **2019**, *9*, 3674. [CrossRef]

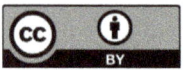

© 2020 by the author. Licensee MDPI, Basel, Switzerland. This article is an open access article distributed under the terms and conditions of the Creative Commons Attribution (CC BY) license (http://creativecommons.org/licenses/by/4.0/).

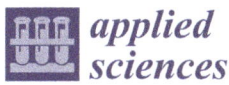

Article

Scaffolds with a High Surface Area-to-Volume Ratio and Cultured Under Fast Flow Perfusion Result in Optimal O_2 Delivery to the Cells in Artificial Bone Tissues

Thanh Danh Nguyen [1], Olufemi E. Kadri [1], Vassilios I. Sikavitsas [2] and Roman S. Voronov [1,*]

1. Otto H. York Department of Chemical and Materials Engineering, New Jersey Institute of Technology, Newark, NJ 07102, USA; dtn9@njit.edu (T.D.N.); ok26@njit.edu (O.E.K.)
2. School of Chemical, Biological and Materials Engineering, University of Oklahoma Norman, OK 73019, USA; vis@ou.edu
* Correspondence: rvoronov@njit.edu; Tel.: +1-973-642-4762

Received: 1 May 2019; Accepted: 7 June 2019; Published: 11 June 2019

Featured Application: Optimization of Scaffold Design and Flow Perfusion Culturing Conditions for Maximal Delivery of Oxygen to the Cells Embedded Deep Inside of Engineered Tissues.

Abstract: Tissue engineering has the potential for repairing large bone defects, which impose a heavy financial burden on the public health. However, difficulties with O_2 delivery to the cells residing in the interior of tissue engineering scaffolds make it challenging to grow artificial tissues of clinically-relevant sizes. This study uses image-based simulation in order to provide insight into how to better optimize the scaffold manufacturing parameters, and the culturing conditions, in order to resolve the O_2 bottleneck. To do this, high resolution 3D X-ray images of two common scaffold types (salt leached foam and non-woven fiber mesh) are fed into Lattice Boltzmann Method fluid dynamics and reactive Lagrangian Scalar Tracking mass transfer solvers. The obtained findings indicate that the scaffolds should have maximal surface area-to-solid volume ratios for higher chances of the molecular collisions with the cells. Furthermore, the cell culture media should be flown through the scaffold pores as fast as practically possible (without detaching or killing the cells). Finally, we have provided a parametric sweep that maps how the molecular transport within the scaffolds is affected by variations in rates of O_2 consumption by the cells. Ultimately, the results of this study are expected to benefit the computer-assisted design of tissue engineering scaffolds and culturing experiments.

Keywords: oxygen delivery; optimization; mass transfer; transport; bone tissue engineering; computational fluid dynamics; Lattice Boltzmann method; scaffold design; culturing protocol; Lagrangian scalar tracking

1. Introduction

Incidences of bone disorders constitute a significant economic burden to societies globally. In the United States alone, the total annual cost (direct and indirect) of treating an estimated 126.6 million people affected by musculoskeletal disorders exceeds $213 billion [1]. Moreover, with an increasingly obese and ageing population, this trend is expected to continue further. Unfortunately, according to U.S Department of Health & Human Services, only ~10% out of the 115,000 people who needed a lifesaving organ transplant in 2018 have actually received it. This is because despite the overwhelming demand, almost no FDA approved [2] artificial tissue products are commercially available today.

A major hurdle standing in the way of producing viable engineered bone is product size limitations. These in turn stem from the inability to deliver sufficient amounts of metabolites (e.g., O_2, nutrients, etc.) to the inner pore spaces of scaffolds, given that the cells consume them in large quantities as they build tissue. Among these, O_2 plays a critical role in the cell growth and proliferation, and thus its high concentrations have been correlated with both increased cellularity [3] and cell viability [4]. Conversely, a deficiency in O_2 can result in a hypoxic cell state, which is commonly associated with decreased metabolic activity and potentially undesirable differentiation behavior [5–7]. Hence, optimal oxygen transport is important in maintaining tissue function and overall survival within the artificial tissues. For that reason, bone tissue engineering scaffolds are typically cultured in perfusion bioreactors, the idea behind which is to facilitate the mass transfer using flow.

However, understanding what scaffold fabrication parameters and flow culturing conditions result in the optimal O_2 delivery to the cells is made difficult by the complexity of the pore network architectures in which they reside. This is because most large scaffolds are not transparent enough for microscopy, and it is also difficult to measure the O_2 concentrations at different locations within the scaffolds. Furthermore, the O_2 uptake rate by the cells changes over time [3]. All these complications make the problem even more difficult to solve manually. For these reasons, computer simulation of the O_2 transport and consumption offers itself as a viable alternative for obtaining insight into the microenvironment, which is experienced by the cells seeded on the surfaces of the scaffold pores.

Yet, modeling of mass transport (and specifically of O_2) within scaffolds is uncommon when compared to flow parameters, such as stimulatory fluid shear stress, permeability, and pressure (see Table II in Ref. [8]). Furthermore, Table 1 below summarizes our overview of the few O_2 models that we did find in literature. From it, it can be seen that the studies commonly use idealized geometries for the scaffolds (e.g., a homogeneous porous medium) instead of realistic image-based. In reality, however, the scaffold architectures may be inhomogeneous. Moreover, many of the models either do not take into account specificities of bone tissue engineering, such as the need for flow perfusion, which generates a stimulatory shear environment natural to the bone canaliculi [9,10]. Instead, many models either target tissue engineering in general, or they may be specific to other tissue engineering disciplines; for example, Ferroni et al. [11] modeled a cardiac scaffold, which is cultured under pulsatile flow (not the case for bone). Finally, few of the models take into account O_2 consumption by the cells. And among those that do, the rate is typically assumed to be constant. Thus, we were not able to find a single bone tissue engineering model that accounted for all of the following: the realistic scaffold structure, O_2 diffusion, convection, and variable consumption rates.

Table 1. Literature overview of O_2 simulations in tissue engineering scaffolds, shows that image-based simulation of convection with diffusion and reaction has not yet been done.

Scaffold Type	Simulated Geometry	O_2 Diffusion	O_2 Convection	O_2 Reaction	Varied Parameter	Citation
45S5 Bioglass-PCL Robocast, Bioactive Glass 70S30C Sol-Gel Foamed and Titania Foam Replicated	Micro-computed Tomography	Yes	No	No	Void Fraction	Fiedler et al. [12]
Cardiac Tissue Eng.	Idealized	Yes	Yes	No	Squeeze Pressure	Ferroni et al. [11]
Microchanneled Hydrogel	Idealized	Yes	No	No	Microchannel Configuration	Arrigoni et al. [13]
Periodically Self-Repeated Representative Volume Element	Idealized	Yes	No	Yes	Geometry of the Repeating Element	Li et al. [14]
Bone Tissue Eng. Molded Tantalum	Idealized	Yes	Yes	Yes	Flow rate	Bergemann et al. [4]
Homogeneous Porous Medium	Idealized	Yes	Yes	Yes	Flow rate, Porosity	Yan et al. [15]

Therefore, in this work we aim to shed insight on how scaffold manufacturing parameters and flow culturing conditions affect the O_2 transport and uptake by the cells in realistic bone tissue engineering scaffolds. To do this, we use two types of commonly-implemented types: the salt leached foam and the non-woven fiber mesh poly-L-lactic acid (PLLA) scaffolds. Their geometries are scanned in 3D using high resolution micro-computed tomography (µCT), and are imported into our image-based Lattice Boltzmann Method (LBM) flow [16–19] and reactive Lagrangian Scalar Tracking (rLST) mass transport [20] solvers. A big advantage of the latter is it can model particles with a range of reactivity, which is informative about how cells that are not necessarily starved for O_2 consume it. In this way, a more complete picture of O_2 transport within the different types of BTE scaffolds can be constructed. The overall computational scheme is depicted in Figure 1.

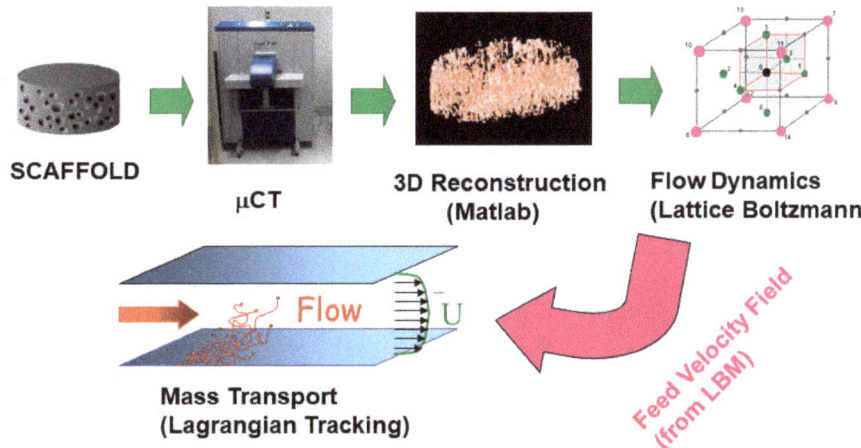

Figure 1. The image-based modeling methodology used in this work; scaffolds are scanned in 3D via high resolution µCT, reconstructed in silico, and the resulting geometries are used by the LBM and rLST solvers.

2. Materials and Methods

2.1. Scaffold Fabrication

The full details of the scaffold preparation protocols can be found in our previous publications [16,17]. Briefly, the scaffolds were non-woven fiber meshes constructed using polymer micro-fibers produced with spunbonding. The polymer used in the production of fibers was poly-L-lactic-acid (grade 6251D, 1.4% D enantiomer 108,500 MW, 1.87 PDI, NatureWorks LLC). A custom Brabender extruder (19.1 mm (0.75 in.) diameter × 381 mm length) was used to pressurize and melt the polymer. A manually circulated collection screen was used to collect a random even layering of fibers. Layers of fibers were stacked and measured until the stack reached a mass of 9.0 ± 0.1 g within an area of 162.8 cm^2. The collected non-woven fiber stack then had a 7 cm center cut sheet obtained from it. Finally, using an 8 mm diameter die, discs were punched from the layered fiber sheets. The resulting scaffolds used in culturing were 8 mm diameter and ~2.3 mm thickness. Average fiber diameter was measured optically, using a Nikon HFX-II microscope.

The porous foam scaffolds were prepared using solvent casting/particulate leaching method [21–24]. Briefly, poly-L-lactic acid (PLLA, 114,500 MW, 1.87 PDI, Birmingham Polymers) was dissolved into chloroform 5% w/v. The solution was then poured over a bed of sodium chloride crystals. Solvent was allowed to evaporate for 24 h. The resulting salt-polymer composite was inserted into an 8 mm diameter cylindrical mold and compressed at 500 psi. During compression, the composite was heated to 130 °C and held at constant temperature and pressure for 30 min. Using a diamond wheel saw (Model 650, South Bay Technology, Inc.), the resulting composite rod was cut into 2.3 mm thick discs. The discs were placed into deionized water (DIH$_2$O) under agitation for 2 days to leach out NaCl. Entire DIH$_2$O volumes were replaced twice per day. Leached discs were then removed from DIH$_2$O and placed under vacuum to remove moisture from the scaffolds. The resulting products were 8 mm diameter, 2.3 mm thick discs. Porosity of scaffolds was determined by measuring the solid volume (mass of the scaffold divided by the density of PLLA) and by comparing it to the total scaffold volume (assuming a cylindrical scaffold shape).

2.2. 3D Imaging and Virtual Reconstruction

The full details of our scanning procedure can be found in our previous publication [16,17,25]. Briefly, scaffolds were then scanned via μCT using a ScanCo VivaCT40 system (ScanCo Medical, Bassersdorf, Switzerland) to obtain 10 μm resolution, 2D intensity image slices at the optimum settings of 88 μA (intensity), and 45 kV (energy). The acquired X-ray images were filtered for noise reduction and assembled into 3D reconstructions of the scaffolds using a custom Matlab code (MathWorks Inc., Natick, MA). The scans were segmented using global thresholding. Threshold values were chosen such that the porosity of scaffolds from 3D reconstructions were within 1% of experimentally calculated porosities. Figure 2 is a typical 3D reconstruction of each scaffold type. Experimental porosities were obtained by measuring the solid volume (mass of the scaffolds divided by the density of scaffold materials) and comparing with total scaffold volume (assuming a cylindrical scaffold) as reported in [16,17,20].

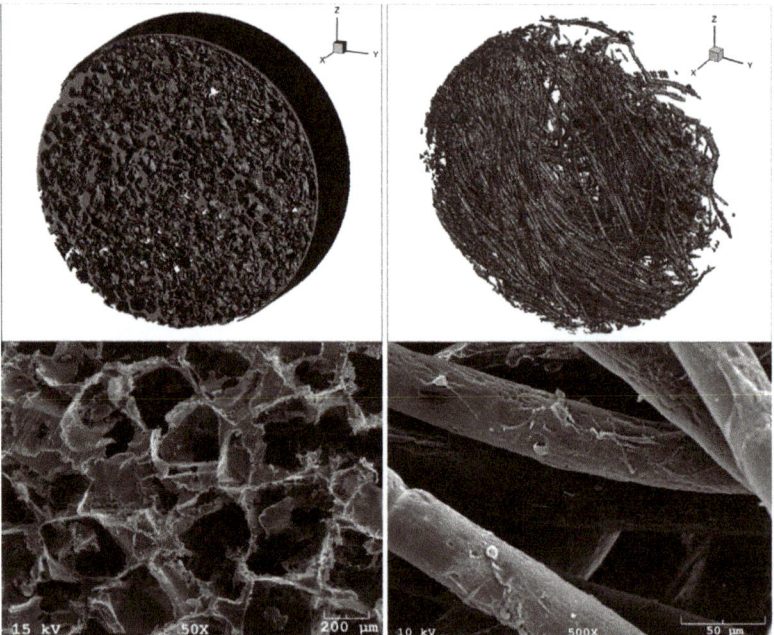

Figure 2. Visual comparison of the two scaffold architecture types used in this study. LEFT COLUMN—Salt-Leached Porous Foam Scaffold; RIGHT COLUMN—Non-woven Fiber Mesh Scaffold. TOP ROW—Three dimensional reconstructions of 8-mm-diameter and 2.3-mm-thickness scaffolds, obtained via μCT imaging (described in our previous works [16,17,25]). BOTTOM ROW—SEM close-ups of representative regions on the scaffolds' surfaces. Images are shown at two different magnifications to illustrate morphological feature scales of the two scaffold types. Both of the scaffolds are made from poly-L-lactic acid.

2.3. Fluid Flow Modeling: Lattice Boltzmann Method (LBM)

LBM was chosen for the present application because it is especially appropriate for modeling pore-scale flow through porous media (such as scaffolds) due to the simplicity with which it handles complicated boundaries [16–18,20,26–29]. This is because LBM uses structured meshes for complex geometries, unlike classical CFD approaches, which will rather utilize unstructured meshes. Another advantage of LBM is that it uses a direct method based on first principles at the mesoscopic scale rather than modeling the terms of the fluid flow governing equations at the macroscopic scale. In addition, the LBM method has gained popularity within the scientific computing community because of the ease with which it can be parallelized on supercomputers [30].

A previously developed custom-written, in-house code was used in this work [16–18,20,26,29,31]. The D3Q15 lattice [32], in conjunction with the single-relaxation time Bhatnagar, Gross, and Krook [33] collision term approximation, was used to perform simulations. The no-slip boundary condition was applied at solid faces using the "bounce-back" technique [34]. To take advantage of the inherent LBM parallelizability, domains were decomposed using message passing interface [18,26]. The code has been validated for several flow cases for which analytical solutions are available: forced flow in a slit, flow in a pipe, and flow through an infinite array of spheres [16,26].

Each simulation domain was composed of a scaffold placed inside of a pipe. This is meant to mimic the cassette holder that typically fixes the scaffold in the perfusion bioreactors. The pipe's length was taken to be approximately 10 times greater than the scaffold thickness, in order to avoid periodicity artifacts, and to ensure that a uniform parabolic profile is developed before the flow reaches the scaffolds. Simulations were performed for flow rates ranging between 0.15–1 mL/min. This is considered a suitable range for culturing bone tissue in typical perfusion bioreactors. Convergence was defined as when the average and highest velocities computed for the simulation domain vary by less than 0.01% for two consecutive time steps.

2.4. Oxygen Transport Modeling: Reactive Lagrangian Scalar Tracking (rLST)

The full details of the rLST code can be found in our prior publications [20,26]. Briefly, the trajectories of the rLST particles are determined by contributions from convection (obtained using the velocity field from the LBM simulations) and diffusion (i.e., Brownian motion obtained from a mesoscopic Monte-Carlo approach). For example, the new X position of a marker at time t+1 is calculated from the previous position at time t as follows:

$$\vec{X}_{t+1} = \vec{X}_t + \vec{U}_t^{(LBM)} \Delta t + \Delta \vec{X}_t^{(random)} \quad (1)$$

where $\vec{U}_t$ is the fluid velocity at the particle's location at time t, as obtained from the LBM solver. On the other hand, the random jump has a standard deviation that is given by $\sigma = \sqrt{2D_0 \Delta t} = \sqrt{2\nu \Delta t / Sc}$, where D_0 is the nominal molecular diffusivity (i.e., the diffusivity that the particles would have if their motion was purely Brownian). It can also be expressed in terms of the dimensionless Schmidt number Sc, which depends on the carrier fluid's viscosity. The molecular diffusivity of O_2 in the cell culture medium (assumed to be an aqueous solution at the physiological temperature of T = 37 °C) was 2.62×10^{-5} cm^2/s, which corresponded to a Schmidt number of 328.14.

The rLST simulations were performed using 1 million particles, which was found to be sufficient to reproduce analytical results from the Taylor–Aris formula, during the validation runs. Their initial positions were distributed uniformly in a release plane at the pipe's entrance. Furthermore, in order to model the O_2 consumption by the cells, each of the rLST particles had a probability 'q' to react upon colliding with the scaffold walls: ranging from q = 0 (non-reactive) to q = 1 (fully reactive).

It was also assumed that the scaffold's surface was uniformly covered with a monolayer of the cells, each of them capable of consuming the O_2. Since second order reactions (reactions between solute particles) were not considered for this model, any interactions between the rLST markers were neglected (i.e., they did not affect each other's path). This approximation is good for a dilute solution. The simulation was allowed to evolve for a total of 10,000-time steps, which were needed to achieve equilibration. The 'Mersenne Twister' random number generator with a cycle of length ($2^{19937} - 1$) was used for all random number generation in the rLST code [35].

3. Results

As previously discussed, efficient delivery of O_2 is vital to the cell survival in the 3D bone tissue engineering scaffolds. Yet, choosing the optimal scaffold manufacturing parameters and the culturing flow conditions is non-trivial, due to the complex transport phenomena occurring in the pore networks of the engineered tissue constructs. For this reason, we have performed image-based simulation of the fluid flow and of the O_2 transport that occur within two common types of bone tissue engineering PLLA scaffolds: the salt-leached foam and the non-woven fiber mesh.

Their geometries were varied by controlling the amount and the size of the leached salt grains for the former, and the fiber diameter for the latter. In order to compare the scaffolds on the same scale, here the results are plotted as a function of the "specific surface area"—defined as the ratio of surface area to total volume (as opposed to just solid volume). Furthermore, in order to analyze how the transport of O_2 is affected by the rate at which it is consumed by the cells, we considered different probabilities with which its molecules can react upon colliding with the scaffold walls. Specifically, we examined the condition of a uniform coverage of the scaffold surfaces with O_2-starved cells in Figures 3–6, while Figure 7 considers the case of the cells not starved for O_2. Namely, the former corresponds to an infinite surface reaction rate (i.e., instantaneous consumption of every O_2 molecule that collides with a scaffold wall). It should be treated as a limiting case scenario, which allows for a comparison of different scaffold structures on an equivalent basis.

Figure 3 is a plot of the O_2 "survival distance" in the stream-wise direction (the X-direction), as a function of the scaffold structure and the cell-culture media perfusion flow rate. The survival distance is defined as the distance that the rLST markers (representing the O_2 molecules) travel on average, until they are "consumed" via a collision with a scaffold wall. From this figure, it is apparent that the survival distance in the stream-wise direction increases as the flow rate goes up. This is consistent with the Taylor–Aris dispersion theory, which states that the effective diffusivity in the stream-wise direction should increase with the square of the Peclet number [20,34]:

$$Pe_m = Re * Sc \qquad (2)$$

where Re is the Reynolds number and Sc is the Schmidt Number. Its physical meaning is the ratio of the transport by advection to transport by diffusion. In this study, Sc is fixed for an O_2 molecule in an aqueous cell culture media at T = 37 °C, as was discussed in the methods section. Hence, according to Equation (2), the Peclet number will increase proportionally with the value of Re, which depends on the velocity of the fluid. This leads to a higher effective diffusivity of the solute in the stream-wise direction, and thus, the O_2 can make it further into the scaffold before it is fully consumed by the cells.

Another trend that is apparent from Figure 3 is that the survival distance of O_2 is also inversely proportional to the specific surface area of the scaffold. This makes sense, because the O_2 molecules have a smaller chance to collide with the scaffold's surface when it has less area exposed. Furthermore, Figure 3 shows that the foam scaffolds have a lower specific surface area than the fiber ones. This leads to noticeably longer survival distances of O_2 in the foam scaffolds.

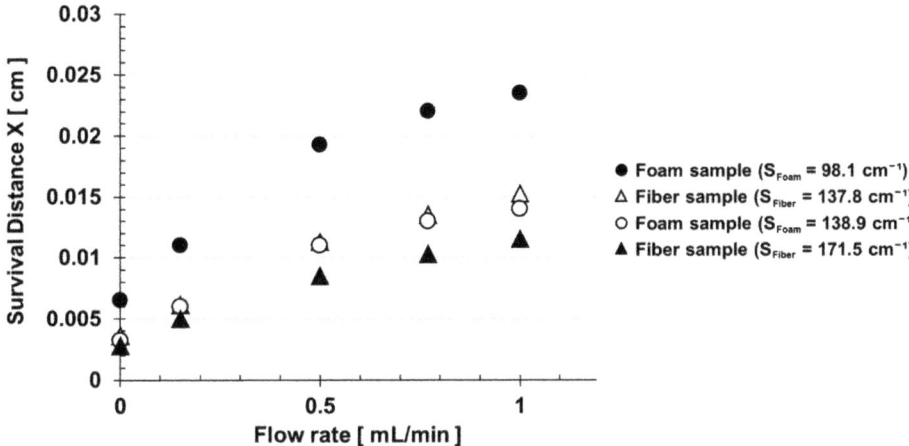

Figure 3. Survival distance in the stream-wise direction as a function of perfusion flow rate and scaffold architecture. Data is plotted for the limiting case of the fully reactive Lagrangian Scalar Tracking (rLST) particles.

Overall, the result demonstrates that it is plausible to modify the scaffold's geometry in order to increase the efficiency of the O_2 transport within its structure. To that end, Equation (3) shows how the surface area-to-total volume ratio 'S' of a fiber mesh scaffold is related to its porosity and fiber diameter (see Supplementary Materials for derivation):

$$S_{Fiber} = \frac{4(1-\varepsilon)}{D_{Fiber}} \quad (3)$$

where D_{Fiber} is the fiber diameter and ε is the scaffold porosity. Similarly, Equation (4) shows how the surface area-to-total volume ratio 'S' of a foam scaffold is related to its porosity and salt grain diameter (see Supplementary Materials for derivation):

$$S_{Foam} = \frac{6\varepsilon}{D_{SaltGrain}} \quad (4)$$

where $D_{SaltGrain}$ is the diameter of the salt grains used for leaching, and ε is the scaffold porosity. Therefore, for a known scaffold porosity and diameter combination, one can relate these geometric parameters to the surface area-to-total volume ratio of the scaffold (and thus, to the results of this manuscript). It is also important to note that while S_{Fiber} goes down with an increasing porosity ε, S_{Foam} displays the opposite behavior, as can be seen from the Equations (3) and (4).

Interestingly, the survival distances in the Y and Z directions (i.e., perpendicular to the flow) go down with the increasing flow rate (see Figure 4). The reason behind this is likely due to the particles becoming entrained by the carrier fluid. Consequently, they move less in the Y and Z directions per time step, relative to their displacement in the X. As a result, there is a smaller probability of collisions with the walls in the former directions. However, since both the Y and Z survival distances are an order of magnitude smaller than those in the X direction, the total survival distance is dominated by the trend displayed by the latter.

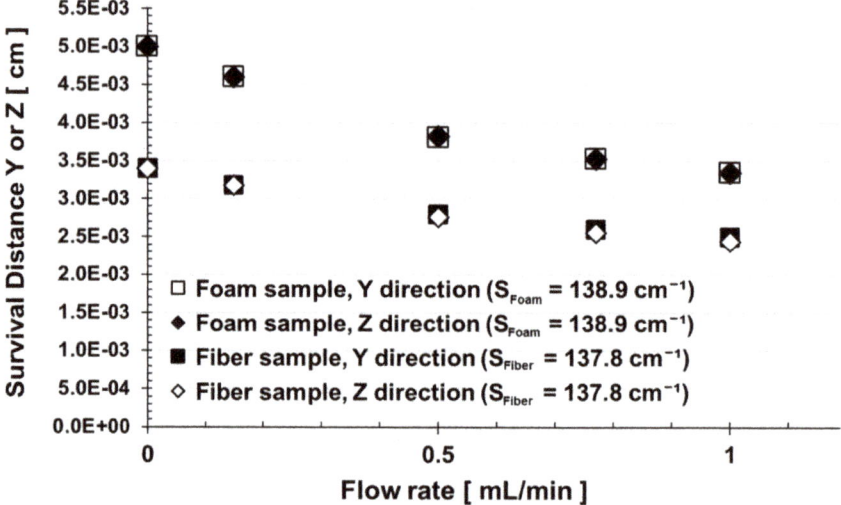

Figure 4. Survival distances in the Y & Z directions, as a function of the scaffold geometry and perfusion flow rate. Data is plotted for the limiting case of the fully reactive rLST particles. Both scaffolds types are chosen to have a similar specific surface area.

Another quantity of interest is the survival time of the O_2 molecules in the scaffolds. Figure 5 plots this quantity as a function of the flow rate and the specific surface area of the scaffolds for the limiting case of fully reactive rLST particles. Conversely to the survival distance in Figure 3, the survival time in Figure 5 decreases with the flow rate, though the effect of the specific surface area remains the same, and the survival time varies inversely-proportionally to it. Combining the results from both of the figures, it becomes apparent that fully reactive molecules get carried to a farther distance by a higher flow rate. However, they take a shorter time to get consumed by the cells on the surface of the scaffolds. This is especially true for the scaffold geometries with a higher exposed surface area.

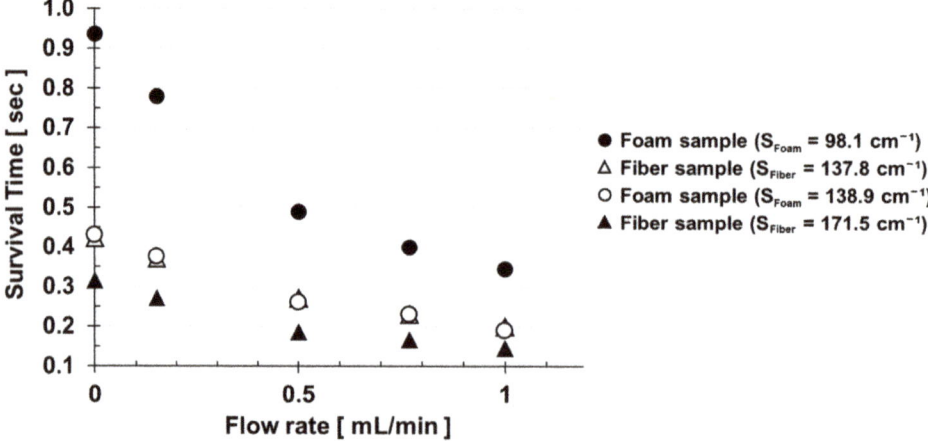

Figure 5. Survival time in the stream-wise direction as a function of perfusion flow rate and scaffold architecture. Data is plotted for the limiting case of the fully reactive rLST particles.

Ultimately, it is of interest to measure the effective first order reaction rate constant k_{eff}, with which the O_2 molecules get consumed in the scaffolds, after accounting for the mass transfer limitations. To that end, Figure 6 is a plot of k_{eff} as a function of the flow rate and specific surface area of the scaffold for the limiting case of an infinitely fast surface consumption of O_2. It reaffirms the previously observed trends, which show that the O_2 is consumed faster in the scaffold structures with the higher surface area-to-solid volume ratios. Furthermore, it also supports the finding that increasing the cell culture media flow rate through the scaffold leads to a faster O_2 consumption in its pores.

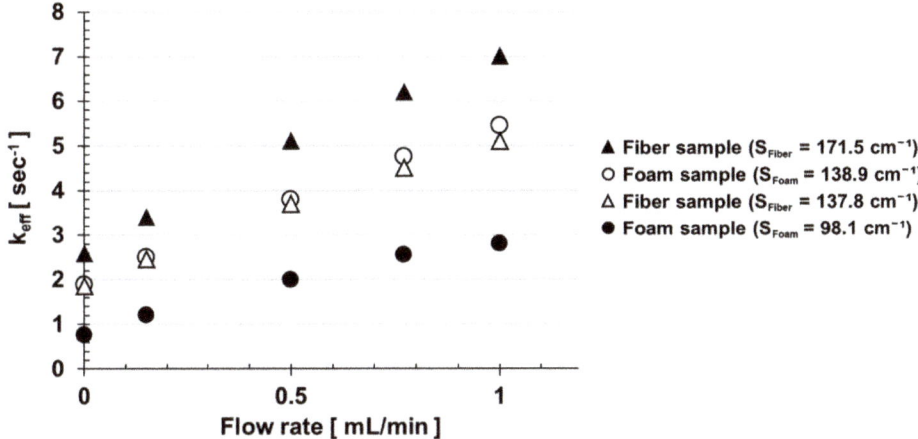

Figure 6. Effective O_2 reaction coefficient k_{eff} as a function of perfusion flow rate and scaffold architecture. Data is plotted for the limiting case of the fully reactive rLST particles.

If the cells are not starved for O_2, however, the rLST particles can be made to have a finite (as opposed to infinite) probability of becoming consumed upon collision with the scaffold walls. Thus, Figure 7 explores the role that the different cell affinities for consuming the O_2 have on its transport in the pores. In this case, the rLST particles with the different reactivities are all released simultaneously, and their survival times are compared as a function of the cell culture media flow rate and the scaffold type.

Two trends are immediately apparent from Figure 7: 1) the O_2 in the fiber scaffolds (solid lines) has a shorter survival time than in the foam ones (dotted lines), regardless of the cells' affinity for its uptake. This is consistent with the trends in the previous section, which showed that the fiber scaffolds have a higher specific surface area than the foams. This makes them more efficient at delivering the O_2 molecules to the cells; and 2) the second trend essentially says that for a given surface reaction rate, the consumption of O_2 will take longer at the slower flows. This is again consistent with a similar trend that was shown in Figure 5, where the survival time increased with the slower flow rate.

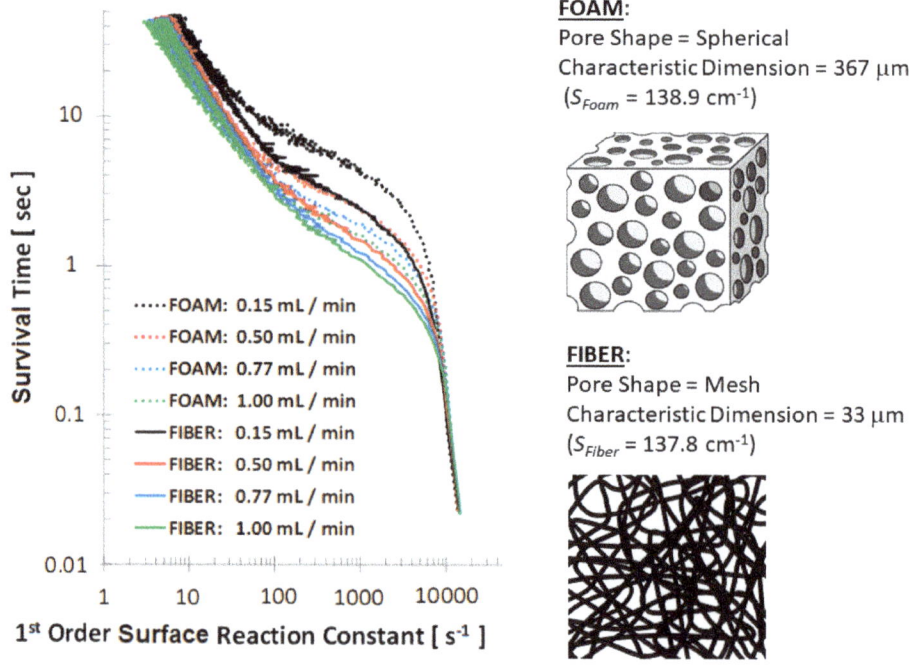

Figure 7. O_2 survival time as a function of the consumption rate by the cells on the scaffold surface. Data is plotted for salt leached foam and non-woven fiber mesh scaffolds at four different flow rates.

4. Discussion

In this manuscript, we carried out a study of how the O_2 mass transfer is affected by the scaffold manufacturing and the flow perfusion culturing parameters in bone tissue engineering scaffolds. The knowledge obtained from the reported results is needed in order to overcome the product-size limitations, which are commonly experienced due to hypoxia and necrosis in the center of large scaffolds. To solve the problem, we used an image-based approach of scanning the true scaffold structures in 3D using a high resolution µCT, and then fed the obtained geometries to our in-house parallelized fluid flow (LBM) and mass transport (rLST) solvers. Two scaffolds commonly used in bone tissue engineering, the salt leached foam and the nonwoven fiber mesh, were used for this study. The O_2 transport results were parametrized as a function of the specific surface area of the scaffold, the flow rate in the bioreactor, and the affinity to consume the molecule by the cells.

The main conclusions from our work are that the scaffolds with the higher specific area (i.e., surface area-to-solid volume ratio) result in more frequent molecular collisions with the cells. This increases the chances of the O_2 uptake by them, which results in a higher consumption (i.e., shorter survival times and distances) of the molecules in the scaffold. Furthermore, by increasing the flow rate in the bioreactor, the O_2 transport can be both facilitated (as seen from the shorter survival time in Figure 4) and delivered deeper into the scaffold (as seen from the longer survival distance in Figure 3). Thus, the overall effective O_2 reaction coefficient k_{eff} can be increased by maximizing both the specific surface area of the scaffold and the flowrate through its pores. This is evident from Figure 6.

Interestingly, the conclusion that an increased flow rate improves the O_2 delivery to the cells has also been reported by Bergemann et al. [4]. However, increasing it indefinitely is not an option because there is a trade-off with the shear forces exerted on the cells by the flow. Specifically, values in the range of 0.1–25 dynes/cm² [36–38] are generally considered to be beneficial because they mimic the natural microenvironment in bone canaliculi [9,10] and have been shown to promote tissue regeneration [39–42]. On the other hand, an excessive shear in the range of 26–54 dynes/cm^2 and higher can cause cell lysing and/or detachment from the scaffold [43,44]. Therefore, there is some optimal flow rate, which was found to be 45 µL/min by the Bergemann et al. study [4]. However, this value is specific to their scaffold-and-cell combination, and it could vary for other alternatives. Therefore, both image-based numerical simulations and cell viability assays are necessary for tuning the optimal conditions for other types of cultures. Whereas, at least the physical understanding provided in our study should be applicable across all scaffold types because they are expressed in terms of the specific surface area.

Finally, Figure 7 in our manuscript provides insight into how the O_2 transport depends on its consumption by the cells. In this case, we are not assuming that the cells are O_2-starved (and as a result take up every oxygen molecule that collides with them). Instead, we vary consumption rate of the O_2 at the scaffold surface in order to measure how this affects its transport in the scaffold. The results reported in this figure allow other researchers to understand the changes in the scaffold's transport microenvironment over time. They also show how the flowrate and specific surface area trends are affected by the cell-specific O_2 consumption rates.

The limitations of our study are that the cells are assumed to have a uniformed coverage on the scaffold surface. In reality, they would likely prefer some areas of the scaffold more than others. Furthermore, the tissue they lay down and the forces they exert on the scaffold would likely alter the internal structure of the scaffold (and in turn the flow field in its pores). Unfortunately, our model does not account for these types of influences by the cells on the mass transfer of O_2. Additionally, the scaffold's structure in the real experiment could change due to wetting forces, fiber flexibility, and the natural degradation of PLLA. The latter produces acidic byproducts, whose removal is facilitated by the fluid flow [45], yet in our study, the scaffold's structure remains static throughout the virtual experiment.

However, the results presented in this manuscript expose qualitative trends that should hold true regardless of the necessary simplifications. Therefore, it is expected that they should contribute significantly to the field of bone tissue engineering scaffold design and experiment optimization.

5. Conclusions

Mass transfer of O_2 in scaffolds cultured in perfusion bioreactors is of interest to the fields of bone and other types of tissue engineering. Specifically, understanding how to control it can be instrumental to resolving product size limitations when it comes to culturing organ-sized scaffolds. Therefore, we performed an image-based simulation study, in which we showed that the scaffolds with the higher surface area-to-solid volume ratio result in a more efficient transfer of O_2. Additionally, we showed that the effect can be increased further by flowing the cell culture media through the scaffold faster. Serendipitously, this also delivers the O_2 deeper into the scaffold pores, which is key to overcoming the product-size limitations mentioned earlier. Furthermore, we provided a parametric sweep over the rates of O_2 consumption by the cells situated on the scaffold surfaces. This visual aid yields insight into how the different cell affinities for consuming the O_2 can affect the molecule's transport through the biological porous media. Finally, the computational framework presented in this study can serve as a viable tool for optimizing the scaffold design and experimental culturing protocols for other types of tissue engineering as well.

Supplementary Materials: The following are available online at http://www.mdpi.com/2076-3417/9/11/2381/s1.

Author Contributions: Conceptualization, S.V.I. and V.R.S.; methodology, N.T.D., K.O.E.; software, V.R.S.; validation, N.T.D., and K.O.E.; formal analysis, N.T.D., and K.O.E.; investigation, N.T.D., and K.O.E.; resources, S.V.I.; data curation, N.T.D.; writing—original draft preparation, N.T.D. and K.O.E.; writing—review and editing, N.T.D., K.O.E., S.V.I. and V.R.S.; visualization, N.TD. and K.O.E.; supervision, V.R.S.; project administration V.R.S.; funding acquisition, V.R.S.

Funding: This research was funded by Gustavus and Louise Pfeiffer Research Foundation Major Research Investment Grant.

Acknowledgments: Financial support from Gustavus and Louise Pfeiffer Research Foundation is gratefully acknowledged. We also acknowledge the computing for this project was performed at the OU Supercomputing Center for Education & Research (OSCER) at the University of Oklahoma (OU) and Texas Advanced Computing Center (TACC) at The University of Texas–Austin. Both have contributed to the research results reported within this paper. URLs: http://www.ou.edu/oscer.html and http://www.tacc.utexas.edu, respectively. This work also used the Extreme Science and Engineering Discovery Environment (XSEDE) [46], which is supported by National Science Foundation grant number ACI-1548562. Allocations: TG-BCS170001 and TG-BIO160074. The Xradia micro-CT scans were made by Mark E. Curtis. Fiber fabrication was performed by Taren Blue, who was studying under the guidance of Prof. Robert L. Shambaugh at OU. Scaffolds were cultured by Sam VanGordon and Cortes Williams also at OU. Finally, the LBM and rLST codes were written under the guidance of Prof. Papavassiliou also at OU. We gratefully acknowledge their expertise and assistance.

Conflicts of Interest: The authors have no competing financial interests to declare.

References

1. American Academy of Orthopaedic Surgeons. One in Two Americans Have a Musculoskeletal Condition. Available online: https://www.sciencedaily.com/releases/2016/03/160301114116.htm (accessed on 13 June 2018).
2. U.S. Food and Drug Administration. Approved Cellular and Gene Therapy Products. Available online: https://www.fda.gov/vaccines-blood-biologics/cellular-gene-therapy-products/approved-cellular-and-gene-therapy-products (accessed on 20 February 2018).
3. Simmons, A.D.; Williams, C.; Degoix, A.; Sikavitsas, V.I. Sensing metabolites for the monitoring of tissue engineered construct cellularity in perfusion bioreactors. *Biosens. Bioelectron.* **2017**, *90*, 443–449. [CrossRef] [PubMed]
4. Bergemann, C.; Elter, P.; Lange, R.; Weissmann, V.; Hansmann, H.; Klinkenberg, E.D.; Nebe, B. Cellular Nutrition in Complex Three-Dimensional Scaffolds: A Comparison between Experiments and Computer Simulations. *Int. J. Biomater.* **2015**, *2015*, 584362. [CrossRef] [PubMed]
5. Gilkes, D.M.; Semenza, G.L.; Wirtz, D. Hypoxia and the extracellular matrix: Drivers of tumour metastasis. *Nat. Rev. Cancer* **2014**, *14*, 430. [CrossRef]
6. Spill, F.; Reynolds, D.S.; Kamm, R.D.; Zaman, M.H. Impact of the physical microenvironment on tumor progression and metastasis. *Curr. Opin. Biotechnol.* **2016**, *40*, 41–48. [CrossRef] [PubMed]
7. Nguyen, T.D.; Song, M.S.; Ly, N.H.; Lee, S.Y.; Joo, S.W. Nanostars on Nanopipette Tips: A Raman Probe for Quantifying Oxygen Levels in Hypoxic Single Cells and Tumours. *Angew. Chem. Int. Ed. Engl.* **2019**, *58*, 2710–2714. [CrossRef]
8. Zhang, S.; Vijayavenkataraman, S.; Lu, W.F.; Fuh, J.Y. A review on the use of computational methods to characterize, design, and optimize tissue engineering scaffolds, with a potential in 3D printing fabrication. *J. Biomed. Mater. Res. Part B Appl. Biomater.* **2018**, *107*, 1329–1351. [CrossRef]
9. Verbruggen, S.W.; Vaughan, T.J.; McNamara, L.M. Fluid flow in the osteocyte mechanical environment: A fluid-structure interaction approach. *Biomech. Model Mechanobiol.* **2014**, *13*, 85–97. [CrossRef]
10. Guyot, Y.; Luyten, F.P.; Schrooten, J.; Papantoniou, I.; Geris, L. A three-dimensional computational fluid dynamics model of shear stress distribution during neotissue growth in a perfusion bioreactor. *Biotechnol. Bioeng.* **2015**, *112*, 2591–2600. [CrossRef]
11. Ferroni, M.; Giusti, S.; Nascimento, D.; Silva, A.; Boschetti, F.; Ahluwalia, A. Modeling the fluid-dynamics and oxygen consumption in a porous scaffold stimulated by cyclic squeeze pressure. *Med. Eng. Phys.* **2016**, *38*, 725–732. [CrossRef]
12. Fiedler, T.; Belova, I.V.; Murch, G.E.; Poologasundarampillai, G.; Jones, J.R.; Roether, J.A.; Boccaccini, A.R. A comparative study of oxygen diffusion in tissue engineering scaffolds. *J. Mater. Sci. Mater. Med.* **2014**, *25*, 2573–2578. [CrossRef]
13. Arrigoni, C.; Bongio, M.; Talò, G.; Bersini, S.; Enomoto, J.; Fukuda, J.; Moretti, M. Rational design of prevascularized large 3D tissue constructs using computational simulations and biofabrication of geometrically controlled microvessels. *Adv. Healthcare Mater.* **2016**, *5*, 1617–1626. [CrossRef] [PubMed]
14. Li, E.; Chang, C.; Zhang, Z.; Li, Q. Characterization of tissue scaffolds for time-dependent biotransport criteria–a novel computational procedure. *Comput. Methods Biomech. Biomed. Eng.* **2016**, *19*, 1210–1224. [CrossRef] [PubMed]

15. Yan, X.; Bergstrom, D.J.; Chen, X.B. Modeling of cell cultures in perfusion bioreactors. *IEEE Trans. Biomed. Eng.* **2012**, *59*, 2568–2575. [CrossRef]
16. Voronov, R.; Vangordon, S.; Sikavitsas, V.I.; Papavassiliou, D.V. Computational modeling of flow-induced shear stresses within 3D salt-leached porous scaffolds imaged via micro-CT. *J. Biomech.* **2010**, *43*, 1279–1286. [CrossRef] [PubMed]
17. VanGordon, S.B.; Voronov, R.S.; Blue, T.B.; Shambaugh, R.L.; Papavassiliou, D.V.; Sikavitsas, V.I. Effects of Scaffold Architecture on Preosteoblastic Cultures under Continuous Fluid Shear. *Ind. Eng. Chem. Res.* **2011**, *50*, 620–629. [CrossRef]
18. Papavassiliou, D.V.; Pham, N.H.; Kadri, O.E.; Voronov, R.S. Chapter 23—Lattice Boltzmann Methods for Bioengineering Applications. In *Numerical Methods and Advanced Simulation in Biomechanics and Biological Processes*; Academic Press: Cambridge, MA, USA, 2018; pp. 415–429.
19. Alam, T.A.; Pham, Q.L.; Sikavitsas, V.I.; Papavassiliou, D.V.; Shambaugh, R.L.; Voronov, R.S. Image-based modeling: A novel tool for realistic simulations of artificial bone cultures. *Technology* **2016**, *4*, 229–233. [CrossRef]
20. Voronov, R.S.; VanGordon, S.B.; Sikavitsas, V.I.; Papavassiliou, D.V. Efficient Lagrangian scalar tracking method for reactive local mass transport simulation through porous media. *Int. J. Numer. Methods Fluids* **2011**, *67*, 501–517. [CrossRef]
21. Lu, L.C.; Peter, S.J.; Lyman, M.D.; Lai, H.L.; Leite, S.M.; Tamada, J.A.; Vacanti, J.P.; Langer, R.; Mikos, A.G. In vitro degradation of porous poly(L-lactic acid) foams. *Biomaterials* **2000**, *21*, 1595–1605. [CrossRef]
22. Alvarez-Barreto, J.F.; Sikavitsas, V.I. Improved mesenchymal stem cell seeding on RGD-modified poly(L-lactic acid) scaffolds using flow perfusion. *Macromol Biosci* **2007**, *7*, 579–588. [CrossRef]
23. Mikos, A.G.; Lyman, M.D.; Freed, L.E.; Langer, R. Wetting of poly(L-lactic acid) and poly(DL-lactic-co-glycolic acid) foams for tissue culture. *Biomaterials* **1994**, *15*, 55–58. [CrossRef]
24. Liu, X.; Ma, P.X. Polymeric scaffolds for bone tissue engineering. *Ann. Biomed. Eng.* **2004**, *32*, 477–486. [CrossRef] [PubMed]
25. Voronov, R.S.; VanGordon, S.B.; Shambaugh, R.L.; Papavassiliou, D.V.; Sikavitsas, V.I. 3D Tissue-Engineered Construct Analysis via Conventional High-Resolution Microcomputed Tomography Without X-Ray Contrast. *Tissue Eng. Part C-Methods* **2013**, *19*, 327–335. [CrossRef] [PubMed]
26. Voronov, R. Fluid Shear Stress and Nutrient Transport effects via Lattice-Boltzmann and Lagrangian Scalar Tracking Simulations of Cell Culture Media Perfusion through Artificial Bone Engineering Constructs Imaged with microCT. Ph.D. Thesis, University of Oklahoma, Norman, OK, USA, 2010.
27. Porter, B.; Zauel, R.; Stockman, H.; Guldberg, R.; Fyhrie, D. 3-D computational modeling of media flow through scaffolds in a perfusion bioreactor. *J. Biomech.* **2005**, *38*, 543–549. [CrossRef] [PubMed]
28. Shakhawath Hossain, M.; Bergstrom, D.J.; Chen, X.B. A mathematical model and computational framework for three-dimensional chondrocyte cell growth in a porous tissue scaffold placed inside a bi-directional flow perfusion bioreactor. *Biotechnol. Bioeng.* **2015**, *112*, 2601–2610. [CrossRef] [PubMed]
29. Williams, C.; Kadri, O.; Voronov, R.; Sikavitsas, V. Time-Dependent Shear Stress Distributions during Extended Flow Perfusion Culture of Bone Tissue Engineered Constructs. *Fluids* **2018**, *3*, 25. [CrossRef]
30. Wang, J.; Zhang, X.; Bengough, A.G.; Crawford, J.W. Domain-decomposition method for parallel lattice Boltzmann simulation of incompressible flow in porous media. *Phys. Rev. E* **2005**, *72*, 016706. [CrossRef] [PubMed]
31. Kadri, O.E.; Williams, C., 3rd; Sikavitsas, V.; Voronov, R.S. Numerical accuracy comparison of two boundary conditions commonly used to approximate shear stress distributions in tissue engineering scaffolds cultured under flow perfusion. *Int. J. Numer. Method Biomed. Eng.* **2018**, *34*, e3132. [CrossRef] [PubMed]
32. Qian, Y.H.; Dhumieres, D.; Lallemand, P. Lattice Bgk Models for Navier-Stokes Equation. *Europhys. Lett.* **1992**, *17*, 479–484. [CrossRef]
33. Bhatnagar, P.L.; Gross, E.P.; Krook, M. A Model for Collision Processes in Gases.1. Small Amplitude Processes in Charged and Neutral One-Component Systems. *Phys. Rev.* **1954**, *94*, 511–525. [CrossRef]
34. Sukop, M.C.; Thorne, D.T.; NetLibrary Inc. *Lattice Boltzmann Modeling an Introduction for Geoscientists and Engineers*; Springer: Berlin, Germany; New York, NY, USA, 2006.
35. Matsumoto, M.; Nishimura, T. Mersenne twister: A 623-dimensionally equidistributed uniform pseudo-random number generator. *ACM Trans. Model. Comput. Simul.* **1998**, *8*, 3–30. [CrossRef]

36. Stolberg, S.; McCloskey, K.E. Can shear stress direct stem cell fate? *Biotechnol. Progr.* **2009**, *25*, 10–19. [CrossRef] [PubMed]
37. Raimondi, M.T.; Moretti, M.; Cioffi, M.; Giordano, C.; Boschetti, F.; Lagana, K.; Pietrabissa, R. The effect of hydrodynamic shear on 3D engineered chondrocyte systems subject to direct perfusion. *Biorheology* **2006**, *43*, 215–222. [PubMed]
38. Kim, K.M.; Choi, Y.J.; Hwang, J.-H.; Kim, A.R.; Cho, H.J.; Hwang, E.S.; Park, J.Y.; Lee, S.-H.; Hong, J.-H. Shear Stress Induced by an Interstitial Level of Slow Flow Increases the Osteogenic Differentiation of Mesenchymal Stem Cells through TAZ Activation. *PLoS ONE* **2014**, *9*, e92427. [CrossRef] [PubMed]
39. Miyashita, S.; Ahmed, N.E.M.B.; Murakami, M.; Iohara, K.; Yamamoto, T.; Horibe, H.; Kurita, K.; Takano-Yamamoto, T.; Nakashima, M. Mechanical forces induce odontoblastic differentiation of mesenchymal stem cells on three-dimensional biomimetic scaffolds. *J. Tissue Eng. Regener. Med.* **2017**, *11*, 434–446. [CrossRef] [PubMed]
40. Zhao, F.; Vaughan, T.J.; McNamara, L.M. Quantification of fluid shear stress in bone tissue engineering scaffolds with spherical and cubical pore architectures. *Biomech. Model. Mechanobiol.* **2016**, *15*, 561–577. [CrossRef] [PubMed]
41. Sikavitsas, V.I.; Bancroft, G.N.; Holtorf, H.L.; Jansen, J.A.; Mikos, A.G. Mineralized matrix deposition by marrow stromal osteoblasts in 3D perfusion culture increases with increasing fluid shear forces. *Proc. Natl. Acad. Sci. USA* **2003**, *100*, 14683–14688. [CrossRef] [PubMed]
42. Yourek, G.; McCormick, S.M.; Mao, J.J.; Reilly, G.C. Shear stress induces osteogenic differentiation of human mesenchymal stem cells. *Regener. Med.* **2010**, *5*, 713–724. [CrossRef]
43. Brindley, D.; Moorthy, K.; Lee, J.-H.; Mason, C.; Kim, H.-W.; Wall, I. Bioprocess Forces and Their Impact on Cell Behavior: Implications for Bone Regeneration Therapy. *J. Tissue Eng.* **2011**, *2011*, 620247. [CrossRef]
44. Alvarez-Barreto, J.F.; Linehan, S.M.; Shambaugh, R.L.; Sikavitsas, V.I. Flow Perfusion Improves Seeding of Tissue Engineering Scaffolds with Different Architectures. *Ann. Biomed. Eng.* **2007**, *35*, 429–442. [CrossRef]
45. Agrawal, C.M.; McKinney, J.S.; Lanctot, D.; Athanasiou, K.A. Effects of fluid flow on the in vitro degradation kinetics of biodegradable scaffolds for tissue engineering. *Biomaterials* **2000**, *21*, 2443–2452. [CrossRef]
46. Towns, J.; Cockerill, T.; Dahan, M.; Foster, I.; Gaither, K.; Grimshaw, A.; Hazlewood, V.; Lathrop, S.; Lifka, D.; Peterson, G.D.; et al. XSEDE: Accelerating Scientific Discovery. *Comput. Sci. Eng.* **2014**, *16*, 62–74. [CrossRef]

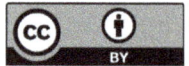

© 2019 by the authors. Licensee MDPI, Basel, Switzerland. This article is an open access article distributed under the terms and conditions of the Creative Commons Attribution (CC BY) license (http://creativecommons.org/licenses/by/4.0/).

Article

Mechanical Behavior of Ti6Al4V Scaffolds Filled with CaSiO₃ for Implant Applications

Ramin Rahmani [1,*], Maksim Antonov [1], Lauri Kollo [1], Yaroslav Holovenko [1] and Konda Gokuldoss Prashanth [1,2,3,*]

[1] Department of Mechanical and Industrial Engineering, Tallinn University of Technology, Ehitajate tee 5, 19086 Tallinn, Estonia; maksim.antonov@taltech.ee (M.A.); lauri.kollo@taltech.ee (L.K.); yaholo@taltech.ee (Y.H.)
[2] Erich Schmid Institute of Materials Science, Austrian Academy of Science, Jahn Straβe 12, A-8700 Leoben, Austria
[3] CBCMT, School of Mechanical Engineering, VIT University, Vellore, Tamil Nadu 632014, India
* Correspondence: ramin.rahmaniahranjani@taltech.ee (R.R.); kgprashanth@gmail.com (K.G.P.)

Received: 30 August 2019; Accepted: 10 September 2019; Published: 13 September 2019

Abstract: Triply periodic minimal surfaces (TPMS) are becoming increasingly attractive due to their biomedical applications and ease of production using additive manufacturing techniques. In the present paper, the architecture of porous scaffolds was utilized to seek for the optimized cellular structure subjected to compression loading. The deformation and stress distribution of five lightweight scaffolds, namely: Rectangular, primitive, lattice, gyroid and honeycomb Ti6Al4V structures were studied. Comparison of finite element simulations and experimental compressive test results was performed to illustrate the failure mechanism of these scaffolds. The experimental compressive results corroborate reasonably with the finite element analyses. Results of this study can be used for bone implants, biomaterial scaffolds and antibacterial applications, produced from the Ti6Al4V scaffold built by a selective laser melting (SLM) method. In addition, Ti6Al4V manufactured metallic lattice was filled by wollastonite ($CaSiO_3$) through spark plasma sintering (SPS) to illustrate the method for the production of a metallic-ceramic composite suitable for bone tissue engineering.

Keywords: Ti6Al4V scaffolds; triply periodic minimal surfaces; selective laser melting; additive manufacturing; biomaterial applications; finite element analysis; spark plasma sintering; wollastonite

---

1. Introduction

Titanium and its alloys have been widely used for biomedical and orthopedic applications, such as hip, knee, femur, vertebra, bone and skull, due to their excellent antibacterial/biocompatibility, strength-to-weight ratio and wear and corrosion resistance in comparison with stainless steel [1–5]. Implants have been made by computer numeric control (CNC) machining, or powder metallurgy, followed by different post-processing procedures. The metallic biomaterial scaffolds are applied for stent placement [6] or bone replacement [7]. Three dimensional (3D) printed porous scaffolds are suitable for seeding cells, delivering drugs, and are able to carry compression/tensile loading [2,3]. Biological activities along the scaffold surface (cell growth) and structural design of the scaffolds for additive manufacturing (AM) are both very important, and extensive research has been conducted [8]. With the use of optimal scaffold material and the suitable design for AM, scaffolds with added functionalities, elastic modulus, and strength matching the human bone can be realized [9].

Triply periodic minimal surfaces (TPMS) are some of the designs that are expected to be optimal candidates for bone tissue engineering applications. Primary simulation of the TPMS are crucial for designing these scaffolds to figure out the stress distribution, deformation and failure mechanism of porous structure [10,11].

Gradient structures, unit cell size, strut diameter, the volume fraction the of sample, plasticity and damage tolerance, as well as the minimizing of cost/time are considered during the computer-aided design (CAD) and simulation. In order to have optimized lightweight structures under loading and in vivo or in vitro conditions, printed scaffolds can be graded axially or radially [12]. Recently, research is focused upon polymeric printing using polyjet/inkjet deposition [13], which is faster with no post-processing, unlike metal printing. However, the low mechanical properties of polymer 3D printed materials make it non-applicable for in vivo conditions. Porous Ti6Al4V structures have yield strength and compressive strength in the range of 90–220 MPa [14]. The computer-aided design (CAD) of porous scaffolds and finite element analysis (FEA) have recently attracted much attention in the tissue engineering field. Fluid permeability [15] and biocompatibility [16] of scaffolds depends directly on the pore geometry and topology [17] of structures. The curved shape, smoothness, good flowability, 3D manufacturability and biocompatibility of Ti6Al4V powder particles makes Ti-based alloy promising for load bearing bone implants [18]. It is well known that the artificial bone scaffolds should have the following characteristics: (1) Biocompatibility with living tissues; (2) mechanical properties for trabecular bone and cortical bone (ranging from 0.7 to 15 MPa till >100 MPa [19]); and (3) porous fabricated structures for osteoporosis diseases. Periodic porous materials like TPMS are potential candidates for biomimetic scaffold architecture [19]. The main advantage of TPMS scaffolds is the open interconnected cell structure, deemed to facilitate cell migration, vitalization and vascularization, while retaining a high degree of structural stiffness [20]. Henceforth, mechanical properties, especially compressive strength, is considered as an important parameter for TPMS scaffolds. In this paper, we have performed compressive tests, where the experimental results are compared with the FEA for the selected promising TPMS structures.

Ti6Al4V is considered as excellent biomaterial because of higher fatigue strength, tensile strength and compressive strength [21–24]. However, it is bioinert, where an improper integration takes place with the host bone, resulting in a weak interfacial bond. As a result, at the bone-implant interface, there can be an accumulation of the necrotic fibrous tissue [25]. Nevertheless, in vivo life of the load bearing scaffolds can be increased by improving the interfacial bond of the bone and the metallic scaffolds. To improve the interfacial bonding, Ti6Al4V scaffolds are filled with wollastonite. Spark plasma sintering (SPS) was used for integrating wollastonite into the cellular Ti6Al4V structure [26]. Highly porous acicular wollastonite ($CaSiO_3$) with micro- or nano-sized pores results in high corrosion resistance and good biocompatibility [27,28].

Hence, the present study aims to fabricate Ti6Al4V scaffolds reinforced with bioactive elements (wollastonite) for the proper integration of the implant to the bone via tissue growth. By reviewing the articles, the deficiency of comparison between the mechanical properties of scaffolds, FEA, and an assortment of them regarding the applications is tangible. Five different Ti6Al4V scaffolds (samples) with identical outside dimensions and similar weight, namely: Rectangular, primitive, lattice, gyroid and honeycomb, were considered. They were chosen based on the desire to provide a continuous surface that is important for the growth/cultivation of viable cells and other aspects of tissue engineering [29]. The rectangular type has vertical available surface, whereas the primitive is made by sequential hollow spheres (proper for fluid permeability and drag delivery). Therefore, scaffolds A and B have vertical flat and spherical areas to flourish the cells. In the case of the lattice type structure, it is possible to specify the size of the cell and the diameter of the strut to figure out the proper cylindrical surface of the metallic rods. It is an intersecting cellular structure that is easy to use during the following of the SPS process, since it can be easily modeled, printed and filled by binder powders, and also allows a larger shrinkage required to produce hard metal-ceramic composites with a low porosity level by SPS [30]. The gyroid-type structure represents irregular continuous curves, and honeycomb considers embedded tubes, which are connected by horizontal washers.

A SolidWorks design and Ansys FEA combination were used to generate these structures and to further anticipate the mechanical behavior of the scaffolds subjected to compressive loading. The results from simulations are compared with the experimental compressive results.

2. Materials and Methods

Five distinct scaffolds were designed by SolidWorks, as shown in Figure 1 (rectangular, primitive, lattice, gyroid and honeycomb, respectively). The names are chosen according to the shape of the structures. These computer-aided design (CAD) models can be used both in finite element analysis (FEA) for the simulation of mechanical properties and the selective laser melting (SLM) process for the fabrication of the real parts. All the five scaffolds were of the following dimensions: A diameter of 20 mm and a height of 15 mm. The weight range of these samples varied between ≈3.8 and 5.5 g. Ti6Al4V powders with size of 10–45 μm (produced by a gas atomization process) from TLS Technik were used as the raw material for the production of triply periodic minimal surfaces (TPMS)-type scaffolds.

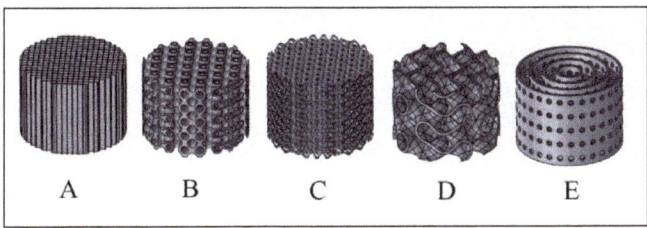

Figure 1. Scaffolds with: (**A**) Rectangular-, (**B**) Primitive-, (**C**) Lattice-, (**D**) Gyroid- and (**E**) Honeycomb-type structures (Dimensions: 20 mm in diameter and with 15 mm height), designed via computer-aided design (CAD) software.

A Realized SLM50 device with a maximum laser power of 120 W was used for the fabrication of the scaffolds. The following parameters were used for the fabrication of Ti6Al4V by SLM: Laser current 3000 mA, exposure time 600 μs, point distance 1 μm and unit cell size 1.5 mm. These are standard parameters that are observed for the fabrication of the Ti6Al4V samples. SLM-SPS processes were combined for producing metal-ceramic hybrid composites, which is suggested for chronic osteomyelitis, Vancomycin local delivery, and infected bones replacement in the field of tissue engineering [9]. The entire spark plasma sintering (SPS) setup is kept under the glovebox, in order to maintain the consolidation process in an inter atmosphere. This also helps in avoiding oxygen contamination during the SPS consolidation process. Microstructure of the samples were observed using scanning electron microscope (SEM), (Zeiss EVO MA 15, Germany)

Structural explicit dynamics using the AUTODYN solver and arbitrary Lagrange-Euler (ALE) method via ANSYS Workbench 17.2 is applied for these simulations. A high-quality finite element analysis (FEA) mesh is generated to gain a high-resolution response. The linearized governing motion equation in cylindrical coordinates (r, θ, z) can be expressed by [31]:

$$\frac{\partial \sigma_{rr}}{\partial r} + \frac{1}{r}\frac{\partial \sigma_{r\theta}}{\partial \theta} + \frac{\partial \sigma_{rz}}{\partial z} + \frac{1}{r}(\sigma_{rr} - \sigma_{\theta\theta}) + F_r = \rho \frac{\partial^2 u_r}{\partial t^2} \quad (1)$$

$$\frac{\partial \sigma_{r\theta}}{\partial r} + \frac{1}{r}\frac{\partial \sigma_{\theta\theta}}{\partial \theta} + \frac{\partial \sigma_{\theta z}}{\partial z} + \frac{2}{r}\sigma_{r\theta} + F_\theta = \rho \frac{\partial^2 u_\theta}{\partial t^2} \quad (2)$$

$$\frac{\partial \sigma_{rz}}{\partial r} + \frac{1}{r}\frac{\partial \sigma_{\theta z}}{\partial \theta} + \frac{\partial \sigma_{zz}}{\partial z} + \frac{2}{r}\sigma_{rz} + F_z = \rho \frac{\partial^2 u_z}{\partial t^2} \quad (3)$$

where, $\sigma_{ij} = \sigma_{ji}$ is the Cauchy stress tensor, u_i is displacement, ρ is density and F_i is body force ($F_r = F_\theta = 0$, F_z = axial compression). In the simulation, compressive punches are assumed rigid (unchanged dimension). Bottom punch is the fixed support and the top punch was kept moving until a maximum force of 100 kN (safe loading of machine), or a maximum deformation of 10 mm (with rate of 2 mm/min), is reached. Both the experimental tests and the numerical simulations have identical boundary conditions. An Instron 8500 apparatus was used for measuring the compression tests of these scaffolds.

3. Biomaterial Production and Characterization

Figure 2 shows the five different TPMS scaffolds with a diameter of 20 mm and a 15 mm height. The five different TPMS scaffold types are: (a) Rectangular with a vertical flat area, (b) primitive, (c) lattice, (which is a very common type of structure produced using SLM [32]), (d) gyroid and (e) honeycomb (which is another common structure that is produced by SLM). Similarly Figures 3–7 exhibits the stress distribution and deformation in the five different TPMS scaffolds.

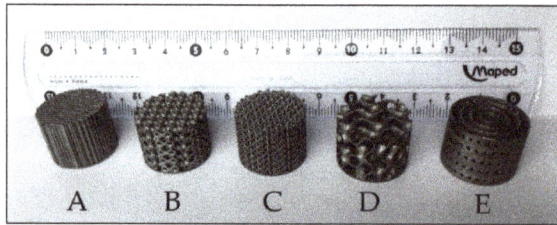

Figure 2. Scaffolds (their weight indicated in parentheses) with: (**A**) Rectangular (3.97 g), (**B**) Primitive (5.35 g), (**C**) Lattice (3.78 g), (**D**) Gyroid (4.04 g) and (**E**) Honeycomb (5.52 g) structures with 20 mm diameter and 15 mm height manufactured by selective laser melting.

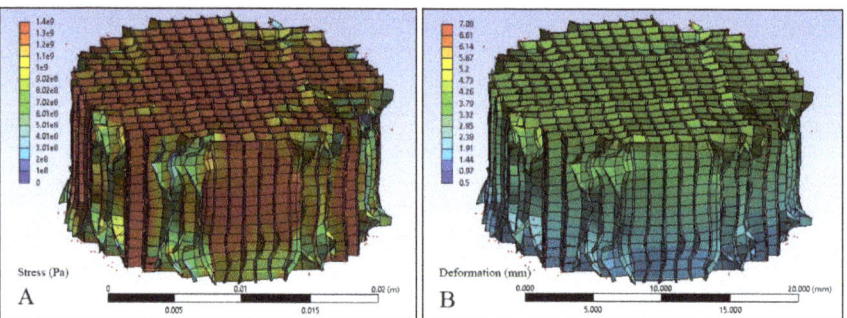

Figure 3. Rectangular scaffold simulation: (**A**) Stress and (**B**) displacement (final height after compression: 15 − 4.26 = 10.74 mm; red dots are separated particles in contact with compressive punches).

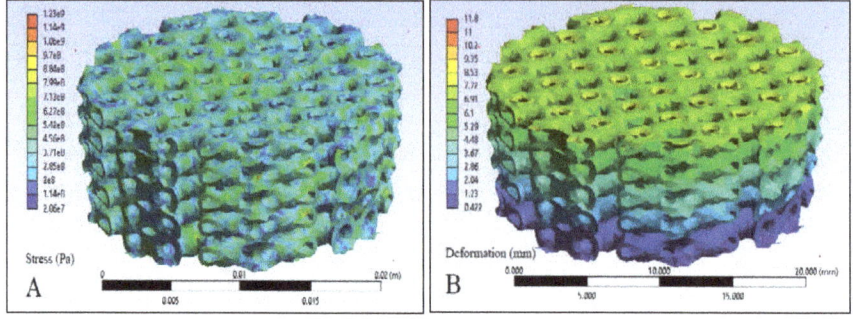

Figure 4. Primitive scaffold simulation: (**A**) Stress and (**B**) displacement (final height after compression 15 − 6.91 = 8.09 mm; the red dots are separated particles in contact with compressive punches).

The 99.9% purity wollastonite ($CaSiO_3$) with a particle size of 1–5 µm (supplied by NYAD, grade 1250) is filled and sintered (frittage) inside an argon-atomized Ti6Al4V cellular lattice structure via an SPS machine (made by FCT Systeme), as shown in Figure 8. The process was performed with an optimal pressure of 30 MPa at a temperature of 1100 °C, with a heating rate of 100 °C/min and a holding time of 5 min [33].

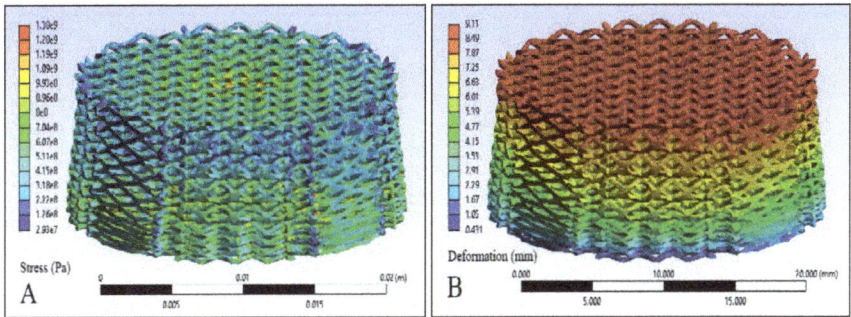

Figure 5. Lattice scaffold simulation: (**A**) Stress and (**B**) displacement (final height after compression 15 − 9.11 = 5.89 mm; red dots are separated particles in contact with compressive punches).

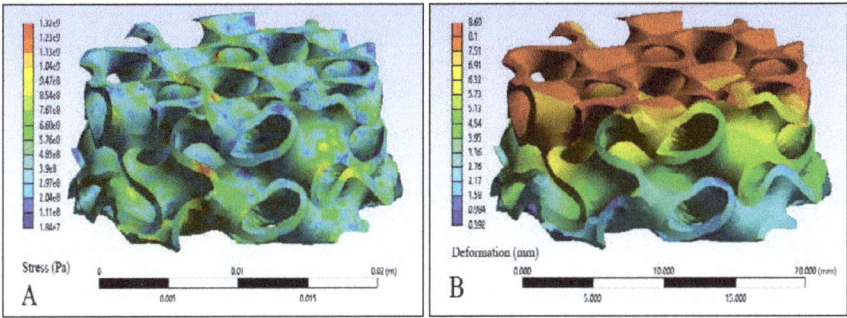

Figure 6. Gyroid scaffold simulation: (**A**) Stress and (**B**) displacement (final height after compression 15 − 8.1 = 6.9 mm; these red dots are separated particles in contact with compressive punches).

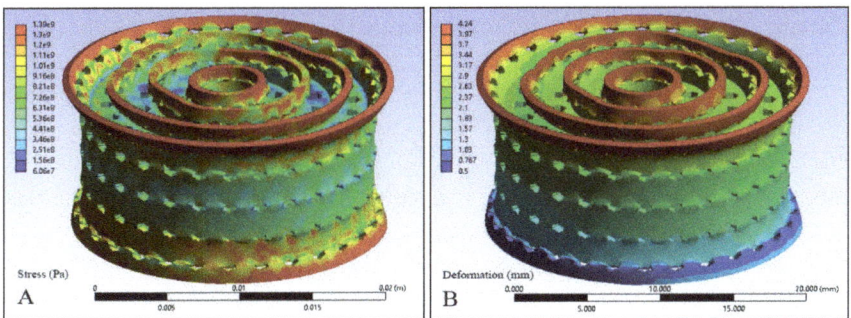

Figure 7. Honeycomb scaffold simulation: (**A**) Stress and (**B**) displacement (final height after compression 15 − 4.24 = 10.76 mm; red dots are separated particles in contact with compressive punches).

Wollastonite composition consists theoretically of 48.28% CaO and 51.72% SiO_2, while usually, the natural mineral may contain small amounts of iron, aluminum, magnesium, potassium and sodium (Figures 8A and 9A). An SLM-manufactured Ti6Al4V lattice with 1 mm cell size filled by $CaSiO_3$ powder and sintered in SPS (Figures 8B and 9B) are shown. The results show a good boundary between ceramic and lattice after SPS and polishing (Figures 8C and 9C).

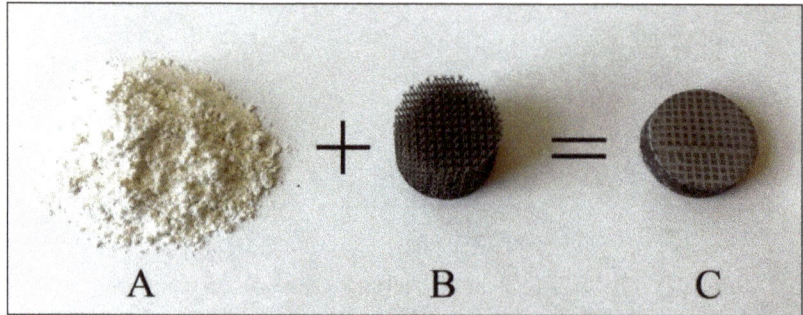

Figure 8. (**A**) Wollastonite ($CaSiO_3$) powder, (**B**) selective laser melting (SLM)-produced Ti6Al4V lattice structure with 1 mm cell size, and (**C**) Sintered sample (dimensions of lattice structure: 20 mm diameter and 15 mm height before spark plasma sintering (SPS) and 6 mm height after SPS and polishing).

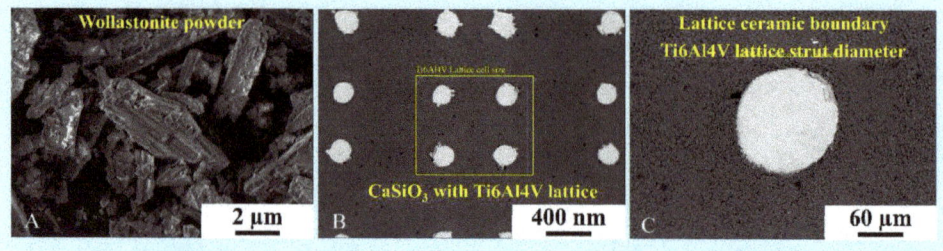

Figure 9. SEM micrographs of (**A**) wollastonite (CaSiO3) powder, (**B**) Sintered $CaSiO_3$ embedded in a Ti6Al4V lattice after SPS, and (**C**) High magnification image of metal-ceramic boundary.

4. Results and Discussion

An in vitro simulation and experimental results are required before an in vivo assessment of any biomaterial. From the literature, the ultimate strength of Ti6Al4V manufactured by SLM or electron beam melting (EBM) can be found between ≈1.0–1.2 GPa [34,35], and this value is applied for simulations in the current research. The rectangular scaffold (Figure 3) exhibits a high compressive strength, and deformation mostly occurs in the top and/or bottom part of the sample. The final height of rectangular and honeycomb after the compression test are similar. Comparison between Figures 3 and 7 present the findings that due to interlayer horizontal sheets, embedded multi-tubes (inspired by multi-walled carbon nanotubes) and hexagonal pores, the honeycomb scaffold has less stress concentration values; it is wrinkled with an expansion in diameter.

As expected, primitive, lattice and gyroid scaffolds (Figures 4–6) exhibited uniform deformation. For these three conditions, adding layers upon layers with a defined unit cell size (for example a lattice with intersecting cellular rods) produce desired structure shapes easily, but will be deformed relatively easily during compressive loading. It shows that cell type, size and alignment together play a pivotal role on their failure mechanism [36]. The experimental stress-strain curves from the compression test are shown in Figure 10. As seen from Figure 10, primitive, lattice and gyroid scaffolds show a more inferior deformation stress than in the case of rectangular scaffolds. In addition, the rectangular scaffold shows uniform plastic deformation allowances, where the stresses were distributed uniformly and the local overloading is completely avoided. It is shown that rectangular (due to vertical channels and fluid permeability) and honeycomb (due to horizontal plates and hexagon pores) are structures can bear high compressive loads. As demonstrated in section views of Figure 11, rectangular scaffolds have vertical thin plates that are resistant against distortion and deformation, whereas, honeycomb is more suitable for alive cell growth due to horizontal plates and continuous open porosity.

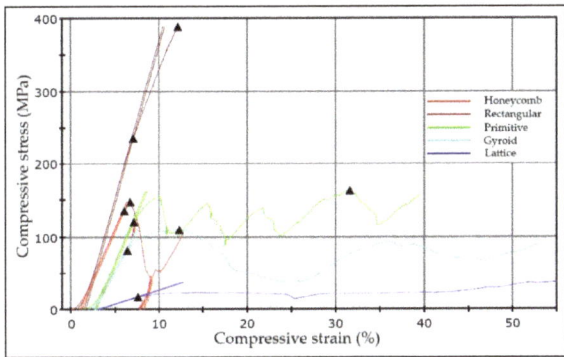

Figure 10. Stress-Strain compression results of scaffolds produced using the selective laser melting.

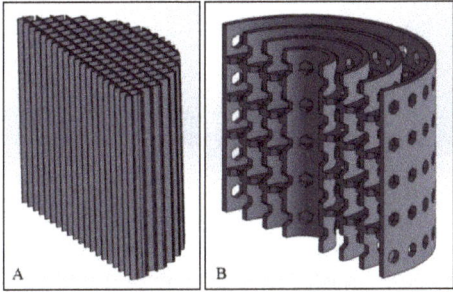

Figure 11. Section view of: (**A**) Rectangular, and (**B**) Honeycomb scaffolds.

The applicability of the porous TPMS scaffolds can be extended to applications related to (1) oxygen transport and/or (2) scaffold permeability [37]. The porous TPMS scaffolds can also contribute to enhanced cell seeding, and at the same time can maintain nutrient transport throughout the whole scaffold during in vitro culturing [16]. Regarding the final height of the deformed samples, the experimental compressive results (Figure 12A–E) are compared with the FEA analytical outcomes (Figures 3B, 4B, 5B, 6B and 7B), which are in good agreement. Regarding the Von Mises stress distribution (Figures 3A, 4A, 5A, 6A and 7A), primitive, lattice and gyroid scaffolds are relatively flexible/deformable structures, while more deformation energy can be absorbed by rectangular and honeycomb structures. Hence, for the rectangular structure, stress concentration and distortion can appear in the upper part of sample, but honeycomb failure started from the bottom of structures. Adding metallic lattice structure (Ti6Al4V) to ceramic reinforcement like wollastonite ($CaSiO_3$) produces a composite with higher wear resistance, damage tolerance and mechanical properties resulting in a higher durability of bones [38,39]. The strut diameter of the lattice is currently ≈ 200 µm, while it could be increased up to 1 mm (Figure 9C). This ability helps to control volume fraction of both Ti6Al4V and $CaSiO_3$ in the composite required to achieve the density and porosity characteristic for bones. Besides, our SLM-SPS combination provides the possibility of making complicated shapes/structures for antibacterial or biomedical applications (Figure 8C). Height of scaffolds after the analytical and experimental compression test are presented in Table 1. Statistical comparison shows a satisfying agreement between them. For Lattice scaffold (1 mm cell size and 0.5 mm strut diameter), the simulation outcomes show relatively lower weight than the experimental results. Such differences between the simulation and experimental results may be attributed to the porosity and unmelted/attached Ti6Al4V particles in the SLM parts [38,40].

Table 1. Compression test data (comparison of finite element analysis (FEA) simulation and experimental results).

Scaffold Type	Weight Before Test (g) (Figure 2)	Volume Fraction (% of Metal)	Height after Simulation (mm) (Figures 3–7)	Height after Experiment (mm) (Figure 8)	Maximum Compressive Load (kN) (Figure 9)
Rectangular	4.0 ± 0.1	19 ± 1	11 ± 1	11 ± 2	100 ± 5
Primitive	5.4 ± 0.2	28 ± 1	8 ± 2	8 ± 2	52 ± 2
Lattice	3.8 ± 0.1	17 ± 2	6 ± 2	8 ± 2	12 ± 1
Gyroid	4.0 ± 0.1	26 ± 2	7 ± 2	8 ± 1	35 ± 2
Honeycomb	5.6 ± 0.1	19 ± 1	11 ± 1	12 ± 3	70 ± 4

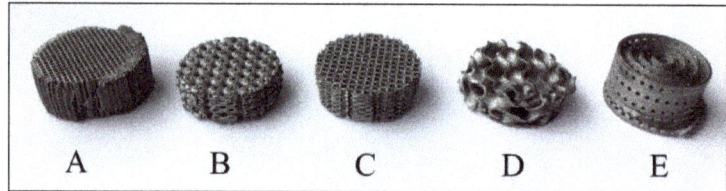

Figure 12. Triply periodic minimal surfaces (TPMS) scaffolds after compressive test with indication of their final height: (**A**) Rectangular −11 mm, (**B**) Primitive −8.4 mm, (**C**) Lattice −8.8 mm, (**D**) Gyroid −7.6 mm and (**E**) Honeycomb −12.1 mm.

Primitive TPMS have the highest volume fraction (28.2%, Table 1), and it might be interesting for biological activities due to a larger specific surface area. Stress distribution was uniform (Figure 4A), and shows a least difference between the simulation and experiment result (Figure 12B). Gyroid shows similar behavior as primitive, but including some broken/separated pieces in the top area because of a curvy cross section surface under compression. Strength of rectangular scaffold (Figure 12A) subjected to compressive loading is presented in Figure 9 and Table 1.

It survived under the maximum test load (100 kN). Comparison between A and Figure 12A shows that middle rectangular sections are less affected during compression, and any major deformation starts from the outer layers. Rectangular structure with rectangular/vertical channels is supposed for cells viability, oxygen transport and fluid permeability, otherwise it can be reinforced by horizontal plates (similar to honeycomb, Figure 11) for higher resistance against shear stress.

5. Conclusions

In this paper, five different Ti6Al4V triply periodic minimal surface structures with different surface areas were created by CAD design, namely rectangular, primitive, lattice, gyroid and honeycomb. The finite element simulation in comparison with 3D additive manufactured experimental results illustrated similar mechanical behaviors when the samples were subjected to compressive loading. They had uniform stress distributions and relatively identical displacements. It was found that ANSYS simulation has a potential to predict the mechanical behavior of additively manufactured scaffolds. Rectangular and honeycomb were novel cellular scaffolds designed for high compressive load-bearing and biological application with vertical and horizontal available surfaces, respectively. Rectangular scaffold is identified as suitable for oxygen transport and fluid permeability, whereas, honeycomb is found to be the best for the growth of cells. SLM-manufactured Ti6Al4V lattice can be sintered via SPS along with $CaSiO_3$ for load bearing bone replacements.

Author Contributions: Conceptualization, R.R. and K.G.P.; methodology, M.A. and L.K.; investigation, R.R. and Y.H.; writing—original draft preparation, R.R.; writing—review and editing, M.A., L.K. and K.G.P.; supervision, M.A. and L.K.; funding acquisition, M.A., L.K. and K.G.P.

Funding: This research was supported by the Estonian Ministry of Education and Research under projects IUT19-29, the European Regional Fund, project number 2014-2020.4.01.16-0183 (Smart Industry Centre), ETAG18012, MOBERC15 and by base finance project B56 and SS427 of Tallinn University of Technology.

Conflicts of Interest: The authors declare no conflict of interest.

References

1. Khan, M.A.; Williams, R.L.; Williams, D.F. In-vitro corrosion and wear of titanium alloys in the biological environment. *Biomaterials* **1996**, *17*, 2117–2126. [CrossRef]
2. Zhuravleva, K.; Boenisch, M.; Prashanth, K.G.; Hempel, U.; Health, A.; Gemming, T.; Caling, M.; Scudino, S.; Schultz, L.; Eckert, J.; et al. Production of porous β-type Ti-40Nb alloy for biomedical applications: Comparison of selective laser melting and hot pressing. *Materials* **2013**, *6*, 5700–5712. [CrossRef] [PubMed]
3. Schwab, H.; Prashanth, K.G.; Loeber, L.; Kuehn, U.; Eckert, J. Selective laser melting of Ti-45Nb alloy. *Metals* **2015**, *5*, 686–694. [CrossRef]
4. Attar, H.; Loeber, L.; Funk, A.; Calin, M.; Zhang, L.C.; Prashanth, K.G.; Scudino, S.; Zhang, Y.S.; Eckert, J. Mechanical behavior of porous commercially pure Ti and Ti-TiB composite materials manufactured by selective laser melting. *Mater. Sci. Eng. A* **2015**, *625*, 350–356. [CrossRef]
5. Attar, H.; Prashanth, K.G.; Zhang, L.C.; Calin, M.; Okulov, I.V.; Scudino, S.; Yang, C.; Eckert, J. Effect of powder particle shape on the properties of in siu Ti-TiB composite powders produced by selective laser melting. *J. Mater. Sci. Technol.* **2015**, *31*, 1001–1005. [CrossRef]
6. Van Lith, R.; Baker, E.; Ware, H.; Yang, J.; Cyrus Farsheed, A.; Sun, C.; Ameer, G. 3D-Printing Strong High-Resolution Antioxidant Bioresorbable Vascular Stents. *Adv. Mater. Technol.* **2016**, *1*, 1600138. [CrossRef]
7. Seitz, H.; Rieder, W.; Irsen, S.; Leukers, B.; Tille, C. Three-dimensional printing of porous ceramic scaffolds for bone tissue engineering. *J. Biomed. Mater. Res.* **2005**, *74*, 782–788. [CrossRef] [PubMed]
8. Wysocki, B.; Idaszek, J.; Szlązak, K.; Strzelczyk, K.; Brynk, T.; Kurzydłowski, K.J.; Święszkowski, W. Post Processing and Biological Evaluation of the Titanium Scaffolds for Bone Tissue Engineering. *Materials* **2016**, *9*, 197. [CrossRef]
9. Kamboj, N.; Rodríguez, M.A.; Rahmani, R.; Prashanth, K.G.; Hussainova, I. Bioceramic scaffolds by additive manufacturing for controlled delivery of the antibiotic vancomycin. *Proc. Est. Acad. Sci.* **2019**, *68*, 185–190. [CrossRef]
10. Afshar, M.; Pourkamali Anaraki, A.; Montazerian, H.; Kadkhodapour, J. Additive manufacturing and mechanical characterization of graded porosity scaffolds designed based on triply periodic minimal surface architectures. *J. Mech. Behav. Biomed. Mater.* **2016**, *62*, 481–494. [CrossRef]
11. Kadkhodapour, J.; Montazerian, H.; Darabi, A.C.; Anaraki, A.P.; Ahmadi, S.M.; Zadpoor, A.A.; Schmauder, S. Failure mechanisms of additively manufactured porous biomaterials: Effects of porosity and type of unit cell. *J. Mech. Behav. Biomed. Mater.* **2015**, *50*, 180–191. [CrossRef]
12. Afshar, M.; Pourkamali Anaraki, A.; Montazerian, H. Compressive characteristics of radially graded porosity scaffolds architectured with minimal surfaces. *Mater. Sci. Eng. C* **2018**, *92*, 254–267. [CrossRef] [PubMed]
13. Abueidda, D.W.; Bakir, M.; Abu Al-Rub, R.K.; Bergström, J.S.; Sobh, N.A.; Jasiuk, I. Mechanical properties of 3D printed polymeric cellular materials with triply periodic minimal surface architectures. *Mater. Des.* **2017**, *122*, 255–267. [CrossRef]
14. Sallica-Leva, E.; Jardini, A.L.; Fogagnolo, J.B. Microstructure and mechanical behavior of porous Ti-6Al-4V parts obtained by selective laser melting. *J. Mech. Behav. Biomed. Mater.* **2013**, *26*, 98–108. [CrossRef] [PubMed]
15. Kapfer, S.C.; Hyde, S.T.; Mecke, K.; Arns, C.H.; Schröder-Turk, G.E. Minimal surface scaffold designs for tissue engineering. *Biomaterials* **2011**, *32*, 6875–6882. [CrossRef]

16. Van Bael, S.; Chai, Y.C.; Truscello, S.; Moesen, M.; Kerckhofs, G.; Van Oosterwyck, H.; Kruth, J.P.; Schrooten, J. The effect of pore geometry on the in vitro biological behavior of human periosteum-derived cells seeded on selective laser-melted Ti6Al4V bone scaffolds. *Acta Biomater.* **2012**, *8*, 2824–2834. [CrossRef] [PubMed]
17. Xiao, D.; Yang, Y.; Su, X.; Wang, D.; Luo, Z. Topology optimization of microstructure and selective laser melting fabrication for metallic biomaterial scaffolds. *Trans. Nonferrous Met. Soc. China* **2012**, *22*, 2554–2561. [CrossRef]
18. Yan, C.; Haob, L.; Hussein, A.; Young, P. Ti-6Al-4V triply periodic minimal surface structures for bone implants fabricated via selective laser melting. *J. Mech. Behav. Biomed. Mater.* **2015**, *51*, 61–73. [CrossRef]
19. Vijayavenkataraman, S.; Zhang, L.; Zhang, S.; Ying Hsi Fuh, J.; Feng Lu, W. Triply Periodic Minimal Surfaces Sheet Scaffolds for Tissue Engineering Applications: An Optimization Approach toward Biomimetic Scaffold Design. *ACS Appl. Bio Mater.* **2018**, *1*, 259–269. [CrossRef]
20. Yoo, D. New paradigms in hierarchical porous scaffold design for tissue engineering. *Mater. Sci. Eng. C* **2013**, *33*, 1759–1772. [CrossRef]
21. Paital, S.R.; Dahotre, N.B. Laser surface treatment for porous and textured Ca-P bio-ceramic coating on Ti-6Al-4V. *Biomed. Mater.* **2007**, *2*, 274. [CrossRef] [PubMed]
22. Prashanth, K.G.; Damodaram, R.; Scudino, S.; Wang, Z.; Prasad Rao, K.; Eckert, J. Friction welding of Al-12Si parts produced by selective laser melting. *Mater. Des.* **2014**, *57*, 632–637. [CrossRef]
23. Qin, P.T.; Damodaram, R.; Maity, T.; Zhang, W.W.; Yang, C.; Wang, Z.; Prashanth, K.G. Friction welding of electron beam melted Ti-6Al-4V. *Mater. Sci. Eng. A* **2019**, *761*, 138045. [CrossRef]
24. Zhang, W.; Qin, P.; Wang, Z.; Yang, C.; Kollo, L.; Grzesiak, D.; Prashanth, K.G. Superior wear resistance in EBM-processed TC4 alloy compared with SLM and forged samples. *Materials* **2019**, *12*, 782. [CrossRef] [PubMed]
25. Bandyopadhyay, A.; Espana, F.; Balla, V.K.; Bose, S.; Ohgami, Y.; Davies, N.M. Influence of porosity on mechanical properties and in vivo response of Ti6Al4V implants. *Acta Biomater.* **2010**, *6*, 1640–1648. [CrossRef] [PubMed]
26. Rahmani, R.; Rosenberg, M.; Ivask, A.; Kollo, L. Comparison of mechanical and antibacterial properties of TiO2/Ag ceramics and Ti6Al4V-TiO2/Ag composite materials using combining SLM-SPS techniques. *Metals* **2019**, *9*, 874. [CrossRef]
27. Papynov, W.K.; Mayorov, V.Y.; Portnyagin, A.S.; Shichalin, O.O.; Kobylyakov, S.P.; Kaidalova, T.A.; Nepomnyashiy, A.V.; Sokol'nitskaya, T.A.; Zub, Y.L.; Avramenko, V.A. Application of carbonaceous template for porous structure control of ceramic composites based on synthetic wollastonite obtained via Spark Plasma Sintering. *Ceramics Int.* **2015**, *41*, 1171–1176. [CrossRef]
28. Xue, W.; Liu, X.; Zheng, X.B.; Ding, C. In vivo evaluation of plasma-sprayed wollastonite coating. *Biomater.* **2005**, *26*, 3455–3460. [CrossRef]
29. Murphy, S.; Atala, A. 3D bioprinting of tissues and organs. *Nat. Biotech.* **2014**, *32*, 773–785. [CrossRef]
30. Rahmani, R.; Antonov, M.; Kollo, L. Wear Resistance of (Diamond-Ni)-Ti6Al4V Gradient Materials Prepared by Combined Selective Laser Melting and Spark Plasma Sintering Techniques. *Adv. Tribol.* **2019**, *2019*, 5415897. [CrossRef]
31. Slaughter, W.S. *The Linearized Theory of Elasticity*; Springer: Berlin/Heidelberg, Germany, 2002.
32. Prashanth, K.G.; Loeber, L.; Klauss, H.-J.; Kuehn, U.; Eckert, J. Characterization of 316L steel cellular dodecahedron structures produced by selective laser melting. *Technologies* **2016**, *4*, 34. [CrossRef]
33. Wan, X.; Hu, A.; Li, M.; Chang, C.; Mao, D. Performances of CaSiO3 ceramic sintered by spark plasma sintering. *Mater. Charact.* **2008**, *59*, 256–260. [CrossRef]
34. Simonelli, M.; Tse, Y.Y.; Tuck, C. Effect of the build orientation on the mechanical properties and fracture modes of SLM Ti-6Al-4V. *Mater. Sci. Eng. A* **2014**, *616*, 1–11. [CrossRef]
35. Murr, L.E.; Esquivel, E.V.; Quinones, S.A.; Gaytan, S.M.; Lopez, M.I.; Martinez, E.Y.; Medina, F.; Hernandez, D.H.; Martinez, E.; Martinez, J.L.; et al. Microstructures and mechanical properties of electron beam-rapid manufactured Ti-6Al-4V biomedical prototypes compared to wrought Ti-6Al-4V. *Mater. Charact.* **2009**, *60*, 96–105. [CrossRef]
36. Maskery, I.; Aboulkhair, N.T.; Aremu, A.O.; Tuck, C.J.; Ashcroft, I.A. Compressive failure modes and energy absorption in additively manufactured double gyroid lattices. *Addit. Manuf.* **2017**, *16*, 24–29. [CrossRef]

37. Truscello, S.; Kerckhofs, G.; Van Bael, S.; Pyka, G.; Schrooten, J.; Van Oosterwyck, H. Prediction of permeability of regular scaffolds for skeletal tissue engineering: A combined computational and experimental study. *Acta Biomater.* **2012**, *8*, 1648–1658. [CrossRef]
38. Li, H.; Chang, J. Fabrication and characterization of bioactive wollastonite/PHBV composite scaffolds. *Biomaterials* **2004**, *25*, 5473–5480. [CrossRef]
39. Rahmani, R.; Antonov, M.; Kollo, L. Selective Laser Melting of Diamond-Containing or Postnitrided Materials Intended for Impact-Abrasive Conditions: Experimental and Analytical Study. *Adv. Mater. Sci. Eng.* **2019**, *2019*, 4210762. [CrossRef]
40. Rahmani, R.; Antonov, M.; Kamboj, N. Modelling of impact-abrasive wear of ceramic, metallic, and composite materials. *Proc. Est. Acad. Sci.* **2019**, *68*, 191–197. [CrossRef]

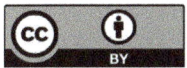 © 2019 by the authors. Licensee MDPI, Basel, Switzerland. This article is an open access article distributed under the terms and conditions of the Creative Commons Attribution (CC BY) license (http://creativecommons.org/licenses/by/4.0/).

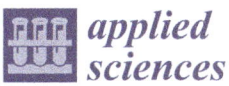

Article

Porous Titanium for Biomedical Applications: Evaluation of the Conventional Powder Metallurgy Frontier and Space-Holder Technique

Sheila Lascano [1,*], Cristina Arévalo [2], Isabel Montealegre-Melendez [2], Sergio Muñoz [2], José A. Rodriguez-Ortiz [2], Paloma Trueba [2] and Yadir Torres [2,*]

[1] Departamento de Ingeniería Mecánica, Universidad Técnica Federico Santa María, Avda. Vicuña Mackenna Poniente N° 3939- San Joaquín, 8320000 Santiago, Chile
[2] Departamento de Ingeniería y Ciencia de los Materiales y del Transporte, E.T.S. de Ingeniería-Escuela Politécnica Superior, Universidad de Sevilla, Camino de los Descubrimientos, s/n. 41092 Sevilla, Spain; carevalo@us.es (C.A.); imontealegre@us.es (I.M.-M.); sergiomunoz@us.es (S.M.); jarortiz@us.es (J.A.R.-O.); ptrueba@us.es (P.T.)
* Correspondence: sheila.lascano@usm.cl (S.L.); ytorres@us.es (Y.T.); Tel.: +56-2-23037262 (S.L.)

Received: 1 February 2019; Accepted: 4 March 2019; Published: 8 March 2019

Abstract: Titanium and its alloys are reference materials in biomedical applications because of their desirable properties. However, one of the most important concerns in long-term prostheses is bone resorption as a result of the stress-shielding phenomena. Development of porous titanium for implants with a low Young's modulus has accomplished increasing scientific and technological attention. The aim of this study is to evaluate the viability, industrial implementation and potential technology transfer of different powder-metallurgy techniques to obtain porous titanium with stiffness values similar to that exhibited by cortical bone. Porous samples of commercial pure titanium grade-4 were obtained by following both conventional powder metallurgy (PM) and space-holder technique. The conventional PM frontier (Loose-Sintering) was evaluated. Additionally, the technical feasibility of two different space holders (NH_4HCO_3 and NaCl) was investigated. The microstructural and mechanical properties were assessed. Furthermore, the mechanical properties of titanium porous structures with porosities of 40% were studied by Finite Element Method (FEM) and compared with the experimental results. Some important findings are: (i) the optimal parameters for processing routes used to obtain low Young's modulus values, retaining suitable mechanical strength; (ii) better mechanical response was obtained by using NH_4HCO_3 as space holder; and (iii) Ti matrix hardening when the interconnected porosity was 36–45% of total porosity. Finally, the advantages and limitations of the PM techniques employed, towards an industrial implementation, were discussed.

Keywords: biomaterials; titanium; powder metallurgy; loose sintering; finite element method; mechanical behaviour

---

1. Introduction

Nowadays, most of the research efforts are focused on the development of metallic biomaterials for bone replacement. Among all biomaterials, it is widely known that titanium and its alloys are the candidates with the best in vitro and in vivo behaviour. However, the stress-shielding phenomenon remains a concern in their use for biomedical applications. The stress shielding is associated with the mismatch between the Young's modulus of bone tissue and titanium (cortical bone around 20–25 GPa and titanium 110 GPa) [1], which causes bone resorption and eventual fracture of the host cortical bone surrounding the implants [2,3].

The design and manufacturing of implants with lower stiffness materials could be a solution for this problem [4] and several works conducted aiming to develop scaffolds with a suitable balance between mechanical and biofunctional behaviour [5–7]. Currently, there are different methods to reduce the stress shielding, such as: (i) Polymer matrix compounds. An example of this kind of biomaterial is the HAPEX®, composed by 40% hydroxyapatite and 60% HDPE (High Density Polyethylene), although it is not used for load-bearing applications due to their limited mechanical properties [8]. (ii) Metastable β-titanium alloys. These materials have lower moduli (55–90 GPa) and have been in development since the 1990s. Even the low moduli monolithic Ti alloys are significantly stiffer than bone [9]. Their medical use is also conditioned for their low wear resistance and limited strength. Important advances in new Ti-Nb-Ta-Mn alloys represent a promising way to solve problems related to stress shielding but still the reduced strength of the samples is considered a concern [10]. (iii) Porous materials. Up to 34 processing routes to fabricate porous materials have been reported [11–13]. The objective of many of these methods is the manufacturing of titanium foams [14–20], in which the porosity percentage must be controlled with the aim to reduce the implant stiffness without any undesirable influence on the mechanical properties [21]. In this context, the limitations in controlling the quantity, size, distribution and morphology of the pores by conventional routes should be considered. Furthermore, the high cost, and the great difficulty in obtaining reproducibility and versatility of the new processing routes (laser sintering, ion beam milling, field-assisted sintering technology (FAST), etc.) should be also contemplated. On the contrary, both the powder-metallurgy processing and the space-holder technique provide a suitable route to obtain Ti porous structures [21]; they also have a remarkable advantage because they are an economical and non-toxic methods, without a toxic agent that can affect cellular functions.

From a powder-technology point of view, porous titanium could be produced by several methods [12,13,17–25]. The performance of porous titanium via conventional Powder Metallurgy (PM) offers flexibility and it is also a cost-effective alternative. Among the different techniques, there are interesting manufacturing processes where low compaction pressures are employed because of higher porosities and a lower Young's modulus can be obtained. Loose sintering (LS) is an attractive method to produce porous specimens. In this process, compaction pressure is not applied. In this way, specimens produced by this technique have higher porosity than specimens fabricated via conventional PM. Despite that, there are not so many works where the porous titanium could be produced at low compaction pressure [1]. In order to solve the limitations of conventional PM, space holder techniques help to control porosity parameters such as pore morphology and percentage [1,15,26–31].

In addition, the effective material response can be determined experimentally or numerically. Although the experimental characterization cannot be replaced entirely by numerical methods, numerical analyses complementing the experimental characterization may serve to reduce the experimental effort significantly, filling gaps in experimentation. In this sense, numerical models have the potential to provide a deeper insight into the underlying microstructural mechanisms of deformation and thus a deeper understanding of the material behaviour. Finite Element Method (FEM) is presented as a useful technique to generate the models of titanium foams in order to obtain mechanical properties [32].

Therefore, within the above context, the aim of the present study is to appraise the feasibility and repeatability of described processing techniques: conventional PM, LS and space-holder technique. In addition, the mechanical properties of porous structures have been assessed by FEM. The results obtained are compared in order to evaluate those different techniques, in terms of advantages and limitations, and the particular features of each fabrication route. The present work has been concluded with a summary of the most favourable technique according to industrial viability, economic benefits and reproducibility, achieving an optimal equilibrium between mechanical properties and biofunctional behaviour.

2. Materials and Methods

Commercially pure titanium (cp Ti) powder produced by a hydrogenation/dehydrogenation process has been used as the starting powder (SE-JONG Materials Co. Ltd., Incheon, Korea).

Its chemical composition is equivalent to cp Ti ASTM F67-00 Grade IV. Two different space holders have been employed: sodium chloride, NaCl (Panreac Química S.A.U., Barcelona, Spain, purity > 99.5%) and ammonium bicarbonate, NH_4HCO_3, (Cymit Química S.L, Barcelona, Spain, with a purity of 99.9%). The space-holder granules, NaCl and NH_4HCO_3, with a large particle size (according to Table 1) were selected to promote a higher degree of interconnectivity of the pores, and a high average size of space holder (>100 μm) would fulfil the requirements to ensure the bone ingrowth.

Table 1. Particle size distribution of materials used.

	$d_{[10]}$, μm	$d_{[50]}$, μm	$d_{[90]}$, μm
Ti powder	9.7	23.3	48.4
NaCl	183.0	384.0	701.0
NH_4HCO_3	73.0	233.0	497.0

In order to obtain the green bodies, conventional PM at low pressure (including its particular limits: loose sintering, LS) and space-holder techniques have been implemented. In an LS route, the metal powder has been poured and vibrated into a cylindrical mould of alumina for 2 min, which has then been heated to the sintering temperature chosen (1000 °C and 1200 °C) under high vacuum (~10^{-5} mbar). In the space-holder technique: (1) the blends of cp Ti powder and space-holder particles [cp Ti+NaCl or cp Ti + NH_4HCO_3], only powder mixtures with 30 and 40 volume percent of space holders were prepared in a Turbula® T2C, blended for 40 min to ensure good homogenization; (2) afterwards, the compaction of the mixture takes place (800 MPa, pressure defined according to the compressibility curve of the material and the results of a previous work [26]), (3) subsequently, regarding to the space holder used, the elimination step has been performed. The NH_4HCO_3 is thermally removed (60 °C + 110 °C; both stages of the thermal treatment are carried out for 10–12 h and at low vacuum conditions 10^{-2} mbar) [26], while the salt has dissolved in distilled water (temperature between 50 and 60 °C, without agitation and during 4–5 immersion cycles) [19]. Sintering was carried out under high vacuum in a CARBOLYTE STF 15/75/450 ceramic furnace with a horizontal tube (2 h at 1250 °C under high vacuum conditions: ~10^{-5} mbar) [26].

The manufacturing parameters have been stablished in order to obtain mechanical properties (Young's modulus, E, and yield strength, σ_y) similar to the cortical bone. The powder mass has been calculated to produce specimens with fit dimensions for compression tests (height/diameter = 0.8). The compaction stage in conventional PM and space-holder technique has been carried out in an INSTRON 5505 machine (Instron, Massachusetts, United State).

Density measurement has been performed out through the Archimedes' method with distilled water impregnation, due to its experimental simplicity and reasonable reliability (ASTM C373-88). Total porosity $P(Arch)$ and interconnected porosity (P_i) have been calculated from the density measurements. For the image analysis, sectioned parts have been prepared by a sequence of conventional metallographic steps (resin mounting and grinding) followed by a mechanic-chemical polishing with magnesium oxide and hydrogen peroxide. The porosity evaluation by image analysis has been performed by using an optical microscope Nikon Epiphot (Nikon, Tokyo, Japan) coupled with a camera Jenoptik Progres C3 (Jenoptik, Jena, Germany), and the software Image-Pro Plus 6.2, Mediacibernetic, Bethesda, MD, USA. Image analysis has been evaluated with 10 pictures of 5× and 20× for each processing condition. The following morphological pore parameters have been estimated by this method: (i) the total porosity $P(IA)$, (ii) equivalent diameter (D_{eq}) defined as the average diameter measured from the pore centroid, (iii) the pore shape factor, $F_f = 4\pi A/(PE)^2$, where A is the pore area and PE is the experimental perimeter of the pore, (iv) the mean free path between the pores is described as the mean size of the necks between the pores, λ, and (v) the pore interconnectivity (C_{pore}) is defined as the fraction of connected pores of the total reference line length. Light Microscopy (LM) has also been used for the basic observation of the microstructural features of the surface samples.

The mechanical compression testing has been achieved according to the recommendations of the Standard ASTM E9-89A, by means of a universal electromechanical Instron machine 5505 applying a strain rate of 0.005 mm/mm·min. All tests have been run up to a strain of 50%. The yield strength (σ_y), relative strength (defined as the ratio between the strength of porous material and the bulk material) and Young's modulus (E_c) have also been determined. Furthermore, dynamic Young's modulus (E_d) measurements by the ultrasound technique have been performed [26,33]. Three specimens have been tested in order to calculate a mean value of dynamic Young's modulus. Previously, the specimens have been characterised by porosity measurements (density) and mechanical compression testing.

Finally, FEM was implemented to conduct the numerical characterization of mechanical properties (Young's modulus, E, and yield strength, σ_y) for the sample with 40 vol.% of porosity developed in this work. For this, a 2D finite element model proposed by the authors [6,34] was used. This numerical model, based on geometries generated from information of the pore morphology, combines a 2D periodic geometry with the information of the pore morphology extracted from image analysis (P(IA), pore size distribution, and elongation factor, F_e).

3. Results

This section may be divided by subheadings. It should provide a concise and precise description of the experimental results, and their interpretation as well as the experimental conclusions that can be drawn.

3.1. Physical and Microstructural Properties

LM micrographs and parameters associated to porosity ($P(IA)$, D_{eq}, F_f, λ and C_{pore}) are shown in Figure 1 and Table 2. These parameters are related to the researched processing routes: conventional PM technique (compaction pressure (0 and 13 MPa) and sintering temperature (1000 and 1200 °C)) and space-holder technique (type (NaCl and NH$_4$HCO$_3$) and space-holder content (30 and 40 vol.%)). For the last route, compaction pressure and sintering temperature have been fixed in 600 MPa and 1250 °C, respectively.

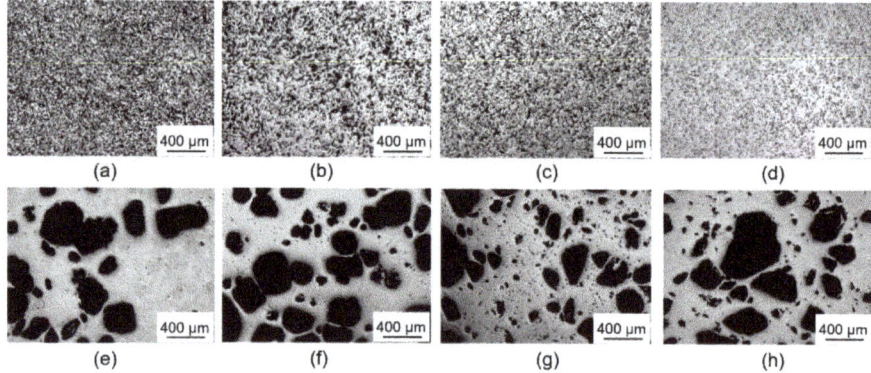

Figure 1. Micrographs corresponding to different processing conditions of evaluated techniques: Loose Sintering, conventional Powder Metallurgy (PM) and space-holder technique: (**a**) 0 MPa and 1000 °C; (**b**) 0 MPa and 1200 °C; (**c**) 13 MPa and 1000 °C; (**d**) 13 MPa and 1200 °C; (**e**) 30 vol.% NaCl; (**f**) 40 vol.% NaCl (**g**) 30 vol.% NH$_4$HCO$_3$; and (**h**) 40 vol.% NH$_4$HCO$_3$. All of the samples have been sintered for 2 h under high vacuum (~10^{-5} bar).

Table 2. Effect of different techniques and processing conditions on the porosity of the samples.

Processing Conditions		Archimedes			Image Analysis			
		P_i, %	$P(Arch)$, %	$P(IA)$, %	D_{eq}, μm	F_f	C_{pore}	λ, μm
Loose Sintering	1000 °C	44.1	44.8	45.3	17	0.70	0.2	25
	1200 °C	28.5	35.2	30.0	15	0.82	0.1	41
13 MPa	1000 °C	28.0	29.3	30.8	14	0.79	0.1	36
	1200 °C	6.2	13.6	13.1	10	0.93	0.0	66
Space holder	30 vol.% NaCl	20.5	28.5	28.4	47.0	0.90	0.3	157
	40 vol.% NaCl	27.5	35.8	35.1	78.0	0.74	0.2	181
	30 vol.% NH_4HCO_3	22.4	27.8	29.1	18.1	0.90	0.3	57
	40 vol.% NH_4HCO_3	29.3	37.6	36.6	32.0	0.84	0.3	80

3.2. Mechanical Properties

In this work, the influence of the manufacturing technique that would lead to obtaining an optimal equilibrium between the mechanical strength and the Young's modulus in order to replace the cortical bone (150–200 MPa and 20–25 GPa, respectively) is analysed. Table 3 summarizes the results of mechanical compression testing and ultrasound technique.

Table 3. Effect of different techniques and processing conditions on mechanical properties of the samples obtained by compression test and ultrasound testing.

Processing Conditions		Experimental		
		σ_y, MPa	E_c, GPa	E_d, GPa
Loose Sintering	1000 °C	67	9.6	29.1
	1200 °C	165	25.1	50.5
13 MPa	1000 °C	200	12.5	50.1
	1200 °C	350	26.1	59.4
Space holder	30 vol.% NaCl	415	4.6	45.1
	40 vol.% NaCl	187	5.3	29.0
	30 vol.% NH_4HCO_3	389	15.9	38.9
	40 vol.% NH_4HCO_3	272	5.8	30.0

In addition, the influence of the total porosity in the Young modulus (by ultrasound technique) is illustrated in Figure 2. As expected, the material stiffness presents a direct relation to the effective area of the titanium matrix (inverse to the porosity). Mathematical models are also added to fit the experimental results: Gibson and Ashby [35], Pabst-Gregorová [36], and Knudsen [37] and Spriggs [38].

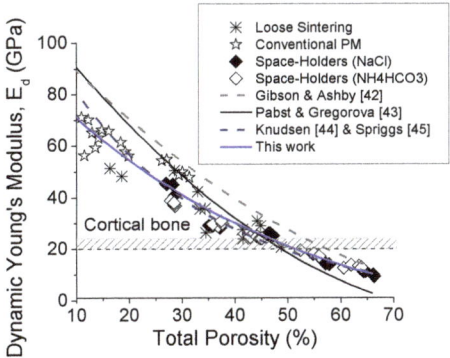

Figure 2. Dynamic Young modulus vs. total porosity: Influence of the manufacturing route.

In the present work, a new and suitable model is proposed in order to represent the experimental results in porous titanium materials from total porosity between 10 and 60 vol.% (see in Equation (1)):

$$E = E_{Ti}\left(e^{-0.02P}\right) - 0.03E_{Ti}, \tag{1}$$

where E_{Ti} is the Young's modulus for bulk titanium and P is the total porosity of the sample.

Moreover, in previous research, different models have been developed to explain the correlation between the relative strength and the density in sintered materials. In the geometric model, spherical pores are assumed [39]. It is based on the geometrical relation between the porosity and the cross section area of the material. In addition, there is a model known as "simple Brick" where the pores with a cubic geometry are supposed [40]. The relative strength is determined in this method, considering the probability of being found a solid part in the tested volume. A correlation between the relative strength vs. density and interconnected porosity of the porous titanium specimens, produced via conventional PM and space-holder techniques, are shown in Figure 3a,b, respectively.

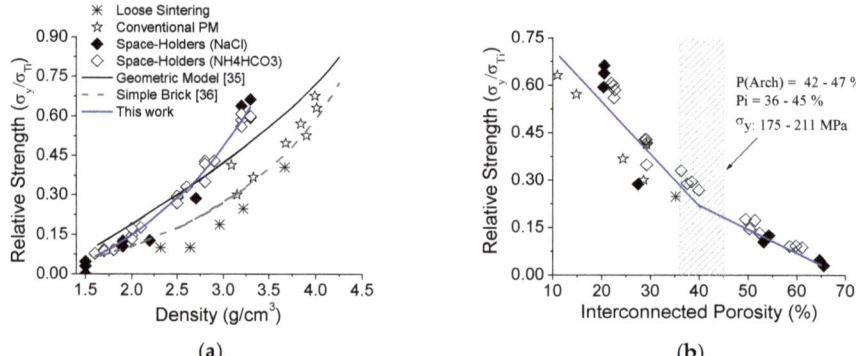

Figure 3. (**a**) Density vs. Relative Strength; (**b**) Interconnected Porosity and Relative Porosity vs. Relative Strength (porous material strength/full dense material strength).

The analysis of mechanical behaviour of specimens produced via conventional PM, could be estimated using the simple brick model; however, the geometrical model is not capable of predicting any tendency. Therefore, in Equation (2), an exponential model is proposed in order to fit successfully the type and range of pores, which are produced by the space -holder technique:

$$\frac{\sigma_y}{\sigma_{Ti}} = \left(1.88\, e^{-3P}\right) - 0.2. \tag{2}$$

3.3. Finite Element Simulation

The case under study chosen in this numerical analysis is the porous compact fabricated following the space holder technique, by using ammonium bicarbonate, NH_4HCO_3, as a space holder and obtaining a 40 vol.% of total porosity. This is the porous compact that has shown the most interesting mechanical properties, with the best balance between stiffness and mechanical integrity and, consequently, the ideal candidate for the use in cortical bone replacement. Following the methodology described by Muñoz et al. [6,34], and making use of the main porosity characteristics extracted from experiments (total porosity, pore size distribution and elongation factor distribution), one finite element geometry has been randomly generated for the porous materials under study: 40 vol.% of total porosity. The simulated microstructure of the porous material is comprised of two different phases: a titanium matrix and a series of pores randomly distributed. The mechanical properties of cp Ti have been used to describe the behaviour of the titanium matrix: a Young's modulus E_{Ti} = 110 GPa, a yield stress

σ_{Ti} = 700 MPa and a Poisson's ratio ν = 0.33. In order to describe the hardening plasticity behaviour of titanium, an isotropic hardening with a very small tangent modulus E_T = 1 GPa has been used. The pore morphology (equivalent diameter, D_{eq}, and elongation factor, F_e) has randomly generated following a normal distribution from the experimental data. The following values have been extracted from experimentation to be used in the pore generation: D_{eq} = 32 µm and F_e = 0.65. In addition, the pore orientation has also been randomly generated following a uniform distribution.

Making use of the FE models, two different compression tests have been simulated. First, with the aim of predicting the mechanical properties of the porous material, a compression test under displacement control up to 1% macroscopic strain has been simulated. Then, the predicted uniaxial stress–strain responses have been obtained. The results in the simulation are summarized in Table 4.

Table 4. Prediction of mechanical properties for the case of study corresponding to a porous compact fabricated by 40 vol.% NH_4HCO_3 space holder.

Properties	Experimental	FEM
E, GPa	31	39
σ_y, MPa	170	153

From the presented results, it can be seen that very good agreement is achieved with the proposed FE model, for both Young's modulus and yield stress.

Second, in order to complete the numerical analysis and for a better understanding of the mechanical behaviour of the porous material, the stress distribution within the porous matrix has been analysed in detail. By using the proposed FE model, a compression test under displacement control was performed until the macroscopic yield is reached (σ_y = 170 MPa, in this case). The results of this virtual test can be seen in Figure 4, where the contour plot of the von Mises stress distribution at macroscopic yield is shown.

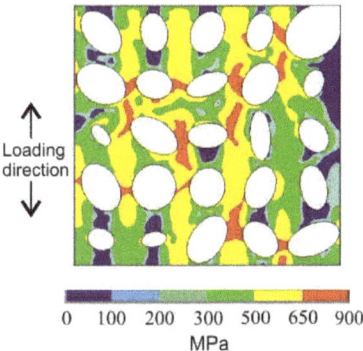

Figure 4. Example of Von Mises stress distribution at macroscopic yield. The case studied corresponding to a porous compact fabricated by a 40 vol.% NH_4HCO_3 space holder.

In Figure 4, it can be observed that, even though the applied macroscopic stress is only 170 MPa, there is a considerable portion of the material with a high stress level, due to stress concentration around the pores, as it could be expected.

4. Discussion

In the present study, potentialities and disadvantages of different processing routes are compared in terms of: viability (cost and potential industrial application), reproducibility (reliability), limitations (porosity range, size, shape and distribution) and transversality of stablished or optimized protocols to other interested emerged and/or higher value added sectors. The framework used to make that comparison is based on the capability to achieve an optimum equilibrium between mechanical (E and σ_y, according according to bone tissue to substitute) and biofunctional behaviour (allowing bone ingrowth and obtaining an inside porous roughness to improve osteointegration and infiltration with bioactive materials).

Concerning to the microstructural results, in conventional PM, compaction pressure and sintering temperature have a significant effect in porosity (see Table 2). In general, temperature has the highest effect over porous morphological parameters as well as final porosity. For the temperature range studied, when temperature increases, an approximately 70% porosity reduction is observed. Porosity range that can be achieved through the implementation of this technique is from 13.6% to 44.8%, reaching the highest values by LS at 1000 °C sintering temperature. In this case, the porosity becomes more interconnected (44.1% at 0 MPa and 28.0% at 13 MPa). As it was expected, when temperature increases: (a) pore size is reduced, a 12% for 0 MPa compaction pressure level and a 29% for the highest pressure value; (b) pores are more rounded (shape factor, F_f, close to one); (c) closed or isolated porosity is higher; (d) porous contiguity decreases until reaching zero value (isolated porosity); and (e) the distance between porous is 2.64 higher. Moreover, in general, compaction pressure effect is lower than the temperature influence.

Regarding to the space-holder technique, the type of space holder used defines the porous morphology (irregular surface), fracture behaviour and plastic deformation of the specimens. These factors could affect, to some extent: (1) preserving the pore size (related to the space-holder volume); (2) the pore walls roughness; (3) increasing of interconnectivity between the pores; (4) the collapse of the porous structure of specimens (structural integrity of the samples during the process of space-holder evacuation); (5) the manufacturing cost of the specimens (time and resources); (6) the reproducibility of the evacuation space-holder process (it depends on the number and control of the process parameters) and (7) the risk of the residual space-holder content, from the point of biomedical view.

In this context, considering the range of compaction pressure, it is observed how the use of space holders allows for achieving higher porosity levels and similar sizes to the original space holder distribution compared to the conventional PM technique.

The total porosity could be controlled by varying space-holder content, although a small proportion of isolated micro-porosity has been observed (Figure 1 and Table 2). This micro-porosity is produced during the sintering of titanium powders.

The role and the comparison of the studied space-holder size (NaCl and NH_4HCO_3) should be analysed by considering the particle size distribution of the starting powders (Table 1). By using 30 vol.% of space-holder content, D_{eq} of the obtained pores is around 2.6 greater employing NaCl. Although the differences between the obtained D_{eq} can lead to a decrease in a 15% using 40 vol.% of space holder. The increasing of interconnectivity (λ) for NH_4HCO_3 implies balances between the differences due to an original space-holder size employed.

Moreover, a round shaped porosity is formed (slightly shape boundary related to the sintering stage). Nevertheless, a small part of the porous, for NaCl as a space-holder, could be preserving the cubic geometry according to the original morphology, whereas the pores are shaped due to the employment of the NH_4HCO_3 showing an elliptical and elongated morphology. Additionally, the porous titanium specimens produced by NH_4HCO_3 manifest a better porous homogeneity distribution than the ones fabricated with NaCl; during the powder compaction, the NaCl is less fractured than the NH_4HCO_3. In spite of that, the NaCl removal is more costly, less repeatable and less feasible to industrial implementation.

Regardless of the nature of the space-holder, increasing their content has some important outcomes: pore shape factor is reduced (irregular morphology of porous boundary); the contiguity (C_{pore}) is kept constant for both cases; interconnected porosity for 30 vol.% of space holder represents the 75% of the total porosity, while 40 vol.% of space holder reaches 78 %. Both values of the interconnected porosity and the suitable size of the pores promote the bone ingrowth. However, its influences on the mechanical behaviour should be considered (see below).

At this point of this reported research, the results and discussion have been focused on the analysis of each fabrication method independently, where the influence of the processing parameters on the porosity has been evaluated. The following stage is now emphasised on a general comparison of both processing routes. A significant difference in morphology and porosity distribution among the specimens produced via conventional PM and a space-holder technique is observed (see in Figure 1). In conventional PM, the obtained pores present an irregular shape and a more homogenous distribution than in the space-holder process, in which the morphology of the pores reproduces the employed space-holder geometry. The D_{eq} obtained by using a space holder are larger than those resulted from the conventional PM (Table 2). These results verify the potential and versatility of the space-holder method to control the shape, the size, the proportion and distribution of the porosity, in order to achieve biofunctional and biomechanical equilibrium of the implants. This notwithstanding, both industrial application viability and low cost of conventional PM routes are well known features.

Within the context of porous implants in contact with bone tissue, some previous papers have reported that a suitable bone ingrowth can be achieved with a mean pore size of around 50 μm [41,42]. However, there are other studies where the optimal bone ingrowth happens for pore size range of 100–200 μm [9,43,44]. Nevertheless, several authors' works show a better infiltration achievement with polymers or bioactive glasses if the pore size overcomes 200 μm [45]. Accordingly, the conventional PM route manifests a drawback and thus only 6% of the pores (0 MPa and 1000 °C), which assures doubtful bone ingrowth, being almost a non-existent possibility to perform infiltration tests. On the other hand, the space-holder method allows for achieving successful results of optimal bone growth and better infiltration of the polymers or bio-glasses in the pores [45].

Considering the mechanical behaviour analysis results (Figure 2), to achieve a suitable stiffness range (20–25 GPa), it is necessary to obtain a total porosity between 40–55%. It could be achieved by using conventional PM, only when temperature and pressure are in the limits of this technique (0 MPa and sintering temperatures 1000 °C and 1100 °C), although there is a notable loss of the mechanical strength (see below). However, the space-holder technique presents a great feasibility to get these values of total porosity and even to lower stiffness values (6–8 GPa at higher porosity), it being possible to replace the trabecular tissue by these obtained results.

Concerning mechanical properties, two different analyses have been made, aiming at the evaluation of the role of the manufacturing route tested in the compression behaviour (Figure 5). Independent of the processing technique used, a parameter is fixed for each comparison: in Figure 5a, Young's modulus close to the cortical bone is set in ~29 GPa (porosity total range between 37.6–44.8%) and the influence of the processing technique on the yield strength (σ_y) of the porous specimens is studied. In order to reach the same Young's modulus, higher porosity is needed for a loose-sintering technique, its compression yield strength being committed (Table 3). This fact is related to the lack of powder compaction step and low sintering temperatures, without ensuring a good strength of the formed neck (also critical to fatigue and flexural requirements).

Yield strength values are fixed in a range from 150 to 200 MPa meeting the requirements of the cortical bone tissue in Figure 5b, evaluating what occurs with the total porosity, the mean size of the pores (Table 2) and the Young's modulus (Table 3). A complete analysis of the results seen in Figure 5b allows for specifying that only samples processed by a space-holder technique with 40 vol.% could be implemented as substitute of the cortical tissue (bio-mechanical balance between stiffness ~20–25 GPa and mechanical strength, ~150–200 MPa). These specimens present a total porosity of ~37%. Two behaviours of losing mechanical efficiency are observed related respectively to: decreasing compaction pressure by a conventional PM route (reduction of cold welding of titanium powders, weaker necks); and increasing the pore size in a space-holder technique.

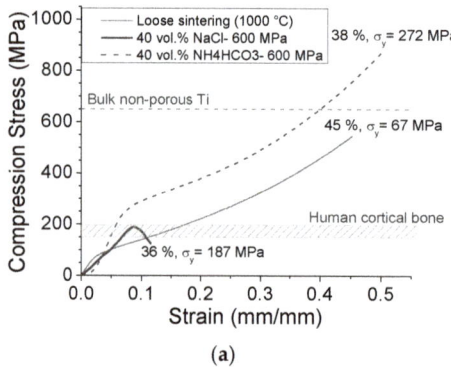 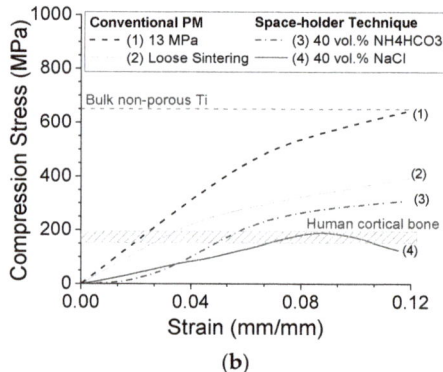

Figure 5. Uniaxial compression tests: (**a**) Young's modulus closed to the cortical bone is set in ~29 GPa (porosity total range between 37.6–44.8%); (**b**) yield strength values are fixed in a range (150–200 MPa) meeting the requirements of the cortical tissue. Compression stress vs. Strain curves of specimens manufactured by different PM routes.

The decreasing trend of the relative strength observed in Figure 3a,b undergoes two different performances (see in the slope curves). A proportional and expected loss of the mechanical strength with the reduction of the load section is observed. Then, a part of the strength decrement regarding the pore content, is compensated by the titanium matrix strengthening (see in the lowest slope); this fact occurs in ratio $P_i/P(\text{Arch}) \geq 0.89$ ($P_i = 40\%$) and it is related to the large stress triaxiality originated by more interconnected porosity, in addition to more roughness contour of pores. This strengthening is not representative to the porosity range achieved via conventional PM. The mechanical requirements of cortical bone tissue could be guaranteed in the shaded area in Figure 3b (175–211 MPa). These results are consistent with that proposed by Kubicki [46]: before the mean stress reaches levels close to the yield strength (approx. 33%), in the surrounding area of the notch, it is produced a triaxiality stress state and local plastic strain. As a consequence in ductile material, the yield strength of a notched specimen is higher than the uniaxial one [47]. Therefore, the local plastic strain involves a macroscopic hardening reflected in the yield strength increment of the material [48]. This aspect was observed in Figure 4, where a localized effect of pores was made evident, but a good balance between the mechanical properties was achieved (Table 4), according to the results obtained by the FE model.

5. Conclusions

The assessing of conventional PM and space holder technique reported here allowed for stating some findings about the influence on both microstructural and mechanical properties of porous Ti for bone replacement:

1. Young's modulus of porous Ti samples could be reached close enough to the cortical bone by conventional PM (29 GPa), in the absence of the compaction pressure stage (loose-sintering technique), with a sintering temperature of 1000 °C, and 2 h under high vacuum. However, the mean pore size (~17 µm) and the mechanical strength (~67 MPa) of the porous titanium do not guarantee the mechanical requirements of biomedical applications. Both increments of compaction pressure and sintering temperature improve the quality of the sintering necks, which imply decreasing of the amount and the size of the pores; consequently, the stiffness is increased (≥ 50.5 GPa) and the capability of bone ingrowth.

2. The space-holder method is the more suitable of the two evaluated routes to reach a biomechanical balance (E and σ_y) and biofunctional equilibrium (bone ingrowth), through the control of the processing parameters, the type of space holder, the compaction pressure and the sintering temperature, according to viability, feasibility and implementation costs in the industrial sector, in

addition to the achievement of the desirable balance. The use of NH_4HCO_3 as space holder (40 vol.% and ~200–300 μm mean particle size distribution) is recommended. The optimal manufacturing parameters proposed are the following ones: firstly, a compaction pressure of 600 MPa, next, in the space-holder elimination stage, 60 °C for 10 h plus 110 °C for 12 h in vacuum (10^{-2} mbar) and sintering conditions at 1250 °C, for 2 h and high vacuum (10^{-5} mbar). These parameters ensure the production of porous titanium where the stress-shielding phenomenon is reduced, and suitable mechanical strength and bone ingrowth are achieved.

Author Contributions: All of the authors have contributed to obtaining a high-quality research work. S.L. has been responsible for the experimental results and analysis of data, C.A. and I.M.-M. performed analysis of the results and writing the original draft, S.M. was responsible of finite element analysis, J.A.R.-O. and Y.T. have been responsible for materials and processing techniques selection, funding acquisition and project administration, P.T. was responsible for the fabrication processes and the discussion of the results.

Funding: This work was supported by the Ministry of Economy and Competitiveness of Spain under Grant MAT2015-71284-P, Junta de Andalucía under Grant No. P12-TEP-1401 and the funding provided by the Comisión Nacional de Investigación, Científica y Tecnológica (CONICYT) of the Chilean government under the project FONDECYT 11160865.

Acknowledgments: The authors dedicate this paper to the memory of Juan J. Pavón Palacio (University of Antioquia, Colombia) for his valuable contribution in the metal biomaterials field, being a pioneer in this sector and an honourable researcher in the group that has performed this work. The authors wish to thank the laboratory technicians Jesús Pinto and Mari Cruz. Martín, Glenda Hernández and Mauricio Reyes-Valenzuela for carrying out the microstructure characterization and mechanical testing.

Conflicts of Interest: The authors declare no conflict of interest.

References

1. Torres, Y.; Trueba, P.; Pavón, J.; Montealegre, I.; Rodríguez-Ortiz, J. Designing, processing and characterisation of titanium cylinders with graded porosity: An alternative to stress-shielding solutions. *Mater. Des.* **2014**, *63*, 316–324. [CrossRef]
2. Niinomi, M.; Nakai, M.; Hieda, J. Development of new metallic alloys for biomedical applications. *Acta Biomater.* **2012**, *8*, 3888–3903. [CrossRef]
3. Xiong, J.; Li, Y.; Wang, X.; Hodgson, P.; Wen, C.E. Mechanical properties and bioactive surface modification via alkali-heat treatment of a porous Ti–18Nb–4Sn alloy for biomedical applications. *Acta Biomater.* **2008**, *4*, 1963–1968. [CrossRef] [PubMed]
4. Schmidutz, F.; Agarwal, Y.; Müller, P.; Gueorguiev, B.; Richards, R.; Sprecher, C. Stress-shielding induced bone remodeling in cementless shoulder resurfacing arthroplasty: A finite element analysis and in vivo results. *J. Biomech.* **2014**, *47*, 3509–3516. [CrossRef] [PubMed]
5. Herrera, A.; Yánez, A.; Martel, O.; Afonso, H.; Monopoli, D. Computational study and experimental validation of porous structures fabricated by electron beam melting: A challenge to avoid stress shielding. *Mater. Sci. Eng. C* **2014**, *45*, 89–93. [CrossRef] [PubMed]
6. Muñoz, S.; Castillo, S.; Torres, Y. Different models for simulation of mechanical behaviour of porous materials. *J. Mech. Behav. Biomed. Mater.* **2018**, *80*, 88–96. [CrossRef] [PubMed]
7. Arabnejad, S.; Johnston, B.; Tanzer, M.; Pasini, D. Fully porous 3D printed titanium femoral stem to reduce stress-shielding following total hip arthroplasty. *J. Orthop. Res.* **2017**, *35*, 1774–1783. [CrossRef] [PubMed]
8. Bonfield, W.; Grynpas, M.D.; Tully, A.E. Hydroxyapatite reinforced polyethylene—A mechanically compatible implant material for bone replacement. *Biomaterials* **1981**, *2*, 185–186. [CrossRef]
9. Geetha, M.; Singh, R.; Asokamani, R.; Gogia, A.K. Ti based biomaterials, the ultimate choice for orthopaedic implants—A review. *Prog. Mater. Sci.* **2009**, *54*, 397–425. [CrossRef]
10. Aguilar, C.; Guerra, C.; Lascano, S.; Guzman, D.; Rojas, P.A.; Thirumurugan, M.; Bejar, L.; Medina, A. Synthesis and characterization of Ti–Ta–Nb–Mn foams. *Mater. Sci. Eng. C* **2016**, *58*, 420–431. [CrossRef]
11. Trueba, P. Desarrollo de titanio con porosidad gradiente radial y longitudinal para aplicaciones biomédicas. Ph.D. Thesis, University of Seville, Seville, Spain, 2017.
12. Naebe, M.; Shirvanimoghaddam, K. Functionally graded materials: A review of fabrication and properties. *Appl. Mater. Today* **2016**, *5*, 223–245. [CrossRef]

13. Singh, S.; Ramakrishna, S.; Singh, R. Material issues in additive manufacturing: A review. *J. Manuf. Process.* **2017**, *25*, 185–200. [CrossRef]
14. Dewidar, M.M.; Lim, J.K. Properties of solid core and porous surface Ti–6Al–4V implants manufactured by powder metallurgy. *J. Alloys Compd.* **2008**, *454*, 442–446. [CrossRef]
15. Wenjuan, N.; Chenguang, B.; GuiBao, Q.; Qiang, W. Processing and properties of porous titanium using space holder technique. *Mater. Sci. Eng. A* **2009**, *506*, 148–151.
16. Yavari, S.A.; van der Stok, J.; Chai, Y.C.; Wauthle, R.; Birgani, Z.T.; Habibovic, P.; Mulier, M.; Schrooten, J.; Weinans, H.; Zadpoor, A.A. Bone regeneration performance of surface-treated porous titanium. *Biomaterials* **2014**, *35*, 6172–6181. [CrossRef] [PubMed]
17. Torres, Y.; Pavón, J.J.; Nieto, I.; Rodríguez, J.A. Conventional Powder Metallurgy Process and Characterization of Porous Titanium for Biomedical Applications. *Metall. Mater. Trans. B* **2011**, *42*, 891–900. [CrossRef]
18. Li, Y.; Yang, C.; Zhao, H.; Qu, S.; Li, X.; Li, Y. New Developments of Ti-Based Alloys for Biomedical Applications. *Materials* **2014**, *7*, 1709–1800. [CrossRef]
19. Torres, Y.; Pavón, J.; Rodríguez, J. Processing and characterization of porous titanium for implants by using NaCl as space holder. *J. Mater. Process. Technol.* **2012**, *212*, 1061–1069. [CrossRef]
20. Wang, X.; Xu, S.; Zhou, S.; Xu, W.; Leary, M.; Choong, P.; Qian, M.; Brandt, M.; Xie, Y.M. Topological design and additive manufacturing of porous metals for bone scaffolds and orthopaedic implants: A review. *Biomaterials* **2016**, *83*, 127–141. [CrossRef]
21. Torres, Y.; Lascano, S.; Bris, J.; Pavón, J.; Rodriguez, J.A. Development of porous titanium for biomedical applications: A comparison between loose sintering and space-holder techniques. *Mater. Sci. Eng. C* **2014**, *37*, 148–155. [CrossRef]
22. Oh, I.H.; Nomura, N.; Masahashi, N.; Hanada, S. Mechanical properties of porous titanium compacts prepared by powder sintering. *Scr. Mater.* **2003**, *49*, 1197–1202. [CrossRef]
23. Ryan, G.; Pandit, A.; Apatsidis, D.P. Fabrication methods of porous metals for use in orthopaedic applications. *Biomaterials* **2006**, *27*, 2651–2670. [CrossRef] [PubMed]
24. Wang, L.; Liu, P.; Wang, L.; Xing, W.; Fan, Y.; Xu, N. Preparation conditions and porosity of porous titanium sintered under positive pressure. *Mater. Manufact. Proce.* **2013**, *28*, 1166–1170. [CrossRef]
25. Kato, K.; Ochiai, S.; Yamamoto, A.; Daigo, Y.; Honma, K.; Matano, S.; Omori, K. Novel multilayer Ti foam with cortical bone strength and cytocompatibility. *Acta Biomater.* **2013**, *9*, 5802–5809. [CrossRef] [PubMed]
26. Torres, Y.; Rodríguez, J.A.; Arias, S.; Echeverry, M.; Robledo, S.; Amigó, V.; Pavón, J.J. Processing, Characterization and biological testing of porous titanium obtained by space-holder technique. *J. Mater. Sci.* **2012**, *47*, 6565–6576. [CrossRef]
27. Wen, C.E.; Mabuchi, M.; Yamada, Y.; Shimojima, K.; Chino, Y.; Asahina, T. Processing of biocompatible porous Ti and Mg. *Scr. Mater.* **2001**, *45*, 1147–1153. [CrossRef]
28. Laptev, A.; Bram, M.; Buchkremer, D.; Stover, D. Green strength of powder compacts provided for production of highly porous titanium parts. *Powder Metall.* **2005**, *48*, 358. [CrossRef]
29. Jia, J.; Siddiq, A.R.; Kennedy, A.R. Porous titanium manufactured by a novel powder tapping method using spherical salt bead space holders: Characterisation and mechanical properties. *J. Mech. Behav. Biomed. Mater.* **2015**, *48*, 229–240. [CrossRef]
30. Kim, S.W.; Jung, H.-D.; Kang, M.-H.; Kim, H.-E.; Koh, Y.-H.; Estrin, Y. Fabrication of porous titanium scaffold with controlled porous structure and net-shape using magnesium as spacer. *Mater. Sci. Eng. C* **2013**, *33*, 2808–2815. [CrossRef]
31. Mansourighasri, A.; Muhamad, N.; Sulong, A.B. Processing titanium foams using tapioca starch as a space holder. *J. Mater. Process. Technol.* **2012**, *212*, 83–89. [CrossRef]
32. Reddy, T.H.; Pal, S.; Kumar, K.C.; Mohan, M.K.; Kokol, V. Finite Element Analysis for Mechanical Response of Magnesium Foams with Regular Structure Obtained by Powder Metallurgy Method. *Procedia Eng.* **2016**, *149*, 425–430. [CrossRef]
33. Kikuchi, M.; Takahashi, M.; Okuno, O. Elastic Moduli of Cast Ti-Au, Ti- Ag, and Ti- Cu alloys. *Dent. Mater.* **2006**, *22*, 641–646. [CrossRef]
34. Muñoz, S.; Pavón, J.; Rodríguez-Ortiz, J.; Civantos, A.; Allain, J.; Torres, Y. On the influence of space holder in the development of porous titanium implants: Mechanical, computational and biological evaluation. *Mater. Charact.* **2015**, *108*, 68–78. [CrossRef]

35. Gibson, L.J.; Ashby, M.F. *Cellular Solids: Structure and Properties*; Cambridge University Press: Cambridge, UK, 1999.
36. Pabst, W.; Gregorová, E. New relation for the porosity dependence of the effective tensile modulus of brittle materials. *J. Mater. Sci.* **2004**, *39*, 3501–3503. [CrossRef]
37. Knudsen, F. Dependence of mechanical strength of brittle polycrystalline specimens on porosity and grain size. *J. Am. Ceram. Soc.* **1959**, *42*, 376–387. [CrossRef]
38. Spriggs, R. Expression for effect of porosity on elastic modulus of polycrystalline refractory materials, particularly aluminum oxide. *J. Am. Ceram. Soc.* **1961**, *44*, 628–629. [CrossRef]
39. Eudier, M. The mechanical properties of sintered low-alloy steels. *Powder Metall.* **1962**, *5*, 278–290. [CrossRef]
40. Fleck, N.; Smith, R. The mechanical properties of sintered low-alloy steels. *Powder Metall.* **1981**, *3*, 121–125. [CrossRef]
41. Itälä, A.; Ylanen, H.; Ekholm, C.; Karlsson, K.; Aro, H. Pore diameter of more than 100 micron is not requisite for bone ingrowth in rabbits. *J. Biomed. Mater. Res.* **2001**, *58*, 679–683. [CrossRef]
42. Stangl, R.; Rinne, B.; Kastl, S.; Hendrich, C. The influence of pore geometry in cp Ti-implants a cell culture investigation. *Eur. Cells Mater.* **2001**, *2*, 1–9. [CrossRef]
43. Götz, H.E.; Müller, M.; Emmel, A.; Holzwarth, U.; Erben, R.G.; Stangl, R. Effect of surface finish on the osseointegration of laser-treated titanium alloy implants. *Biomaterials* **2004**, *25*, 4057–4064. [CrossRef] [PubMed]
44. Lewis, G. Properties of open-cell porous metals and alloys for orthopaedic applications. *J. Mater. Sci. Mater. Med.* **2013**, *24*, 2293–2325. [CrossRef]
45. Boccaccini, A.R.; Gil, E.; Torres, Y.; Cordero-Arias, L.; Pavón, J.; Rodríguez-Ortiz, J.A.; Borjas, S. Optimization of electrophoretic deposition and characterization of CHITOSAN/45S5 BIOGLASS© composite coatings on porous titanium for biomedical applications. In Proceedings of the International Conference on Electrophoretic Deposition V: Fundamentals and Applications (EPD 2014), Hernstein, Austria, 5–10 October 2014.
46. Kubicki, B. Stress concentration at pores in sintered materials. *Powder Metall.* **1995**, *38*, 295–298. [CrossRef]
47. Dieter, G. *Mechanical Metallurgy*; McGraw-Hill Book Company: New York, NY, USA, 1988.
48. Straffelini, G. Strain hardening behaviour of powder metallurgy alloys. *Powder Metall.* **2005**, *48*, 189–192. [CrossRef]

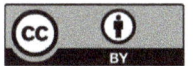

© 2019 by the authors. Licensee MDPI, Basel, Switzerland. This article is an open access article distributed under the terms and conditions of the Creative Commons Attribution (CC BY) license (http://creativecommons.org/licenses/by/4.0/).

Article

Electrical Stimulation through Conductive Substrate to Enhance Osteo-Differentiation of Human Dental Pulp-Derived Stem Cells

Yu-Che Cheng [1,2,3,†], Chien-Hsun Chen [4,†], Hong-Wei Kuo [1,5], Ting-Ling Yen [6], Ya-Yuan Mao [1] and Wei-Wen Hu [5,*]

1. Proteomics Laboratory, Department of Medical Research, Cathay General Hospital, Taipei 10630, Taiwan; yccheng@cgh.org.tw (Y.-C.C.); ggarbage2000@yahoo.com.tw (H.-W.K.); yoyo790520@gmail.com (Y.-Y.M.)
2. Department of Biomedical Sciences and Engineering, National Central University, Zhongli District, Taoyuan City 32001, Taiwan
3. School of Medicine, Fu Jen Catholic University, New Taipei City 24205, Taiwan
4. Department of Periodontics, Cathay General Hospital, Taipei 10630, Taiwan; s82028@yahoo.com.tw
5. Department of Chemical and Materials Engineering, National Central University, Zhongli District, Taoyuan City 32001, Taiwan
6. Department of Medical Research, Cathay General Hospital, Taipei 10630, Taiwan; d119096015@tmu.edu.tw
* Correspondence: huweiwen@cc.ncu.edu.tw; Tel.: +886-3-4227151 (ext. 34246); Fax: +886-3-4252296
† These two authors contributed equally.

Received: 12 August 2019; Accepted: 16 September 2019; Published: 19 September 2019

Abstract: Human dental pulp-derived stem cells (hDPSCs) are promising cellular sources for bone healing. The acceleration of their differentiation should be beneficial to their clinical application. Therefore, a conductive polypyrrole (PPy)-made electrical stimulation (ES) device was fabricated to provide direct-current electric field (DCEF) treatment, and its effect on osteo-differentiation of hDPSCs was investigated in this study. To determine the optimal treating time, electrical field of 0.33 V/cm was applied to hDPSCs once for 4 h on different days after the osteo-induction. The alizarin red S staining results suggested that ES accelerated the mineralization rates of hDPSCs. The quantification analysis results revealed a nearly threefold enhancement in calcium deposition by ES at day 0, 2, and 4, whereas the promotion effect in later stages was in vain. To determine the ES-mediated signaling pathway, the expression of genes in the bone morphogenetic protein (BMP) family and related receptors were quantified using qPCR. In the early stages of osteo-differentiation, the mRNA levels of BMP2, BMP3, BMP4, and BMP5 were increased significantly in the ES groups, indicating that these genes were involved in the specific signaling routes induced by ES. We are the first using DCEF to improve the osteo-differentiation of hDPSCs, and our results promise the therapeutic applications of hDPSCs on cell-based bone tissue engineering.

Keywords: human dental pulp stem cells; substrate-mediated electrical stimulation; direct current electric field; osteo-differentiation; bone morphogenesis proteins

1. Introduction

Mesenchymal stem cells (MSCs) are one of the promising stem cell types due to their availability and relatively simple requirements for in vitro expansion and genetic manipulation [1]. In addition to the well-characterized MSCs derived from bone marrow, increasing evidence suggests that human dental pulp contains a substantial amount of stem cells, i.e., human dental pulp stem cells (hDPSCs) [2]. These cells demonstrate proliferation and differentiation properties similar to those of MSCs [3]. Unlike bone marrow stem cells, the harvest of hDPSCs does not require additional clinical procedures, making them a promising source of stem cells for tissue regeneration [4]. In addition to the application of generating dentin-like structures [5], hDPSCs also exhibit proliferative ability in vitro and can be induced to differentiate into numerous cell types, such as neurons, osteoblasts, and adipocytes [6–8]. Therefore, hDPSCs have been applied in several regenerative studies including ischemia [9], muscular dystrophy [10], neurological diseases [11], and diseases of bone and cartilages [12,13].

Bone is a specialized connective tissue that develops through the differentiation of osteo-progenitor cells, primarily osteoblasts, towards gradual ossification, i.e., osteogenesis [14]. Osteoblasts produce amorphously fibrous tissue that gradually becomes densely packed to form core bone matrix through adhesion between the secreted extracellular matrices (ECM) followed by calcium phosphate crystal deposition, which is known as bone mineralization [15]. When the stem cells were cultured in vitro, they could be osteo-induced by chemicals, including dexamethasone, 2-phospho-L-ascorbic acid, and β-glycerophosphate [16]. Because osteogenic growth factors, such as bone morphogenetic proteins (BMPs) and their receptors, can modulate the proliferation and differentiation of implanted osteogenic cells [17], another induction method is to transfect cells with certain kind of BMPs genes to increase their osteogenic capability [18]. Due to multiple functions of BMPs in postnatal bone growth and bone homeostasis [19], they are highly required for osteoblast differentiation and bone formation during embryonic development. Therefore, BMPs are broadly applied for bone regeneration to attract precursor cells from the host to invade scaffolds and induce osteoblastic differentiation.

In addition to chemical and biological inductions, physical cues are also applied for bone tissue engineering. Electrical stimulation (ES) has been proven to influence numerous cellular processes, including migration (via TORC2/PI3K), cell cycle, cell proliferation, and angiogenesis [20–22]. Therefore, different tissues, such as nerves, muscles, and cartilage, have been guided by ES to promote their development and regeneration [23]. Actually, hDPSCs have been administrated in vivo combing pulsed electrical magnetic field (PEMF) treatment for healing injured nerves, however, there was no difference when comparing to the PEMF only group [24]. In contrast, electrodes have been inserted to medium to directly stimulate hDPSCs, which significantly improved the expression of osteocalcin [25], suggesting that direct-current electric field (DCEF) may facilitate the differentiation of hDPSCs compared to the PEMF treatment. Regarding the bone repair, Wolff's law indicates that bone regeneration always adapts to the loading. Because collagen in bone tissue demonstrates piezoelectricity, it has been hypothesized that mechanical signals delivered to cells may be mediated by electrical current generated by bone matrix [26]. Therefore, ES may be a potential treatment to promote differentiation of stem cells.

Although the insertion of electrodes to culture medium may easily provide DCEF treatment, this method may elicit unwanted redox reactions of the medium ingredients as well as the faradaic reaction and corrosion of the electrodes [27]. Therefore, we have previously fabricated a conductive polypyrrole (PPy) film to construct an ES device [28]. Different from 3D conductive scaffolds, 2D conductive films allow us to easily monitor cells [29,30]. These PPy films were applied for direct-current electric field (DCEF) treatment to rat bone marrow stromal cells (rBMSCs) [28]. Although these PPy films were not examined in vivo, rBMSCs demonstrated good adhesion and proliferation on these PPy films because of their good biocompatibility [31,32]. Our results revealed that the mineralization of rBMSCs can be highly promoted by DCEF treatment, and the improvement highly depended on the ES treating time [33].

Although our study indicated that DCEF may facilitate osteogenesis of rBMSCs, whether this ES provides similar effects on hDPSCs is still unclear. Therefore, ES devices fabricated using conductive PPy films were applied in this study to investigate the promotion effect of substrate-mediated ES treatment on osteo-differentiation of hDPSCs in vitro. Mineralization levels were illustrated by alizarin red S staining and quantified by the calcium-(ocresolphthalein complexone) (Ca-OCPC) complex method. The expression profiles of genes in the BMP family were also evaluated by qPCR. In addition, stimulations at different time points were performed to determine the temporal influences of ES on osteogenesis.

2. Materials and Methods

2.1. Materials

Fetal bovine serum (FBS) and trypsin-EDTA were obtained from Gibco/Thermo Fisher Scientific (Waltham, MA, USA). The DPSC BulletKit was obtained from Lonza (Basal, Switzerland). Pyrrole, ammonium persulfate, dexamethasone, 2-phospho-L-ascorbic acid trisodium salt, β-glycerophosphate disodium salt hydrate, Triton X-100, and glutaraldehyde were purchased from Sigma-Aldrich (St Louis, MO, USA).

2.2. Cell Culture of Human Dental Pulp Stem Cells (hDPSCs) and Osteogenesis Induction

Human dental pulp stem cells (hDPSCs) were obtained from Lonza (Basel, Switzerland), which were isolated from adult third molars collected during the extraction of a donor's "wisdom" teeth. These cells express CD105, CD166, CD29, CD90, and CD73, and they do not express CD34, CD45, and CD133 markers. After being thawed from cryopreserved tubes, the cells were maintained in DPSC BulletKit medium with 10% FBS. The osteogenesis of hDPSCs was induced by adding osteogenic supplements (100 μm ascorbic-2-phosphate, 10 mM β-glycerophosphate, and 100 nM dexamethasone) to the DPSC BulletKit medium.

2.3. The Preparation of Polypyrrole (PPy) Films and the Fabrication of the Electrical Stimulation Device

The fabrication of PPy films was performed following our previous publication [20] with slight modifications. Tissue culture polystyrene (TCPS) dishes with diameters of 10 cm were used as the substrates for PPy film deposition. First, 15 mL each of 0.1, 0.3, or 0.5 M of pyrrole and ammonium persulfate at 0.2 equivalent concentrations (i.e., 0.02, 0.06, and 0.1 M, respectively) were added to the dishes and gently mixed for 15 min at 4 °C to facilitate film formation. Afterward, the film was rinsed with deionized water and dried in an oven at 37 °C. The sheet resistances of these PPy films were examined using four-point probe (EverBeing, Hsinchu, Taiwan) analysis. To ensure coating uniformity, each film was examined at 20 different points in different regions. Afterward, the fabricated PPy films were trimmed to rectangles with dimensions of 60 mm × 58 mm. Polypropylene rings with diameters of 10 mm and heights of 8 mm were glued onto the PPy films to create wells for the cell culture (Figure 1). The opposite ends of the films were covered with tin foil paper as electrodes and fixed with stainless steel clips. The device was sterilized under UV light for 30 min. The culture areas were washed with phosphate-buffered saline (PBS) followed by culture medium. These ES devices were placed in polystyrene culture dishes with diameters of 15 cm for insulation, and the electrodes were connected in parallel to a DC power supply (Regulated DC power supply, Hola, Taiwan). In addition, these ES devices were examined by DCEF procedure for 12 h to ensure their electrical stability.

2.4. Culture of hDPSCs on the Electrical Stimulation Devices and the Induction of Osteogenesis

For the DCEF treatment, the cells were seeded in regular culture medium on the PPy films at a density of 15,000 cells/cm^2 for one day. Afterward, the medium was replaced with osteogenic medium, and the DCEF treatment with an electric field of 0.33 V/cm was immediately applied for 4 h, which was determined according to our previous study [28,33]. The medium was changed every three days.

2.5. Lactate Dehydrogenase (LDH) Assay

Cell numbers were quantified using the CytoTox 96 Non-Radioactive Cytotoxicity Assay (Promega, Madison, WI, USA) by measuring cytosolic lactate dehydrogenase (LDH) activity. Prior to the analysis, 100 μL of fresh medium was replaced to each well, and 15 μL of lysis buffer was added to release LDH from the live cells. After transferring 50 μL of LDH-releasing medium to 96-well microplates, 50 μL of LDH reagent was added and incubated for 30 min at room temperature. Finally, 50 μL of stop solution was added per well, and the absorbance at a wavelength of 490 nm was measured. A standard curve was generated using known cell amounts to calculate the cell numbers of the samples.

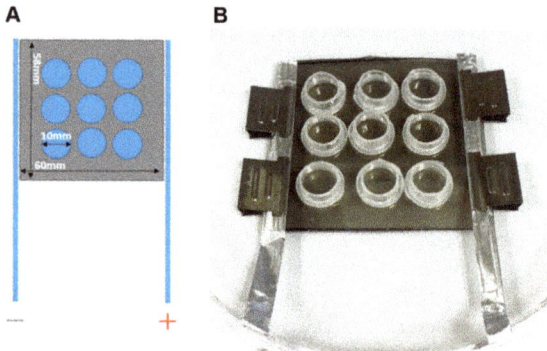

Figure 1. The layout of the electrical stimulation (ES) device and the actual fabrication format. (**A**) The design of substrate-mediated ES device. The polypyrrole (PPy) films were deposited on the tissue culture polystyrene (TCPS) dishes and trimmed to rectangles with dimensions of 60 mm × 58 mm. Nine polypropylene rings with diameters of 10 mm were glued onto PPy films to constrain the area of cell culture. Two electrodes were placed at the opposite ends of the PPy films and were connected in parallel to an external DC power source. (**B**) The actual photo of the ES device.

2.6. RNA Extraction and Real-Time Quantitative PCR (qPCR)

Cells in each experimental group were collected, and their mRNAs were extracted using TRIzol reagent (Life Technologies/Thermo Fisher Scientific, Waltham, MA, USA). The collected mRNA was reversely transcribed to cDNA using the SuperScript III First-Strand Synthesis System (Invitrogen/Thermo Fisher Scientific, Waltham, MA, USA). The relative mRNA levels were quantified using qPCR in the presence of a TaqMan probe and the TaqMan Master Mix (Roche Diagnostics GmbH, Mannheim, Germany), according to the manufacturer's instructions. The primers used for the amplification of each gene are listed in Table 1. The expression levels of the target genes were normalized to that of GAPDH. The LightCycler Software (Version 4.05, Roche Diagnostics GmbH) was used to generate the quantitative data.

2.7. Alizarin Red S Staining

The cells were washed with PBS, and then 70% ethanol was added to fix the cells at 4 °C for 1 h. Next, cells were washed with PBS, and the staining solution (40 mM alizarin red S, pH 4.2) was added at room temperature for 5 min. The staining solution was subsequently discarded, and then the cells were washed three times with distilled water. The stained images were visualized using a Nikon Eclipse 80i fluorescence microscope and captured using a cooled CCD apparatus (Nikon Instruments, Tokyo, Japan).

2.8. Quantitative and Qualitative Analyses of Calcium Deposition in the Extracellular Matrix (ECM)

The Ca-OCPC complex method was used to quantify the level of calcium deposition. Before the assay, the medium was removed from the well, which was washed twice with PBS. Next, 100 μL of 0.5 N acetic acid was added to release the calcium. Then, 10 μL of the calcium-released sample was added to 200 μL of calcium-binding reagent (0.1 mg/mL of o-cresolphthalein complexone (OCPC) and 1 mg/mL of 8-hydroxyquinoline) and 200 μL of buffer reagent (1.6 M 2-amino-2-methyl-1-propanol, pH 10.7). After 15 min incubation, 100 μL of purple-colored Ca-OCPC complex was collected for the measurement of absorbance at a wavelength of 575 nm, and these reads were compared to those of the $CaCl_2$ standard solutions for quantification.

Table 1. Primers for qPCR analysis.

Gene	Primers
GAPDH	5'-CTCTGCTCCTCCTGTTCGAC 3'-ACGACCAAATCCGTTGACTC
BMP1	5'-ACCCTGGGCAGCTACAAGT 3'-TGAGGAATCCGCCACAAG
BMP2	5'-CAGACCACCGGTTGGAGA 3'-CCCACTCGTTTCTGGTAGTTCT
BMP3	5'-CCCAAGTCCTTTGATGCCTA 3'-TCTGGATGGTAGCATGATTTGA
BMP4	5'-CTTTACCGGCTTCAGTCTGG 3'-TGGGATGTTCTCCAGATGTTC
BMP5	5'-AACCGCAATAAATCCAGCTC 3'-TTTTGCTCACTTGTGTTATAATCTCC
BMP6	5'-ACATGGTCATGAGCTTTGTGA 3'-ACTCTTTGTGGTGTCGCTGA
BMP7	5'-ACCACTGGGTGGTCAATCC 3'-CAACTTGGGGTTGATGCTCT
BMPR1A	5'-GGACGAAAGCCTGAACAAAA 3'-GCAATTGGTATTCTTCCACGA
BMPR1B	5'-CGAATGTAATAAAGACCTACACCCTA 3'-GTGTATAGGTCCATCAACAAAATCTC
BMPR2	5'-TCTGGATCTTTCAGCCACAA 3'-TGCCATCTTGTGTTGACTCAC

2.9. Statistical Analysis

The statistical analyses were performed using a two-tailed Student's *t*-test to make comparison, and the errors were reported as standard deviations.

3. Results

3.1. Osteogenic Potential of Human Dental Pulp Stem Cells on Conductive PPy Films

For treatment of skeletal defects, osteo-conductive materials are critical to promote bone healing [34]. To determine whether PPy is a suitable substrate for cell culture in vitro, hDPSCs were seeded on PPy films. The morphology of the hDPSCs on PPy was maintained as spindle-like, which was similar to that of cells grown on TCPS (Figure 2A). The results of lactose dehydrogenase (LDH) assay revealed that there was nearly no difference in the proliferation rates of hDPSCs cultured on TCPS and PPy, suggesting the good biocompatibility of PPy (Figure 2B).

To investigate the effects of conductivity of cell substrate on osteogenesis, differentiation concentrations of pyrrole were used to prepare PPy films. Four-point probe analysis was applied to measure sheet resistances of PPy films, and the results indicate that electrical resistances decreased with increasing pyrrole concentrations (Table 2), suggesting that the conductivity of PPy films can be easily manipulated. These PPy films were then applied as substrates to examine their effects on osteo-differentiation of hDPSCs. These seeded cells were induced by osteogenic medium, and alizarin red S staining was applied on day 14 to determine the level of calcium deposition (Figure 2C). The results showed that cells grown on PPy films with lower electrical resistances demonstrated higher levels of mineralization.

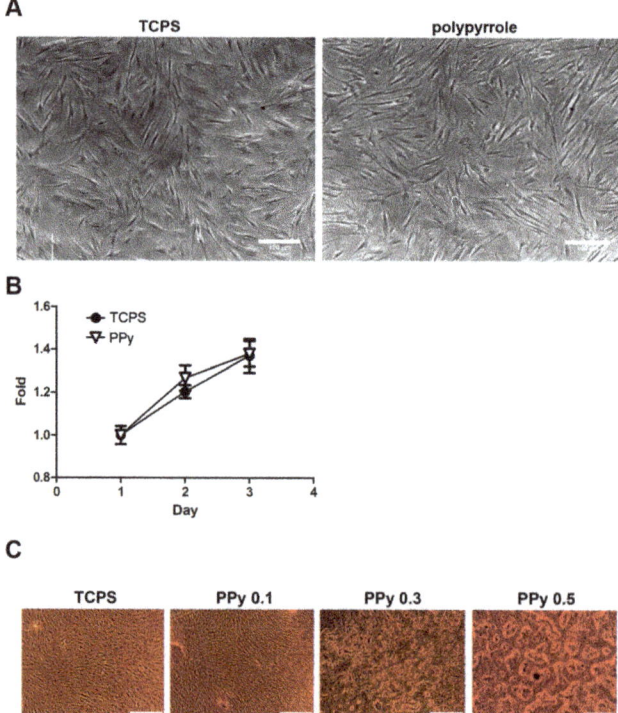

Figure 2. (**A**) Phase contrast images of human dental pulp stem cells (hDPSCs) on TCPS (left) and PPy films (right). The hDPSCs were cultivated on TCPS or PPy for 3 days. The cells on both materials exhibited almost the same typical fibroblast-like morphology with comparable confluency, indicating that cell adhesion and extension were similar on these two surfaces (scale bar = 100 μm). (**B**) The LDH assays were applied to quantify the amounts of hDPSCs on TCPS or PPy films. All cell numbers were compared to those in day 1. The results showed comparable cell viability and proliferation between two surfaces, suggesting the good biocompatibility of PPy films ($n = 3$). (**C**) Alizarin red S staining was performed to evaluate the level of mineralization. The hDPSCs were seeded on PPy films prepared by pyrrole solutions in concentrations of 0.1, 0.3, and 0.5 M, respectively. The photos were taken 14 days after osteo-induction, which indicated that PPy films prepared in higher concentrations of pyrroles resulted in the better mineralization (scale bar = 500 μm).

Table 2. The sheet resistances of PPy films prepared by different concentrations of pyrrole.

Solutions for PPy Preparation	Sheet Resistances of PPy Films (kΩ/Square)
0.1 M pyrrole	25.72 ± 1.52
0.3 M pyrrole	10.58 ± 0.65
0.5 M pyrrole	7.83 ± 0.47

3.2. Analysis of Gene Expression of the BMP Family and BMP Receptors in hDPSCs under Electrical Stimulation

Because PPy films were not only suitable but also beneficial to osteogenesis, these conductive substrates were further applied to investigate the potential of ES on facilitating hDPSCs differentiation. Bone morphogenetic proteins (BMPs) are well-known signal proteins in osteogenesis [35]; thus, the gene expression profiles of the BMP family and BMP receptors were evaluated in this study. After seeding hDPSCs on PPy films for one day, these cells were osteo-induced by replacing the culture medium with osteogenetic medium (day 0) and ES was immediately performed once for 4 h. The mRNAs were extracted from the hDPSCs with or without ES treatment on different days for qPCR analysis. Gene expressions were investigated from day 0 to day 6 because genes affected in early stage of differentiation may participate in the ES-driven signaling pathways. The qPCR results demonstrated increasing expression levels of BMP2, BMP3, BMP4, BMP5, and BMPR1B in the ES group (Figure 3). Among these up-regulated genes, the differences were significant for BMP2 on day 0 and 1, BMP3 on day 0 and day 4, BMP4 on day 0 and 1, BMP5 on day 0 and 2, and BMPR1B on day 0. It is worth noting that the expression of BMP2 on day 1 exhibited 7.7-fold increase, BMP3 on day 0 exhibited 3.9-fold increase, BMP4 on day 1 exhibited 2-fold increase, BMP5 on day 2 exhibited a nearly 2-fold increase, and BMPR1B on day 0 exhibited 2.2-fold increase by ES, compared to those of the control group. These significant changes suggested that these genes may be directly influenced by ES. The expression levels of BMP1, BMP6, and BMPR2 did not demonstrate significant difference between two groups. The gene expressions of BMP7 and BMPR1-A were also evaluated; however, the expressions of these two genes were undetectable in hDPSCs.

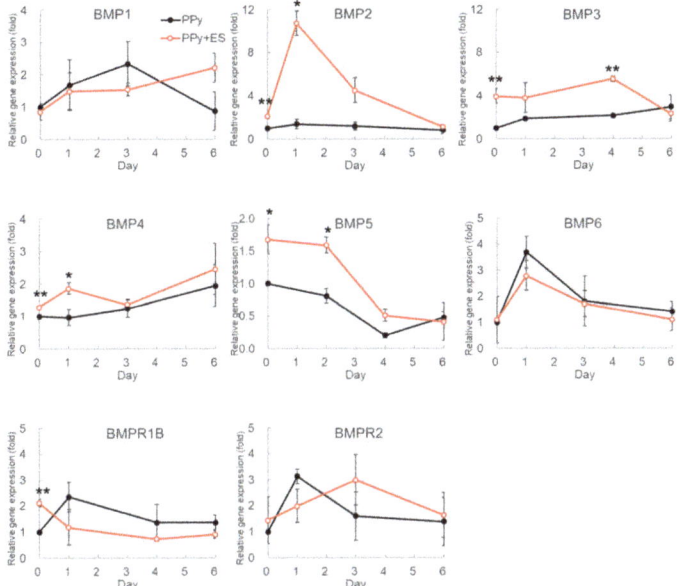

Figure 3. Gene expressions of bone morphogenesis proteins (BMPs) and BMP receptors family in osteogenesis-induced hDPSCs under ES. To determine the ES effects on gene expressions during osteo-differentiation, hDPSCs were seeded to PPy films for 1 day and then were induced by osteogenic medium. In the same time, one-time DCEF treatment was performed for 4 h to stimulate cells immediately after medium replacement (day 0). The mRNAs were harvested from differentiated hDPSCs on different days, and the transcriptional levels of BMP family were determined using quantitative real-time PCR (qPCR). All relative results were compared to those from undifferentiated hDPSCs, and the red and black circles represent the relative gene expression levels of hDPSCs with or without DCEF treatment, respectively. Each value is the average ± SD of three independent experiments ($n = 3$; *: $p < 0.05$, **: $p < 0.01$).

3.3. Electrical Stimulation Enhanced the Calcium Deposition of hDPSCs on PPy Films Under Osteogenesis Induction

The qPCR results indicated that some of BMPs were up-regulated by ES treatment in the early osteogenesis stage. It is essential to evaluate whether these up-regulated BMPs indeed promoted osteo-differentiation and eventually improved bone matrix formation. In addition, the optimal ES treating time is still undetermined.

To investigate the temporal effects of ES on osteogenesis, hDPSCs were stimulated by DCEF once for 4 h at different time points after the induction with osteogenic medium. Mineralized matrix was stained by alizarin red S (Figure 4), and the deposited calcium was analyzed using Ca-OCPC complex method on day 12, day 14, and day 21 after osteo-induction (Figure 5).

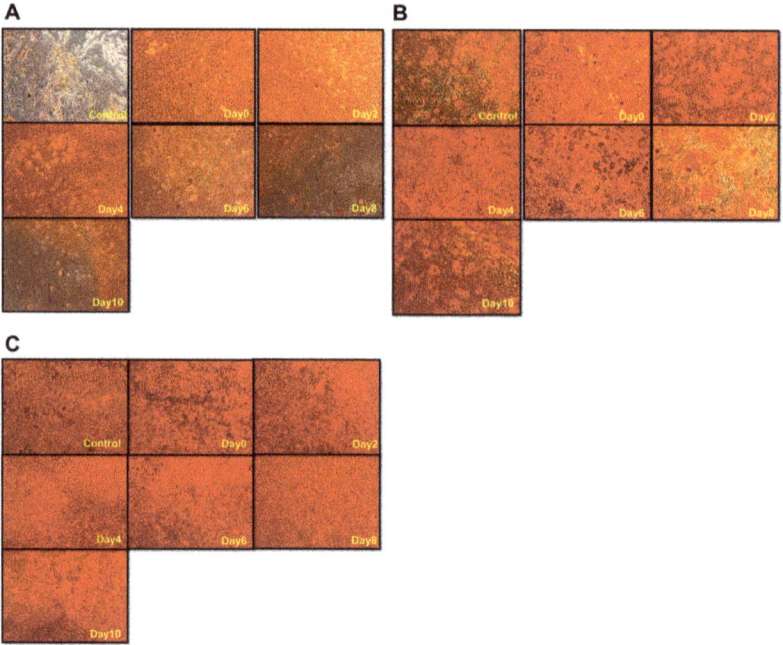

Figure 4. The levels and distributions of mineralization of hDPSCs treated with direct-current electric field (DCEF) on different days during osteo-differentiation. After the induction of osteogenic medium, hDPSCs were stimulated by DCEF on different days (indicated by yellow words at the bottom-right corner of each image). Alizarin red S staining was performed on (**A**) day 12, (**B**) day 14, and (**C**) day 21 after osteo-induction to visualize the mineralization condition.

The alizarin red S results demonstrated that DCEF highly improved mineralization (Figure 4). For the day 12 results, hDPSCs treated with DCEF on day 0, 2, and 4 all exhibited great enhancement in calcium deposition compared to that of the control group (no ES) (Figure 4A). However, the promotion effects were reduced when the ES was performed after day 6 or later. The results evaluated on day 14 demonstrated a similar trend (Figure 4B). These results indicate that the ES seemed to work mainly on the early stage of osteogenesis. However, when the alizarin red S staining was performed on day 21, there was almost no difference among groups (Figure 4C).

In addition to qualitative alizarin red S staining, Ca-OCPC complex method was also applied to measure the deposited calcium in ECM to quantitatively evaluate the level of mineralization (Figure 5). The results of day 12 and day 14 both indicated that hDPSCs treated with DCEF before day 6 exhibited a trend of gradual enhancement in calcium deposition compared to the control with statistical significance, and the optimum enhancement appeared on day 4 (Figure 5A,B). In addition, the calcium content reached a plateau by day 21 (Figure 5C). These results were consistent with the alizarin red S staining, suggesting that the ES-triggered pathways were likely involved in the early stages of the osteogenesis process, and the mineralization was therefore accelerated.

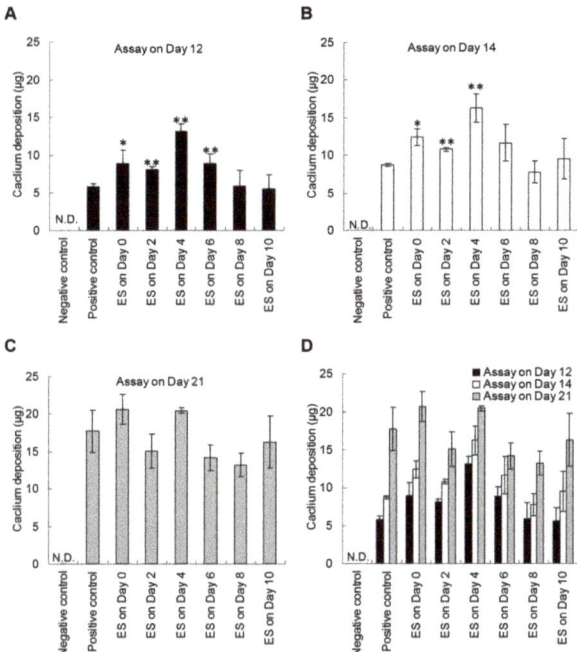

Figure 5. The calcium deposition of hDPSCs under DCEF treatment on different days during osteo-differentiation. To determine the temporal effects of ES on mineralization, hDPSCs seeded on PPy films were treated with DCEF (0.33 V/cm) for 4 h on different days after the induction with osteogenic medium. The calcium deposition of cells was evaluated using calcium-(ocresolphthalein complexone) (Ca-OCPC) complex method on (**A**) day 12, (**B**) day 14, and (**C**) day 21 after osteo-induction. (**D**) The overall results were grouped to better understand the efficacy of ES. The negative and positive control groups were hDPSCs cultured on PPy films using normal or osteogenic media, respectively. These two control groups were not treated by DCEF. ($n = 3$; *: $p < 0.05$, **: $p < 0.01$ compared with the positive control group) (N.D.: Non-detectable).

3.4. Enhanced Potential Derived from ES in the Process of Osteogenesis

Although our results demonstrated that the DCEF treatment effectively promoted mineralization, it was unclear whether the augment in calcium deposition was due to enhanced osteogenesis or an increase in cell number. To address this question, we quantified the cells by the LDH assay to determine the osteo-differentiation potential as Ca^{2+} content normalized with cell number. The level of mineralization in the early stage was analyzed on day 12, and the results showed that ES treatment before day 8 increased the differentiation potential twofold compared with the positive control group (Figure 6A). The results of assay on day 14 also showed the same trends (Figure 6B). However, when the analysis was performed on day 21, i.e., the late stage of mineralization, there was no difference between the experimental and positive control groups, indicating that ES plays a role in accelerating the rate of osteogenesis rather than in increasing the numbers of differentiated cells in our study model (Figure 6C). Again, there was no observed effect on the rate of osteogenesis when ES was applied after day 6, suggesting that the effect of ES on accelerating osteo-differentiation should mainly trigger the early pathways in the osteogenesis progress.

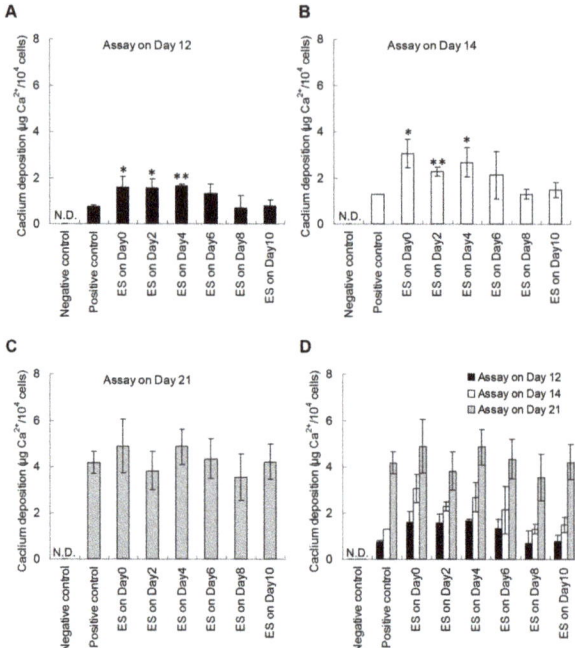

Figure 6. The normalized quantification of calcium deposition of hDPSCs under DCEF treatment at different stages of osteo-differentiation. To distinguish whether the calcium deposition results were affected by cell proliferation, the quantification results in Figure 5 were divided by cell numbers for normalization. Cells were lysed and the released LDH were evaluated to determine cell numbers. The normalized results were evaluated on (**A**) day 12, (**B**) day 14, and (**C**) day 21 after osteo-induction. (**D**) The results from all experimental groups were grouped to better understand the efficacy of ES. The negative and positive control groups were hDPSCs cultured on PPy films using normal or osteogenic media, respectively. These two control groups were not treated by DCEF. ($n = 3$; *: $p < 0.05$, **: $p < 0.01$ compared with the positive control group) (N.D.: Non-detectable).

4. Discussion

Human dental pulp stem cells (hDPSCs) are a kind of mesenchymal stem cells derived from the pulp of human tooth. Because hDPSCs demonstrate the capacity of self-renewal and multilineage differentiation, they have therapeutic potentials similar to those of bone marrow stem cells [36]. In addition, hDPSCs can be extracted from teeth recovered during routine dental procedures, making them a convenient source of stem cells for cell-based therapy. Furthermore, the multilineage differentiation of hDPSCs makes them an alternative strategy for treating various human diseases, rather than limiting to the treatment of dental-related problems [37].

Although the application of biochemical cues is the gold standard to induce cell differentiation, the promising promotion effects of physical stimulations, especially electrical stimulation (ES), have also been proven. For example, neural differentiation of PC12 cells in the presence of nerve growth factor (NGF) can be significantly enhanced by ES treatment [38]. Mobini et al. also demonstrated that ES improves osteogenic-related gene expression at specific time points with different gene expression patterns between bone marrow and adipose-derived MSCs [39]. These findings suggest that ES may regulate the physiology of the cell and the differentiation potential of stem cells.

To date, the promotion effect of ES on the hDPSCs differentiation is rare. Im et al. have inserted electrodes in culture medium to stimulate hDPSCs by electrical current, and their results showed that this fluid-mediated ES treatment seems to improve cell proliferation, and the expression of OCN is slightly enhanced [25]. However, whether ES may promote osteo-differentiation, especially the level of mineralization, is still unclear. In addition, the exact role of electrical signals in regulating the biosynthetic activity and homeostasis of osteogenesis remains elusive.

In our previous study, conductive PPy films have been developed for ES to significantly improve the osteo-differentiation of rBMSCs [28]. These PPy films can be deposited onto various substrates, such as culture dishes, glass plates, and even metal devices. In addition, the electrical resistances of PPy films can be easily adjusted to meet specific requirements. These properties suggest that PPy-mediated ES treatment is a feasible approach to promote tissue regeneration [33].

Here, we demonstrated that hDPSCs could adhere on conductive PPy films with comparable proliferation rate to those on TCPS (Figure 2b). In addition, the lower resistances of PPy films resulted in the higher level of mineralization of hDPSCs (Figure 2c), which were in accordance with our previous finding of rBMSCs, suggesting that osteo-differentiation of hDPSCs can be improved by the conductivity of scaffolds [28].

Regarding the DCEF treatment, it can be either constant or in different waveforms, and the frequency of the electrical current may influence the biological effects [22]. Therefore, our previous study has treated rBMSCs using DCEF in different modes, including DCEF in constant and square waves in different frequency, offset, amplitude, and duty cycle [33]. Although these systematic examinations are helpful for optimization, we only applied 0.33 V/cm of continuous DCEF in this study because the goal of this study is to determine whether ES treatment may promote osteo-differentiation, and this constant electric field has been proven to stably improve osteo-differentiation of rBMSCs [28,33]. The DCEF treatment of hDPSCs not only enhanced osteogenic capacity but also promoted mineralization. In addition, only ES performed before day 6 resulted in increasing calcium deposition and mineralization. Therefore, we conclude that ES mainly triggers pathways in the early stages of osteo-differentiation.

Gene regulation plays an important role in osteogenesis. It has been shown that mesenchymal stem cells and osteo-progenitor cells can be differentiated into osteoblasts by certain key cytokines and functional proteins, including proteins in the BMP family, Runx2, and certain ECM proteins [40,41]. Bone morphogenesis proteins (BMPs) belong to the transforming growth factor-β (TGF-β) superfamily. Because BMPs comprise a group of proteins participating in bone formation [42], they are important in adult tissue homeostasis [43]. BMPs may initiate Smad-dependent or non-canonical pathways via binding to type I and type II heterotetrameric receptors [44]. According to a previous sequence alignment analysis, BMP2/4 and BMP5/6/7 are two groups of structurally related proteins; however, BMP1 and BMP3 are more distantly related [42]. BMP1 exhibits no sequence similarity to BMP2/4 or BMP5/6/7 because BMP1 is a metalloprotease that participates in collagen maturation and is therefore independent of BMP-mediated pathways [45]. In our study model, there was a 3.9-fold up-regulation in the expression of BMP3 on day 0. Although BMP3 has been shown to be a negative regulator of osteogenesis [46], it also has been reported that BMP3 expression in the perichondrium of chick limbs may regulate cartilage cell proliferation to ensure proper ossification [47]. Therefore, we speculate that the up-regulated expression of BMP3 by ES may play a role in modulating the levels of other BMP signaling, thereby enhancing mineralization. However, further experiments are needed to confirm this hypothesis.

The expression levels of BMP1 and BMP6 in our study model fluctuated in both control and ES-treated groups during the experimental time period, indicating that these BMPs may not be involved in ES-stimulated osteogenesis. BMP7 was reported to participate in eye and kidney development [48], but its expression is undetectable in hDPSCs. BMP2 has been studied extensively in osteogenesis [49], and numerous evidence indicates that BMP2 plays a crucial role in osteogenesis via its modulation of RUNX2 expression, especially in the early stages of osteogenesis [50]. In our study model, the expression of BMP2 was up-regulated 7.7-fold by ES on day 1. It was a significant change because no other BMPs exhibited such a profound up-regulation by ES in the early stages of osteogenesis. Therefore, we deduce that the ES-induced promotion of osteogenesis may be directly modulated via BMP2.

There are two types of BMP receptors, i.e., type I and type II, and these receptors participate in BMP-mediated signal transduction [51]. When these serine/threonine kinase receptors are triggered by a ligand, they form a heterotetrameric complex in which the type II receptor transphosphorylates the type I receptor, and the signal conducts though Smads to the nucleus [52]. In hDPSCs, the expression of BMPR1-A was undetectable with qPCR; therefore, we assume that BMPR1-B and BMPR2 are expressed in hDPSCs as heterotetramers to accept BMP protein-ligands.

In this study, we comprehensively investigated mRNA of BMPs and their receptors through qPCR analysis because BMPs are the most well-known growth factors to initiate osteo-differentiation. However, these qPCR results did not represent the corresponding protein expression levels. Further analysis such as Western blotting or ELISA should be performed to specifically determine ES effects on protein expressions. In addition, if BMPs induce osteo-differentiation of hDPSCs, relative outcome markers, such as Runx2, collagen I, alkaline phosphatase activity/expression, osteocalcin, and osteonectin, should thus be up-regulated [33]. Therefore, our future study will also focus on exploring the profiles of these outcome markers of osteogenic differentiation. As shown in Figures 4 and 5, when the assay was performed on day 21, i.e., the late stage of osteo-differentiation, there was no difference between the experimental and positive control groups, suggesting that ES plays a role in accelerating but not increasing the level of mineralization. Similarly, it has been reported that the mineralization of rat bone marrow stromal cells may only be improved when ES is applied at early stage of osteo-differentiation [33]. However, Srirussamee et al. have applied ES to pre-osteoblasts (MC3T3-E1), and their results showed that the level of Runx2 expression remains unchanged during the early stage [27]. Because pre-osteoblasts are committed cells, their results implied that ES may mainly promote stem cell differentiation to therefore accelerate mineralization.

The promotion effect of ES treatment on osteogenesis has also been reported by Zhang et al. [53]. They seeded adipose-derived mesenchymal stem cells (AD-MSCs) to electrically conductive scaffold, and DCEF was applied to treat these seeded cells. Blockers of different voltage-gated ion channels were applied before ES treatment, and their results showed that the promotion effect of ES on AD-MSCs highly related to voltage-gated calcium channels. According to this study, we speculate that ES may promote the influx of calcium to bind calmodulin, by which CaM kinase is activated to regulate transcription factor of BMPs [54,55].

5. Conclusions

In this study, hDPSCs were successfully induced by osteo-differentiation, suggesting their potential use in bone regeneration. In addition, the differentiation levels were enhanced as hDPSCs were seeded on PPy films, indicating that the conductive substrates were favorable to osteogenesis. When these PPy films were applied to treat DCEF on hDPSCs, the mRNA levels of BMPs were significantly up-regulated. Therefore, the in vitro experiment showed that the calcium deposition of hDPSCs was effectively improved when DCEF was applied in the early stage of osteo-differentiation, which suggested that ES treatment can accelerate the mineralization of hDPSCs. To the best of our knowledge, this study is the first to use substrate-mediated ES treatment to enhance the osteo-differentiation and mineralization of hDPSCs, and our results should be beneficial for tissue engineering application.

Author Contributions: Conceptualization, W.-W.H.; Methodology, Y.-C.C.; Resources, C.-H.C.; Investigation, H.-W.K. and Y.-Y.M.; Formal analysis, H.-W.K. and T.-L.Y.; Writing—original draft preparation, C.-H.C. and Y.-C.C.; Writing—review and editing, W.-W.H.

Funding: This study was supported, in part, by research grants from the Ministry of Science and Technology in Taiwan (MOST 108-2628-E-008-002-MY3 and MOST 106-2314-B-281-001-MY3) and the Cathay General Hospital (CGH-MR-10210), and a joint grant from the National Central University and the Cathay General Hospital (104 CGH-NCU-A2), Taiwan.

Conflicts of Interest: The authors declare no conflict of interest.

References

1. Grayson, W.L.; Bunnell, B.A.; Martin, E.; Frazier, T.; Hung, B.P.; Gimble, J.M. Stromal cells and stem cells in clinical bone regeneration. *Nat. Rev. Endocrinol.* **2015**, *11*, 140–150. [CrossRef] [PubMed]
2. Campanella, V. Dental stem cells: Current research and future applications. *Eur. J. Paediatr. Dent.* **2018**, *19*, 257. [PubMed]
3. Ballini, A.; De Frenza, G.; Cantore, S.; Papa, F.; Grano, M.; Mastrangelo, F.; Tete, S.; Grassi, F.R. In vitro stem cell cultures from human dental pulp and periodontal ligament: New prospects in dentistry. *Int. J. Immunopathol. Pharmacol.* **2007**, *20*, 9–16. [CrossRef] [PubMed]
4. Garzon, I.; Martin-Piedra, M.A.; Alaminos, M. Human dental pulp stem cells. A promising epithelial-like cell source. *Med. Hypotheses* **2015**, *84*, 516–517. [CrossRef] [PubMed]
5. Gronthos, S.; Mankani, M.; Brahim, J.; Robey, P.G.; Shi, S. Postnatal human dental pulp stem cells (dpscs) in vitro and in vivo. *Proc. Natl. Acad. Sci. USA* **2000**, *97*, 13625–13630. [CrossRef] [PubMed]
6. Karaoz, E.; Demircan, P.C.; Saglam, O.; Aksoy, A.; Kaymaz, F.; Duruksu, G. Human dental pulp stem cells demonstrate better neural and epithelial stem cell properties than bone marrow-derived mesenchymal stem cells. *Histochem. Cell Biol.* **2011**, *136*, 455–473. [CrossRef]
7. Li, J.H.; Liu, D.Y.; Zhang, F.M.; Wang, F.; Zhang, W.K.; Zhang, Z.T. Human dental pulp stem cell is a promising autologous seed cell for bone tissue engineering. *Chin. Med. J. (Engl.)* **2011**, *124*, 4022–4028.
8. Hilkens, P.; Gervois, P.; Fanton, Y.; Vanormelingen, J.; Martens, W.; Struys, T.; Politis, C.; Lambrichts, I.; Bronckaers, A. Effect of isolation methodology on stem cell properties and multilineage differentiation potential of human dental pulp stem cells. *Cell Tissue Res.* **2013**, *353*, 65–78. [CrossRef]
9. Iohara, K.; Zheng, L.; Wake, H.; Ito, M.; Nabekura, J.; Wakita, H.; Nakamura, H.; Into, T.; Matsushita, K.; Nakashima, M. A novel stem cell source for vasculogenesis in ischemia: Subfraction of side population cells from dental pulp. *Stem Cells* **2008**, *26*, 2408–2418. [CrossRef]
10. Yang, R.; Chen, M.; Lee, C.H.; Yoon, R.; Lal, S.; Mao, J.J. Clones of ectopic stem cells in the regeneration of muscle defects in vivo. *PLoS ONE* **2010**, *5*, e13547. [CrossRef]
11. Apel, C.; Forlenza, O.V.; de Paula, V.J.; Talib, L.L.; Denecke, B.; Eduardo, C.P.; Gattaz, W.F. The neuroprotective effect of dental pulp cells in models of alzheimer's and parkinson's disease. *J. Neural Transm. (Vienna)* **2009**, *116*, 71–78. [CrossRef] [PubMed]
12. Machado, E.; Fernandes, M.H.; Gomes Pde, S. Dental stem cells for craniofacial tissue engineering. *Oral Surg. Oral Med. Oral Pathol. Oral Radiol.* **2012**, *113*, 728–733. [CrossRef] [PubMed]
13. Mao, J.J.; Giannobile, W.V.; Helms, J.A.; Hollister, S.J.; Krebsbach, P.H.; Longaker, M.T.; Shi, S. Craniofacial tissue engineering by stem cells. *J. Dent. Res.* **2006**, *85*, 966–979. [CrossRef] [PubMed]
14. Gong, T.; Heng, B.C.; Lo, E.C.; Zhang, C. Current advance and future prospects of tissue engineering approach to dentin/pulp regenerative therapy. *Stem Cells Int.* **2016**, *2016*, 9204574. [CrossRef] [PubMed]
15. Chang, Y.L.; Stanford, C.M.; Keller, J.C. Calcium and phosphate supplementation promotes bone cell mineralization: Implications for hydroxyapatite (ha)-enhanced bone formation. *J. Biomed. Mater. Res.* **2000**, *52*, 270–278. [CrossRef]
16. Cheng, C.C.; Chung, C.A.; Su, L.C.; Chien, C.C.; Cheng, Y.C. Osteogenic differentiation of placenta-derived multipotent cells in vitro. *Taiwan J. Obstet. Gynecol.* **2014**, *53*, 187–192. [CrossRef] [PubMed]
17. Reddi, A.H.; Reddi, A. Bone morphogenetic proteins (bmps): From morphogens to metabologens. *Cytokine Growth Factor Rev.* **2009**, *20*, 341–342. [CrossRef]
18. Rogers, M.B.; Shah, T.A.; Shaikh, N.N. Turning bone morphogenetic protein 2 (bmp2) on and off in mesenchymal cells. *J. Cell. Biochem.* **2015**, *116*, 2127–2138. [CrossRef]
19. Xie, H.; Cui, Z.; Wang, L.; Xia, Z.; Hu, Y.; Xian, L.; Li, C.; Xie, L.; Crane, J.; Wan, M.; et al. Pdgf-bb secreted by preosteoclasts induces angiogenesis during coupling with osteogenesis. *Nat. Med.* **2014**, *20*, 1270–1278. [CrossRef]
20. McCaig, C.D.; Song, B.; Rajnicek, A.M. Electrical dimensions in cell science. *J. Cell Sci.* **2009**, *122*, 4267–4276. [CrossRef]
21. Jeon, T.J.; Gao, R.; Kim, H.; Lee, A.; Jeon, P.; Devreotes, P.N.; Zhao, M. Cell migration directionality and speed are independently regulated by rasg and gbeta in dictyostelium cells in electrotaxis. *Biol. Open* **2019**, *8*, bio-042457. [CrossRef] [PubMed]

22. Beugels, J.; Molin, D.G.M.; Ophelders, D.; Rutten, T.; Kessels, L.; Kloosterboer, N.; Grzymala, A.A.P.; Kramer, B.W.W.; van der Hulst, R.; Wolfs, T. Electrical stimulation promotes the angiogenic potential of adipose-derived stem cells. *Sci. Rep.* **2019**, *9*, 12076. [CrossRef] [PubMed]
23. Peckham, P.H.; Knutson, J.S. Functional electrical stimulation for neuromuscular applications. *Annu. Rev. Biomed. Eng.* **2005**, *7*, 327–360. [CrossRef] [PubMed]
24. Kim, Y.T.; Hei, W.H.; Kim, S.; Seo, Y.K.; Kim, S.M.; Jahng, J.W.; Lee, J.H. Co-treatment effect of pulsed electromagnetic field (pemf) with human dental pulp stromal cells and fk506 on the regeneration of crush injured rat sciatic nerve. *Int. J. Neurosci.* **2015**, *125*, 774–783. [CrossRef] [PubMed]
25. Im, A.-L.; Kim, J.; Lim, K.; Seonwoo, H.; Cho, W.; Choung, P.-H.; Chung, J.H. Effects of micro-electrical stimulation on regulation of behavior of electro-active stem cells. *J. Biosyst. Eng.* **2013**, *38*, 113–120. [CrossRef]
26. Shamos, M.H.; Lavine, L.S.; Shamos, M.I. Piezoelectric effect in bone. *Nature* **1963**, *197*, 81. [CrossRef] [PubMed]
27. Srirussamee, K.; Mobini, S.; Cassidy, N.J.; Cartmell, S.H. Direct electrical stimulation enhances osteogenesis by inducing bmp2 and spp1 expressions from macrophages and pre-osteoblasts. *Biotechnol. Bioeng.* **2019**. [CrossRef]
28. Hu, W.W.; Hsu, Y.T.; Cheng, Y.C.; Li, C.; Ruaan, R.C.; Chien, C.C.; Chung, C.A.; Tsao, C.W. Electrical stimulation to promote osteogenesis using conductive polypyrrole films. *Mater. Sci. Eng. C Mater. Biol. Appl.* **2014**, *37*, 28–36. [CrossRef]
29. Shi, Z.; Gao, X.; Ullah, M.W.; Li, S.; Wang, Q.; Yang, G. Electroconductive natural polymer-based hydrogels. *Biomaterials* **2016**, *111*, 40–54. [CrossRef]
30. Lu, H.; Zhang, N.; Ma, M. Electroconductive hydrogels for biomedical applications. *Wiley Interdiscip. Rev. Nanomed. Nanobiotechnol.* **2019**, e1568. [CrossRef]
31. Mao, J.; Zhang, Z. Polypyrrole as electrically conductive biomaterials: Synthesis, biofunctionalization, potential applications and challenges. *Adv. Exp. Med. Biol.* **2018**, *1078*, 347–370. [PubMed]
32. Li, C.; Hsu, Y.-T.; Hu, W.-W. The regulation of osteogenesis using electroactive polypyrrole films. *Polymers* **2016**, *8*, 258. [CrossRef]
33. Hu, W.W.; Chen, T.C.; Tsao, C.W.; Cheng, Y.C. The effects of substrate-mediated electrical stimulation on the promotion of osteogenic differentiation and its optimization. *J. Biomed. Mater. Res. B Appl. Biomater.* **2019**, *107*, 1607–1619. [CrossRef]
34. Dawson, E.R.; Suzuki, R.K.; Samano, M.A.; Murphy, M.B. Increased internal porosity and surface area of hydroxyapatite accelerates healing and compensates for low bone marrow mesenchymal stem cell concentrations in critically-sized bone defects. *Appl. Sci.* **2018**, *8*, 366. [CrossRef]
35. Kugimiya, F.; Ohba, S.; Nakamura, K.; Kawaguchi, H.; Chung, U.I. Physiological role of bone morphogenetic proteins in osteogenesis. *J. Bone Miner. Metab.* **2006**, *24*, 95–99. [CrossRef]
36. Struys, T.; Moreels, M.; Martens, W.; Donders, R.; Wolfs, E.; Lambrichts, I. Ultrastructural and immunocytochemical analysis of multilineage differentiated human dental pulp- and umbilical cord-derived mesenchymal stem cells. *Cells Tissues Organs* **2011**, *193*, 366–378. [CrossRef] [PubMed]
37. Potdar, P.D.; Jethmalani, Y.D. Human dental pulp stem cells: Applications in future regenerative medicine. *World J. Stem Cells* **2015**, *7*, 839–851. [CrossRef] [PubMed]
38. Liu, X.; Gilmore, K.J.; Moulton, S.E.; Wallace, G.G. Electrical stimulation promotes nerve cell differentiation on polypyrrole/poly (2-methoxy-5 aniline sulfonic acid) composites. *J. Neural Eng.* **2009**, *6*, 065002. [CrossRef]
39. Mobini, S.; Leppik, L.; Thottakkattumana Parameswaran, V.; Barker, J.H. In vitro effect of direct current electrical stimulation on rat mesenchymal stem cells. *PeerJ* **2017**, *5*, e2821. [CrossRef]
40. Fakhry, M.; Hamade, E.; Badran, B.; Buchet, R.; Magne, D. Molecular mechanisms of mesenchymal stem cell differentiation towards osteoblasts. *World J. Stem Cells* **2013**, *5*, 136–148. [CrossRef]
41. Terhi, J.H.; Teuvo, A.H. Differentiation of osteoblasts and osteocytes from mesenchymal stem cells. *Curr. Stem Cell Res. Ther.* **2008**, *3*, 131–145.
42. Wang, R.N.; Green, J.; Wang, Z.; Deng, Y.; Qiao, M.; Peabody, M.; Zhang, Q.; Ye, J.; Yan, Z.; Denduluri, S.; et al. Bone morphogenetic protein (bmp) signaling in development and human diseases. *Genes Dis.* **2014**, *1*, 87–105. [CrossRef] [PubMed]
43. Carreira, A.C.; Alves, G.G.; Zambuzzi, W.F.; Sogayar, M.C.; Granjeiro, J.M. Bone morphogenetic proteins: Structure, biological function and therapeutic applications. *Arch. Biochem. Biophys.* **2014**, *561*, 64–73. [CrossRef] [PubMed]

44. Rahman, M.S.; Akhtar, N.; Jamil, H.M.; Banik, R.S.; Asaduzzaman, S.M. Tgf-β/bmp signaling and other molecular events: Regulation of osteoblastogenesis and bone formation. *Bone Res.* **2015**, *3*, 15005. [CrossRef] [PubMed]
45. Ge, G.; Greenspan, D.S. Developmental roles of the bmp1/tld metalloproteinases. *Birth Defects Res. C Embryo Today* **2006**, *78*, 47–68. [CrossRef] [PubMed]
46. Daluiski, A.; Engstrand, T.; Bahamonde, M.E.; Gamer, L.W.; Agius, E.; Stevenson, S.L.; Cox, K.; Rosen, V.; Lyons, K.M. Bone morphogenetic protein-3 is a negative regulator of bone density. *Nat. Genet.* **2001**, *27*, 84. [CrossRef] [PubMed]
47. Gamer, L.W.; Ho, V.; Cox, K.; Rosen, V. Expression and function of bmp3 during chick limb development. *Dev. Dyn. Off. Publ. Am. Assoc. Anat.* **2008**, *237*, 1691–1698. [CrossRef] [PubMed]
48. Dudley, A.T.; Lyons, K.M.; Robertson, E.J. A requirement for bone morphogenetic protein-7 during development of the mammalian kidney and eye. *Genes Dev.* **1995**, *9*, 2795–2807. [CrossRef]
49. Nguyen, V.; Meyers, C.A.; Yan, N.; Agarwal, S.; Levi, B.; James, A.W. Bmp-2-induced bone formation and neural inflammation. *J. Orthop.* **2017**, *14*, 252–256. [CrossRef]
50. Shahrul Hisham Zainal, A.; Thanaletchumi, M.; Intan Zarina Zainol, A.; Rohaya Megat Abdul, W.; Sahidan, S. A perspective on stem cells as biological systems that produce differentiated osteoblasts and odontoblasts. *Curr. Stem Cell Res. Ther.* **2017**, *12*, 247–259.
51. Yadin, D.; Knaus, P.; Mueller, T.D. Structural insights into bmp receptors: Specificity, activation and inhibition. *Cytokine Growth Factor Rev.* **2016**, *27*, 13–34. [CrossRef] [PubMed]
52. Wu, M.; Chen, G.; Li, Y.P. Tgf-beta and bmp signaling in osteoblast, skeletal development, and bone formation, homeostasis and disease. *Bone Res.* **2016**, *4*, 16009. [CrossRef] [PubMed]
53. Zhang, Y.; Liu, Y.; Hang, A.; Phan, E.; Wildsoet, C.F. Differential gene expression of bmp2 and bmp receptors in chick retina & choroid induced by imposed optical defocus. *Vis. Neurosci.* **2016**, *33*, E015. [PubMed]
54. Siddappa, R.; Martens, A.; Doorn, J.; Leusink, A.; Olivo, C.; Licht, R.; van Rijn, L.; Gaspar, C.; Fodde, R.; Janssen, F.; et al. Camp/pka pathway activation in human mesenchymal stem cells in vitro results in robust bone formation in vivo. *Proc. Natl. Acad. Sci. USA* **2008**, *105*, 7281–7286. [CrossRef] [PubMed]
55. Zayzafoon, M. Calcium/calmodulin signaling controls osteoblast growth and differentiation. *J. Cell. Biochem.* **2006**, *97*, 56–70. [CrossRef] [PubMed]

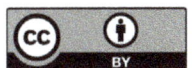

© 2019 by the authors. Licensee MDPI, Basel, Switzerland. This article is an open access article distributed under the terms and conditions of the Creative Commons Attribution (CC BY) license (http://creativecommons.org/licenses/by/4.0/).

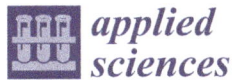

Article

Potential Marker Genes for Predicting Adipogenic Differentiation of Mesenchymal Stromal Cells

Masami Kanawa [1], Akira Igarashi [2,3], Katsumi Fujimoto [3,4], Veronica Sainik Ronald [3,5], Yukihito Higashi [6], Hidemi Kurihara [7], Yukio Kato [3] and Takeshi Kawamoto [3,8,*]

1. Natural Science Center for Basic Research and Development, Hiroshima University, Hiroshima 734-8533, Japan
2. Department of Advanced Technology and Development, BML, Inc., Saitama 350-1101, Japan
3. Department of Dental and Medical Biochemistry, Institute of Biomedical & Health Sciences, Hiroshima University, Hiroshima 734-8533, Japan
4. Department of Molecular Biology and Biochemistry, Graduate School of Biomedical & Health Sciences, Hiroshima University, Hiroshima 734-8533, Japan
5. Cancer Research Centre, Institute for Medical Research, Kuala Lumpur 50588, Malaysia
6. Research Center for Radiation Genome Medicine, Research Institute for Radiation Biology and Medicine, Hiroshima 734-8533, Japan
7. Departments of Periodontal Medicine, Graduate School of Biomedical & Health Sciences, Hiroshima University, Hiroshima 734-8533, Japan
8. Writing Center, Hiroshima University, Higashi-Hiroshima 739-8512, Japan
* Correspondence: tkawamo@hiroshima-u.ac.jp; Tel.: +81-82-424-6207

Received: 24 June 2019; Accepted: 19 July 2019; Published: 23 July 2019

Abstract: Mesenchymal stromal cells (MSCs) are a promising source for tissue engineering of soft connective tissues. However, the differentiation capacity of MSCs varies among individual cell lines. Here, we show marker genes to predict the adipogenic potential of MSCs. To clarify the correlation between gene expression patterns before adipogenic induction and the differentiation level of MSCs after differentiation, we compared mRNA levels of 95 genes and glycerol-3-phosphate dehydrogenase (GPDH) activities in 15 MSC lines (five jaw and 10 ilium MSCs) from 15 donors. Expression profiles of 22 genes before differentiation significantly correlated with GPDH activities after differentiation. Expression levels of 11 out of the 22 genes in highly potent ilium MSCs were at least three times higher compared with jaw MSCs, which have limited differentiation potential. Furthermore, three-dimensional scatter plot for mRNA expression of ITGA5, CDKN2D, and CD74 could completely distinguish highly potent MSCs from poorly potent MSCs for adipogenesis. The treatment of MSC cultures with the anti-ITGA5 antibody reduced adipogenic differentiation of MSCs. Collectively, these results suggest that the three genes play a role in adipogenesis before induction and can serve as predictors to select potent MSCs for adipogenic differentiation.

Keywords: adipogenesis; bone marrow; MSCs; prediction marker

1. Introduction

Mesenchymal stromal cells (MSCs) can be used in regenerative medicine to treat various tissue defects [1–3]. Adipose tissue engineering was developed to reconstruct soft tissue with defects caused by trauma or resection of tumors. Since adipose tissue transplantation did not provide promising results, stem cell transplantation is now gaining support as another strategy for restoring soft tissue defects [4]. Although stem cells such as MSCs can proliferate and differentiate into various types of cells, MSCs obtained from different sources may differ in potential or direction of differentiation [5–7]. For the reconstruction of soft connective tissues, cells capable of differentiating into adipocytes are essential. Thus, there is an urgent need for effective strategies to select suitable MSCs. Recent studies have described cell surface markers that predict the potential of MSCs to differentiate into chondrocytes or osteoblasts [8,9]. However, prediction markers for the adipogenic potential of MSCs have not yet been identified.

Recently, we identified marker genes to predict the chondrogenic differentiation potential of MSCs [7]. The mRNA levels of the prediction markers before differentiation showed significant correlations with the protein levels of glycosaminoglycan, a chondrogenic marker, in MSC cultures after chondrogenic differentiation. The combined analysis of three marker genes presented an excellent predictive ability for screening MSCs with high differentiation potential for chondrogenesis.

Here we report potential prediction markers for the selection of potent MSCs for adipogenesis. By comparing expression profiles of 95 genes in 15 undifferentiated MSCs with glycerol-3-phosphate dehydrogenase (GPDH) activities in the same MSCs after adipogenic induction, 22 genes were selected for further analysis. Combined three-dimensional (3D) analysis of mRNA expression of these genes showed the complete separation of highly potent ilium MSCs from jaw MSCs with limited differentiation capacity.

2. Materials and Methods

2.1. Cells

Human MSCs were obtained from the iliac crest or jaw bone marrow of 15 patients at Hiroshima University Hospital as described previously [7]. Patient information is listed in Table S1. The protocol was approved by the Hiroshima University Ethics Committee (Permit Number: Epd-D88-4).

2.2. Adipogenic Differentiation of MSCs

After four passages, MSCs were seeded at 3×10^3 cells per cm^2 in 24-well plates and maintained to 90% confluence in Dulbecco's modified Eagle's medium (DMEM; Sigma) supplemented with 10% fetal bovine serum (FBS, Hyclone), 100 U/mL penicillin G (Sigma), and 100 mg/mL streptomycin (Sigma). For adipogenic induction, the MSCs were maintained in DMEM (high glucose) (Sigma) containing 10% FBS, 10 mg/mL insulin (Wako), 0.2 mM indomethacin (Wako), 0.5 mM 3-isobutyl-1-methyl-xanthine (Wako), and 1 mM dexamethasone (Sigma) (adipogenic induction medium) for three days, followed by a 4-day incubation with DMEM containing 10% FBS and 10 mg/mL insulin (maintenance medium). The adipogenic treatment was repeated four times. GPDH activities were determined at 28 days using a GPDH activity assay kit (Hokudo), as previously described [10]. GPDH activities were normalized using genomic DNA content, which was determined by the PicoGreen fluorescence assay (Invitrogen).

2.3. Osteogenic Differentiation of MSCs

Confluent MSCs were maintained in DMEM supplemented with 10% FBS, 100 nM dexamethasone, 10 mM β-glycerophosphate (Tokyo-Kasei-Kogyo), 50 mg/mL ascorbic 2-phosphate (Sigma), 100 U/mL penicillin G, and 100 mg/mL streptomycin (osteogenic induction medium) for 28 days. Calcium content was determined using Calcium C Test (Wako) as described previously [11] and normalized to the content of genomic DNA (Figure S1).

2.4. Quantitative RT-PCR

The selection of 95 genes as candidate markers and the measurement of mRNA expression by a TaqMan low-density array (Applied Biosystems) with the ABI Prism 7900 Sequence Detection System (Applied Biosystems) has been described previously [7,10]. Relative mRNA levels were normalized to those of β-actin. The gene names and the probe set IDs for primers, and TaqMan probes are summarized in Table S2.

2.5. 3D Scatter Plot

Scatter plots of the relative mRNA expression of CDKN2D, ITGA5, and CD74 in 15 MSC lines were generated using SPSS 24.0. (IBM Corp.). Distances between the origin and each point were measured to compare differences among the MSC lines.

2.6. Effects of Anti-ITGA5 Antibody on Adipogenesis

To examine the effects of anti-ITGA5 antibody on adipogenic differentiation, anti-ITGA5 (BioLegend, #328004) or control IgG (BioLegend, #400348) was added to the adipogenic induction medium and maintenance medium of ilium MSCs (Riken BRC) for 21 days. Cultures were washed with PBS and incubated with oil red O dye (Wako, 0.3% in isopropanol) for 15 min at 37 °C [12]. The percent of the stained area of cells was quantified using ImageJ software [13].

2.7. Statistical Analysis

Statistical analyses were conducted using SPSS. Correlation between mRNA expression levels and GPDH activities was identified using the Pearson correlation coefficient as described previously [7]. The statistical significance between two groups was determined by Student's t-test. One-way ANOVA was used for multiple comparisons. A p value of less than 0.05 was considered statistically significant.

3. Results

3.1. Correlational Analysis between Gene Expression before Differentiation and GPDH Activity after Adipogenic Differentiation

The ability of MSCs to differentiate into a distinct type of cells, such as adipocytes, is thought to vary among MSCs isolated from different tissues and/or donors. To confirm this assumption, we measured the activity of GPDH, an adipogenic differentiation marker, in 15 different MSCs (five jaw and 10 ilium MSCs) from 15 donors at 28 days after induction of adipogenesis. As expected, GPDH activities significantly varied across the MSC lines (Figure 1, $p < 0.001$, one-way ANOVA). However, the GPDH activity of ilium MSCs was 18 times higher than that of jaw MSCs (Figure S1a). On the other hand, after osteogenic differentiation, calcium content, an osteogenic differentiation marker, was not significantly different between jaw and ilium MSCs (Figure S1b).

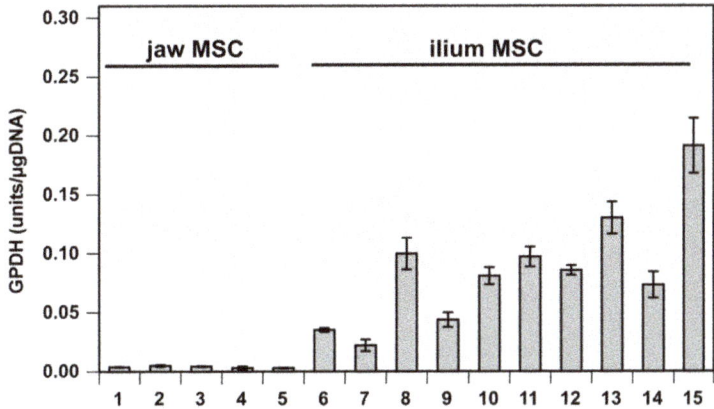

Figure 1. Adipogenic differentiation levels of bone marrow mesenchymal stromal cells (MSCs) evaluated by glycerol-3-phosphate dehydrogenase (GPDH) activity at 28 days after adipogenic induction. The activity was normalized using genomic DNA content to show means ± standard error ($n = 3$). 1–15, donor ID numbers; 1–5, jaw MSCs; 6–15, ilium MSCs.

To screen candidate markers for predicting the adipogenic differentiation ability of MSCs before adipogenic induction, we investigated the correlation between GPDH activities described above and mRNA expression of 95 genes in undifferentiated MSCs using the data from low-density arrays of previous studies [7,10] (Table S2). The expression patterns of 22 out of 95 genes in the 15 MSCs before differentiation significantly positively related to the GPDH activities in the same MSC lines after adipogenic differentiation (Table 1 and Table S2).

Table 1. Candidate genes whose mRNA expression in MSCs before differentiation showing positive correlation with GPDH activities after adipogenic differentiation.

Symbol	Gene Name	Correlation (r)
ITGA5	integrin subunit alpha 5	0.826 ***
MCAM	melanoma cell adhesion molecule	0.812 ***
GPR37	G protein-coupled receptor 37	0.782 **
PSMC5	proteasome 26S subunit, ATPase 5	0.769 **
ACLY	ATP citrate lyase	0.737 **
DNCI1	dynein cytoplasmic 1 intermediate chain 1	0.732 **
P4HA2	prolyl 4-hydroxylase subunit alpha 2	0.720 **
LIF	leukemia inhibitory factor	0.708 **
ZNF185	zinc finger protein 185 with LIM domain	0.708 **
CDKN2D	cyclin dependent kinase inhibitor 2D	0.703 **
DPYSL3	dihydropyrimidinase like 3	0.664 **
INPP5E	inositol polyphosphate-5-phosphatase E	0.650 **
UBE2C	ubiquitin conjugating enzyme E2 C	0.612 *
E2F1	E2F transcription factor 1	0.608 *
CCNB1	cyclin B1	0.598 *
CD74	CD74 antigen	0.561 *
COL7A1	collagen type VII alpha 1 chain	0.561 *
AURKB	aurora kinase B	0.556 *
AMD1	adenosylmethionine decarboxylase 1	0.545 *
CDC20	cell division cycle 20	0.526 *
SLC2A1	solute carrier family 2 member 1	0.526 *
MCM7	minichromosome maintenance complex component 7	0.517 *

r: Pearson correlation coefficient; * $p < 0.05$, ** $p < 0.01$, *** $p < 0.001$.

3.2. Combined Evaluation of mRNA Expression of Candidate Genes

Since GPDH activity was much higher in ilium MSCs relative to jaw MSCs (Figure S1a), the mRNA expression of the isolated 22 candidates in ilium MSCs was compared with that in jaw MSCs (Table 2). We found that 18 of the 22 genes in ilium MSCs were expressed at significantly higher levels compared with jaw MSCs, whereas the remaining four genes were not significantly higher in ilium MSCs. In addition, mRNA levels of 11 genes in ilium MSCs were at least three times higher than those in jaw MSCs.

The levels of the 11 genes in individual jaw MSCs were lower than those in most, but not all, ilium MSCs (Figure S2), although mean levels of these genes in jaw MSCs were at least three times lower than those in ilium MSCs (Table 2). The highest value of each gene in jaw MSC lines is higher than the lowest value in ilium MSC lines. This inconsistency is because the expression levels of the 11 genes greatly varied across MSC lines even in the same group. To reduce the effect of the inter-individual variation, we performed a combined 3D analysis of gene expression (Figure 2). In this analysis, we chose CD74 and CDKN2D, the expression levels of which were approximately 20 times higher in ilium MSCs compared with jaw MSCs (Table 2). We also chose ITGA5, which showed the highest correlation coefficient of 0.826 in the correlation analysis (Table 1). The 3D scatter plot for CDKN2D, ITGA5, and CD74 mRNA expression showed the complete separation between ilium MSCs and jaw MSCs. The values in all ilium MSC lines were more than three times higher than those in any jaw MSC line (Figure 2b).

Table 2. Comparison of mRNA levels of candidate prediction markers between jaw and ilium MSCs before adipogenic induction. Relative mRNA levels means ± standard errors, $n = 5$ and $n = 10$ for jaw and ilium MSCs.

Gene	Relative mRNA Levels	
	Jaw	Ilium
CDKN2D	1.00 ± 0.16	22.09 ± 4.09 **
CD74	1.00 ± 0.41	18.02 ± 5.05 **
MCAM	1.00 ± 0.64	13.44 ± 2.94 **
DNCI1	1.00 ± 0.23	4.52 ± 0.61 ***
GPR37	1.00 ± 0.65	4.32 ± 0.83 **
P4HA2	1.00 ± 0.43	4.31 ± 0.91 **
ACLY	1.00 ± 0.15	4.14 ± 0.49 ***
SLC2A1	1.00 ± 0.17	3.78 ± 0.44 ***
ITGA5	1.00 ± 0.13	3.72 ± 0.42 ***
LIF	1.00 ± 0.39	3.66 ± 0.53 **
AURKB	1.00 ± 0.26	3.09 ± 0.70 *
E2F1	1.00 ± 0.12	2.38 ± 0.40 **
COL7A1	1.00 ± 0.23	2.21 ± 0.42 *
UBE2C	1.00 ± 0.20	2.15 ± 0.45 *
CDC20	1.00 ± 0.23	2.02 ± 0.40 *
PSMC5	1.00 ± 0.08	1.98 ± 0.31 *
MCM7	1.00 ± 0.10	1.81 ± 0.27 *
INPP5E	1.00 ± 0.24	1.79 ± 0.26 *
ZNF185	1.00 ± 0.06	1.79 ± 0.69
CCNB1	1.00 ± 0.16	1.69 ± 0.36
DPYSL3	1.00 ± 0.17	1.35 ± 0.16
AMD1	1.00 ± 0.11	1.22 ± 0.16

Student's t-test; * $p < 0.05$, ** $p < 0.01$, *** $p < 0.001$.

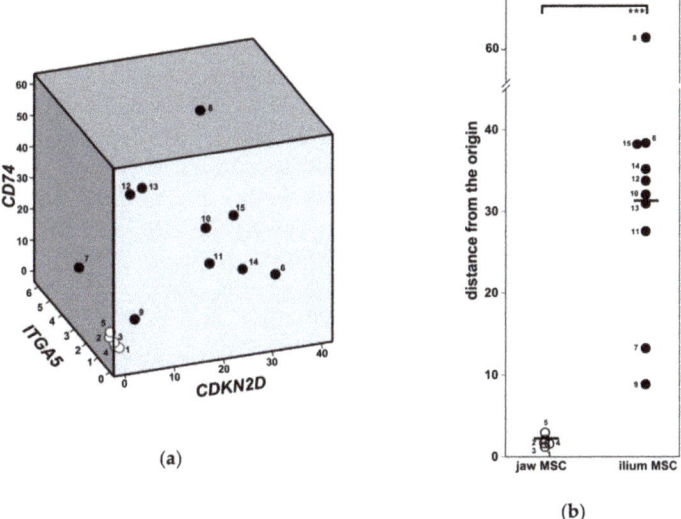

(a)

(b)

Figure 2. Three-dimensional (3D) scatter plots to analyze CDKN2D, ITGA5, and CD74 mRNA expression. (**a**) Using SPSS, the scatter plots showing expression levels of CDKN2D (x-axis), ITGA5 (y-axis), and CD74 (z-axis) were drawn. (**b**) Distances between the origin and each point of ilium MSCs (closed circles, 6–15) were compared with those of jaw MSCs (open circles, 1–5). Mean values are indicated by bars. Student's t-test, *** $p < 0.001$.

3.3. Effects of Anti-ITGA5 Antibody on Adipogenic Differentiation of Ilium MSCs

To explore the potential role of ITGA5, whose correlation coefficient was the highest of all 95 genes examined (Table 1), we investigated the effects of the anti-ITGA5 antibody on the adipogenic differentiation of ilium MSCs. Treatment with the anti-ITGA5 antibody significantly suppressed the adipogenic differentiation of MSCs as compared with control IgG (Figure 3).

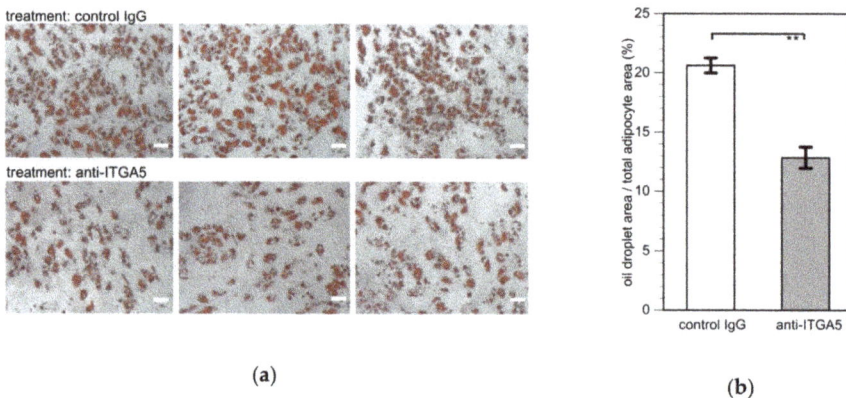

Figure 3. Effects of the anti-ITGA5 antibody on adipogenic differentiation of ilium MSCs. (**a**) MSCs were treated with the anti-ITGA5 or control IgG for 21 days during adipogenic induction and stained with oil red O (scale bar, 70 μm). (**b**) Oil droplet area was quantified by using ImageJ software. Data are presented as mean percent area ± standard error ($n = 3$). Student's *t*-test, ** $p < 0.01$.

4. Discussion

In our previous study, we selected 95 genes as candidate MSC marker genes based on microarray analysis data [10]. Although the 95 genes may not be enough to identify useful markers, and other genes may serve as more reliable markers, these 95 genes can be a promising starting point for further analysis. In this study, we correlated mRNA expression levels in MSCs before induction with GPDH activities after adipogenic differentiation in order to identify marker genes for MSCs with high adipogenic potential. Twenty-two out of the 95 genes showed the expression profiles significantly correlated with GPDH activities. Expression levels of 11 out of the 22 genes in ilium MSCs, which show high differentiation potential, were more than three times higher than those in jaw MSCs, which have only limited potential. We selected the 11 genes, ITGA5, MCAM, GPR37, ACLY, DNCI1, P4HA2, LIF, CDKN2D, CD74, AURKB, and SLC2A1, as potential markers. Although none of these genes accurately distinguished ilium MSCs from jaw MSCs, combined 3D analysis of CDKN2D, ITGA5, and CD74 mRNA expression allowed us to completely separate the two types of MSCs. Thus, the 3D analysis can provide an effective strategy to select MSCs with high adipogenic potential.

All 11 genes identified in the present study are involved in cell growth and/or cell cycle regulation [14–24]. ITGA5 codes the important adhesion molecule involved in adipogenesis [14], and ACLY codes a key enzyme in fat synthesis [17,25]. MCAM (CD146) regulates the proliferation and differentiation of MSCs [15] and serves as a cell surface marker for predicting the potential of MSCs to differentiate into chondrocytes [8]. Although our results suggest that ITGA5 plays a role in the differentiation of MSCs at the early stage of adipogenesis, the exact function of these genes in adipogenesis remains to be investigated in future studies.

The differentiation potential and direction of MSCs seems to differ depending on their origins, although MSCs can be obtained from various tissues, including the bone marrow, adipose tissue, synovium, and dental pulp. Matsubara et al. [5] found that MSCs derived from alveolar bone marrow have poor adipogenic or chondrogenic differentiation potential, but high osteogenic differentiation potential similar to ilium MSCs. On the other hand, MSCs from synovium are superior to ilium MSCs in both adipogenesis and chondrogenesis [26]. In this study, we also found bone marrow MSCs obtained from the jaw to have a limited capacity to differentiate into adipocytes as compared with bone marrow MSCs from the ilium, although jaw MSCs have a high ability to become osteoblasts. Furthermore, Mohamed-Ahmed et al. [27] demonstrated that MSCs from adipose tissues have a higher adipogenic ability than MSCs from bone marrow. In contrast, bone marrow MSCs showed a higher ability to differentiate into osteoblasts and chondrocytes than adipose MSCs. However, differentiation levels determined by oil red O staining varied widely among donors of MSCs. In addition, MSCs obtained from adipose tissues have a reduced proliferative capacity [28,29]. Since MSCs from the ilium bone marrow have a high proliferative and multipotent capacity to differentiate into various types of cells, we speculate that ilium bone marrow MSCs have a high adipogenic differentiation potential, and can serve as materials for soft tissue engineering, although their differentiation potential varies among cell lines.

In most previous studies, preadipocytes have been used for tissue engineering of soft connective tissues [30]. However, the precursor cells already committed to certain lineages have only limited proliferative activity [4,31]. MSCs derived from adipose tissues have also been shown to have an ability to differentiate into various types of cells including adipocytes, as described above [27–29]. However, the difference between preadipocytes and MSCs is not clear. Further studies are warranted to evaluate the potential of preadipocytes and MSCs.

In our previous study, we found eight gene markers capable of predicting the potential to differentiate into chondrocytes [7]. In this study, five out of the eight genes were also identified as marker genes for predicting adipogenic differentiation. In addition, we identified the gene for MCAM (CD146), a cell surface marker capable of isolating potent MSCs for chondrogenesis [8], as a prediction marker for adipogenesis. These findings suggest the existence of a common genetic basis for chondrogenesis and adipogenesis. Accordingly, a significant correlation of differentiation marker levels after induction was observed between chondrocytes and adipocytes derived from 17 ilium MSCs [11].

In the present study, we selected CDKN2D, ITGA5, and CD74 for 3D analysis. As we described above, the expression levels of CDKN2D and CD74 in ilium MSCs were approximately 20 times higher than those in jaw MSCs (Table 2), making them promising candidates. Although ITGA5 showed the highest correlation coefficient (Table 1), there is another candidate for 3D analysis. When MCAM, whose expression levels were 13.4 times higher in ilium MSCs (Table 2), was used instead of ITGA5, the 3D analysis showed similar results (Figure S3). CDKN2D and CD74 used for the 3D analysis in this study were also used for the 3D analysis for chondrogenic potential in the previous study [7]. However, the third chondrogenic prediction marker gene, TGM2, was not identified even as a candidate gene in this study. Therefore, two types of 3D analysis with different combinations of the four genes (CDKN2D, ITGA5, CD74, and TGM2) can be used to predict the differentiation of MSCs for adipogenesis as well as chondrogenesis.

5. Conclusions

The 3D analysis of CDKN2D, ITGA5, and CD74 mRNA expression may offer a novel strategy to identify MSCs with the potential to differentiate into adipocytes. This strategy could be useful to improve clinical outcomes for soft tissue regeneration using MSCs.

Supplementary Materials: The following are available online at http://www.mdpi.com/2076-3417/9/14/2942/s1, Figure S1: Comparison of differentiation levels between jaw and ilium MSCs, Figure S2: Comparison of expression levels between jaw and ilium MSCs of the predictor genes before adipogenic induction, Figure S3: 3D analysis of CDKN2D, CD74 and MCAM mRNA expression, Table S1: Donor information, Table S2: Correlation between gene expression levels before induction and GPDH activities after adipogenic induction in 15 MSCs.

Author Contributions: Conceptualization, M.K., Y.K. and T.K.; methodology, M.K., A.I., K.F., Y.H., H.K., Y.K. and T.K.; investigation, M.K., A.I. and V.S.R.; resources, Y.H., H.K.; writing—original draft preparation, M.K. and T.K.; writing—review and editing, K.F. and Y.K.; visualization, M.K., A.I. and T.K.; supervision, H.K., Y.K. and T.K.; funding acquisition, M.K.

Funding: This research was funded by JSPS KAKENHI, grant number JP17K11541.

Conflicts of Interest: The authors declare no conflict of interest.

References

1. Wang, X.; Gao, L.; Han, Y.; Xing, M.; Zhao, C.; Peng, J.; Chang, J. Silicon-Enhanced Adipogenesis and Angiogenesis for Vascularized Adipose Tissue Engineering. *Adv. Sci.* **2018**, *5*, 1800776. [CrossRef] [PubMed]
2. Janderova, L.; McNeil, M.; Murrell, A.N.; Mynatt, R.L.; Smith, S.R. Human mesenchymal stem cells as an in vitro model for human adipogenesis. *Obes. Res.* **2003**, *11*, 65–74. [CrossRef]
3. Samsonraj, R.M.; Raghunath, M.; Nurcombe, V.; Hui, J.H.; van Wijnen, A.J.; Cool, S.M. Concise Review: Multifaceted Characterization of Human Mesenchymal Stem Cells for Use in Regenerative Medicine. *Stem Cells Transl. Med.* **2017**, *6*, 2173–2185. [CrossRef] [PubMed]
4. Choi, Y.S.; Park, S.N.; Suh, H. Adipose tissue engineering using mesenchymal stem cells attached to injectable PLGA spheres. *Biomaterials* **2005**, *26*, 5855–5863. [CrossRef] [PubMed]
5. Matsubara, T.; Suardita, K.; Ishii, M.; Sugiyama, M.; Igarashi, A.; Oda, R.; Nishimura, M.; Saito, M.; Nakagawa, K.; Yamanaka, K.; et al. Alveolar bone marrow as a cell source for regenerative medicine: Differences between alveolar and iliac bone marrow stromal cells. *J. Bone Miner. Res.* **2005**, *20*, 399–409. [CrossRef] [PubMed]
6. Bearden, R.N.; Huggins, S.S.; Cummings, K.J.; Smith, R.; Gregory, C.A.; Saunders, W.B. In-vitro characterization of canine multipotent stromal cells isolated from synovium, bone marrow, and adipose tissue: A donor-matched comparative study. *Stem Cell Res. Ther.* **2017**, *8*, 218. [CrossRef] [PubMed]
7. Kanawa, M.; Igarashi, A.; Fujimoto, K.; Higashi, Y.; Kurihara, H.; Sugiyama, M.; Saskianti, T.; Kato, Y.; Kawamoto, T. Genetic Markers Can Predict Chondrogenic Differentiation Potential in Bone Marrow-Derived Mesenchymal Stromal Cells. *Stem Cells Int.* **2018**, *2018*, 9530932. [CrossRef] [PubMed]
8. Wu, C.C.; Liu, F.L.; Sytwu, H.K.; Tsai, C.Y.; Chang, D.M. $CD146^+$ mesenchymal stem cells display greater therapeutic potential than CD146- cells for treating collagen-induced arthritis in mice. *Stem Cell Res. Ther.* **2016**, *7*, 23. [CrossRef]
9. Shi, Y.; He, G.; Lee, W.C.; McKenzie, J.A.; Silva, M.J.; Long, F. Gli1 identifies osteogenic progenitors for bone formation and fracture repair. *Nat. Commun.* **2017**, *8*, 2043. [CrossRef] [PubMed]
10. Igarashi, A.; Segoshi, K.; Sakai, Y.; Pan, H.; Kanawa, M.; Higashi, Y.; Sugiyama, M.; Nakamura, K.; Kurihara, H.; Yamaguchi, S.; et al. Selection of common markers for bone marrow stromal cells from various bones using real-time RT-PCR: Effects of passage number and donor age. *Tissue Eng.* **2007**, *13*, 2405–2417. [CrossRef]
11. Kanawa, M.; Igarashi, A.; Ronald, V.S.; Higashi, Y.; Kurihara, H.; Sugiyama, M.; Saskianti, T.; Pan, H.; Kato, Y. Age-dependent decrease in the chondrogenic potential of human bone marrow mesenchymal stromal cells expanded with fibroblast growth factor-2. *Cytotherapy* **2013**, *15*, 1062–1072. [CrossRef] [PubMed]
12. Warnke, I.; Goralczyk, R.; Fuhrer, E.; Schwager, J. Dietary constituents reduce lipid accumulation in murine C3H10 T1/2 adipocytes: A novel fluorescent method to quantify fat droplets. *Nutr. Metab. (Lond.)* **2011**, *8*, 30. [CrossRef] [PubMed]
13. Girish, V.; Vijayalakshmi, A. Affordable image analysis using NIH Image/ImageJ. *Indian J. Cancer* **2004**, *41*, 47. [PubMed]
14. Wang, H.; Li, J.; Zhang, X.; Ning, T.; Ma, D.; Ge, Y.; Xu, S.; Hao, Y.; Wu, B. Priming integrin alpha 5 promotes the osteogenic differentiation of human periodontal ligament stem cells due to cytoskeleton and cell cycle changes. *J. Proteom.* **2018**, *179*, 122–130. [CrossRef] [PubMed]
15. Stopp, S.; Bornhauser, M.; Ugarte, F.; Wobus, M.; Kuhn, M.; Brenner, S.; Thieme, S. Expression of the melanoma cell adhesion molecule in human mesenchymal stromal cells regulates proliferation, differentiation, and maintenance of hematopoietic stem and progenitor cells. *Haematologica* **2013**, *98*, 505–513. [CrossRef]
16. Liu, F.; Zhu, C.; Huang, X.; Cai, J.; Wang, H.; Wang, X.; He, S.; Liu, C.; Yang, X.; Zhang, Y.; et al. A low level of GPR37 is associated with human hepatocellular carcinoma progression and poor patient survival. *Pathol. Res. Pract.* **2014**, *210*, 885–892. [CrossRef]
17. Granchi, C. ATP citrate lyase (ACLY) inhibitors: An anti-cancer strategy at the crossroads of glucose and lipid metabolism. *Eur. J. Med. Chem.* **2018**, *157*, 1276–1291. [CrossRef]

18. Kardon, J.R.; Vale, R.D. Regulators of the cytoplasmic dynein motor. *Nat. Rev. Mol. Cell Biol.* **2009**, *10*, 854–865. [CrossRef]
19. Xiong, G.; Deng, L.; Zhu, J.; Rychahou, P.G.; Xu, R. Prolyl-4-hydroxylase alpha subunit 2 promotes breast cancer progression and metastasis by regulating collagen deposition. *BMC Cancer* **2014**, *14*, 1. [CrossRef]
20. Li, X.; Yang, Q.; Yu, H.; Wu, L.; Zhao, Y.; Zhang, C.; Yue, X.; Liu, Z.; Wu, H.; Haffty, B.G.; et al. LIF promotes tumorigenesis and metastasis of breast cancer through the AKT-mTOR pathway. *Oncotarget* **2014**, *5*, 788–801. [CrossRef]
21. Wang, Y.; Jin, W.; Jia, X.; Luo, R.; Tan, Y.; Zhu, X.; Yang, X.; Wang, X.; Wang, K. Transcriptional repression of CDKN2D by PML/RARalpha contributes to the altered proliferation and differentiation block of acute promyelocytic leukemia cells. *Cell Death Dis.* **2014**, *5*, e1431. [CrossRef] [PubMed]
22. Cheng, S.P.; Liu, C.L.; Chen, M.J.; Chien, M.N.; Leung, C.H.; Lin, C.H.; Hsu, Y.C.; Lee, J.J. CD74 expression and its therapeutic potential in thyroid carcinoma. *Endocr. Relat. Cancer* **2015**, *22*, 179–190. [CrossRef] [PubMed]
23. Kim, D.S.; Lee, M.W.; Yoo, K.H.; Lee, T.H.; Kim, H.J.; Jang, I.K.; Chun, Y.H.; Kim, H.J.; Park, S.J.; Lee, S.H.; et al. Gene expression profiles of human adipose tissue-derived mesenchymal stem cells are modified by cell culture density. *PLoS ONE* **2014**, *9*, e83363. [CrossRef] [PubMed]
24. Xiao, H.; Wang, J.; Yan, W.; Cui, Y.; Chen, Z.; Gao, X.; Wen, X.; Chen, J. GLUT1 regulates cell glycolysis and proliferation in prostate cancer. *Prostate* **2018**, *78*, 86–94. [CrossRef] [PubMed]
25. Katsurada, A.; Fukuda, H.; Iritani, N. Effects of dietary nutrients on substrate and effector levels of lipogenic enzymes, and lipogenesis from tritiated water in rat liver. *Biochim. Biophys. Acta* **1986**, *878*, 200–208. [CrossRef] [PubMed]
26. Sakaguchi, Y.; Sekiya, I.; Yagishita, K.; Muneta, T. Comparison of human stem cells derived from various mesenchymal tissues: Superiority of synovium as a cell source. *Arthritis Rheum.* **2005**, *52*, 2521–2529. [CrossRef] [PubMed]
27. Mohamed-Ahmed, S.; Fristad, I.; Lie, S.A.; Suliman, S.; Mustafa, K.; Vindenes, H.; Idris, S.B. Adipose-derived and bone marrow mesenchymal stem cells: A donor-matched comparison. *Stem Cell Res. Ther.* **2018**, *9*, 168. [CrossRef] [PubMed]
28. Woo, D.H.; Hwang, H.S.; Shim, J.H. Comparison of adult stem cells derived from multiple stem cell niches. *Biotechnol. Lett.* **2016**, *38*, 751–759. [CrossRef] [PubMed]
29. Secunda, R.; Vennila, R.; Mohanashankar, A.M.; Rajasundari, M.; Jeswanth, S.; Surendran, R. Isolation, expansion and characterisation of mesenchymal stem cells from human bone marrow, adipose tissue, umbilical cord blood and matrix: A comparative study. *Cytotechnology* **2015**, *67*, 793–807. [CrossRef] [PubMed]
30. Patrick, C.W., Jr. Adipose tissue engineering: The future of breast and soft tissue reconstruction following tumor resection. *Semin. Surg. Oncol.* **2000**, *19*, 302–311. [CrossRef]
31. Entenmann, G.; Hauner, H. Relationship between replication and differentiation in cultured human adipocyte precursor cells. *Am. J. Physiol.* **1996**, *270*, C1011–C1016. [CrossRef] [PubMed]

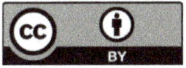

© 2019 by the authors. Licensee MDPI, Basel, Switzerland. This article is an open access article distributed under the terms and conditions of the Creative Commons Attribution (CC BY) license (http://creativecommons.org/licenses/by/4.0/).

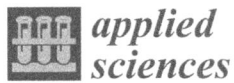

Article

A Radiological Approach to Evaluate Bone Graft Integration in Reconstructive Surgeries

Carlo F. Grottoli [1], Riccardo Ferracini [2,*], Mara Compagno [3], Alessandro Tombolesi [4], Osvaldo Rampado [4], Lucrezia Pilone [1,5], Alessandro Bistolfi [6], Alda Borrè [4], Alberto Cingolani [1] and Giuseppe Perale [1,2,7,*]

1. Industrie Biomediche Insubri SA, Via Cantonale 67, 6805 Mezzovico-Vira, Switzerland; carlo.grottoli@ibi-sa.com (C.F.G.); lucrezia.pilone@gmail.com (L.P.); alberto.cingolani@ibi-sa.com (A.C.)
2. Department of Surgical Sciences, Orthopaedic Clinic-IRCCS A.O.U. San Martino, 16132 Genova, Italy
3. Center for Research and Medical Studies, A.O.U. Città della Salute e della Scienza, 10129 Torino, Italy; mcompagno@cittadellasalute.to.it
4. Radiologia Diagnostica Presidio CTO, Azienda Ospedaliero-Universitaria Città della Salute e della Scienza di Torino, 10129 Torino, Italy; atombolesi@cittadellasalute.to.it (A.T.); orampado@cittadellasalute.to.it (O.R.); aborre@cittadellasalute.to.it (A.B.)
5. Department of Mechanical and Aerospace Engineering, Politecnico di Torino, Corso Duca degli Abruzzi 24, 10129 Torino, Italy
6. Department of Traumatology and Rehabilitation, C.T.O. Hospital-A.O.U. Città della Salute e della Scienza, 10129 Torino, Italy; abistolfi@cittadellasalute.to.it
7. Biomaterials Laboratory, Institute for Mechanical Engineering and Materials Technology, University of Applied Sciences and Arts of Southern Switzerland, Via Cantonale 2C, 6928 Manno, Switzerland
* Correspondence: riccardoferraciniweb@gmail.com (R.F.); giuseppe@ibi-sa.com (G.P.); Tel.: +41-(0)91-930-6640 (G.P.)

Received: 23 January 2019; Accepted: 1 April 2019; Published: 8 April 2019

Featured Application: This protocol allows tracking new bone formation after implantation of a xenohybrid bone graft (SmartBone®), without invasive histological samples.

Abstract: (1) Background: Bone tissue engineering is a promising tool to develop new smart solutions for regeneration of complex bone districts, from orthopedic to oral and maxillo-facial fields. In this respect, a crucial characteristic for biomaterials is the ability to fully integrate within the patient body. In this work, we developed a novel radiological approach, in substitution to invasive histology, for evaluating the level of osteointegration and osteogenesis, in both qualitative and quantitative manners. (2) SmartBone®, a composite xeno-hybrid bone graft, was selected as the base material because of its remarkable effectiveness in clinical practice. Using pre- and post-surgery computed tomography (CT), we built 3D models that faithfully represented the patient's anatomy, with special attention to the bone defects. (3) Results: This way, it was possible to assess whether the new bone formation respected the natural geometry of the healthy bone. In all cases of the study (four dental, one maxillo-facial, and one orthopedic) we evaluated the presence of new bone formation and volumetric increase. (4) Conclusion: The newly established radiological protocol allowed the tracking of SmartBone®effective integration and bone regeneration. Moreover, the patient's anatomy was completely restored in the defect area and functionality completely rehabilitated without foreign body reaction or inflammation.

Keywords: bone tissue regeneration; computed tomography; Xenografts

1. Introduction

In the last 50 years, remarkable advances have been made in the biomaterials field in general, including those for bone regeneration purposes [1]. In this respect, natural and synthetic materials [2] have evolved and are now able to properly replicate complex tissue structures, playing an active role in the repair and regeneration of bone defects [3,4].

Different approaches have been developed to mimic native tissue function [5,6]. One of the most successful one, is the use of porous scaffolds [7] that allow, initially, cell migration and nutrients diffusion, and afterwards provide structural support [8]. This way, cells can grow in the correct shape and location [9,10]. In this respect, certainly the usage of trabecular bone itself (i.e., bone grafts [11–14]) as a template, represent a major strategy, as its porous structure is already naturally suited for cell colonization [15,16]. Moreover, ideal scaffolds, together with biocompatibility, osteocompatibility, osteoconduction, osteoinduction, and neovasculogenic profile [17] should be resorbed or replaced once new bone has formed and they are no longer needed [14]. Apart from bone grafts, other resorbable scaffold constructs are generally composed of a collagen matrix [18], hyaluronan [19], and polymer-based [20,21] materials. If properly formulated [22], they also ensure, together with resorption profile that can be tailored to desired timeframe [23,24], adequate mechanical support [11,16,25] and promoted interactions between growth factors and progenitor cells allowing their proliferation and differentiation into various types [26,27].

In our study, we used SmartBone® (SB), a xeno-hybrid heterologous bone scaffold proved to have osteoconductive abilities [28–30] available on the market since 2012 as a CE-marked class III medical device (according to Directive 93/42/EEC of the European Union). Initially used only in the oral field [31–33], its integration with natural bone resulted to be efficient enough (averagely about one millimeter per month in the complex microenvironment of the mouth, characterized by high concentration of bacteria, which theoretically could limit its osteointegration and cell differentiation [34]) to be successfully extended to other areas [35,36]. As a matter of fact, nowadays, SB is used in the orthopedic field as well.

Together with post-marketing surveillance, in general, advanced clinical and biological analysis are of utmost importance in evaluating an implantable medical device's performance (European Commission guideline Med.Dev 2.7.1, Rev.4, June 2016). This way, in the case of resorbable grafts, it is possible to track whether natural restructuring has allowed the creation of biological tissue with optimized microstructure, according to the physiological function [37,38]. In this respect, certainly histological examinations represent a crucial analysis [39]. This technique involves tissue biopsy, which requires the collection of bone material from the patient [29,31,35]. As a consequence, it results to be an invasive practice and, although it can be carried out fairly smoothly in the oral field, it becomes rather difficult in the skull region or in the orthopedic one [40]. Another very important analysis is represented by in vitro studies that allow directly tracking the cell growth within the scaffold framework [30,41]. On the other hand, they have the limitation of being only partially representative of the actual performance upon implantation into the patient body.

Similar studies have already been performed on SB [29,30,41], providing a complete and detailed explanation of its integration mechanism over time on an averaged base, though not allowing the evaluation of each patient's specific situations. This was mostly due to the aforementioned difficulty in collecting tissue samples from the implantation site. In this respect, we focused, therefore, in developing a non-invasive method that allows an objective and quantitative analysis on the performance of the implanted SB without the surgical procedure for histological samples harvesting. That is, radiographically assessing the new bone formation and its volumetric increase directly in the graft site. Indeed, this can be nicely imaged through computed tomography (CT) [42,43], because native bone and SB have different densities. Therefore, they can be distinguished, and such differences measured by Hounsfield unit (HU).

We here developed a bioinformatical approach to build 3D models by CT scans and validated it evaluating bone regeneration in six individual patients, pre- and post- SB grafting, taking advantage of CT. This represents a non-invasive method based on radiological examination only, used in compliance with the radioprotection principles of justification and optimization. This approach allowed patient-specific analysis of new bone formation over time, objectively and quantitatively: by overlapping CT models, we calculated the volumetric increase of new bone formation, recording higher volumes with respect to grafts after an average of 7 months post-surgery in all dental cases. Finally, apart from this quantitative analysis, we also investigated the density of the newly generated bone, as a read-out of bone quality: the obtained data shows that an average of 80% of bone remodeling occurs already after an average of 9 weeks post-surgery, hence, confirming the excellent performance of SB.

2. Materials and Methods

2.1. Scaffold Preparation

The bovine-derived xenohybrid composite bone scaffold SB was sourced as previously described, being certified for human use and of BSE/TSE (i.e., Bovine Spongiform Encephalopathy / Transmissible Spongiform Encephalopathy) free origin [44]. SB standard blocks, as well as custom-made SB blocks, were used in the surgical interventions, being the latter one also commercially traded under the name SmartBone® on Demand™ (SBoD) [35].

2.2. Clinical Investigations

Six patients were analyzed, and all of them underwent a surgical procedure with SB, receiving either standard blocks or custom-made blocks (Industrie Biomediche Insubri S/A, Mezzovico-Vira, Switzerland). Specifically, four patients underwent dental implants, one case underwent cranio-maxillo-facial (CMF) skull implants, and one case underwent orthopedic implant. Each case is described in detail hereby:

- Case #1: The first patient, 60-year-old female, showed hypodontia in the lower dental arch (three teeth in region 45, 46, 47 missing) and lack of a bone portion at diagnosis by Cone Beam CT (*a.k.a.* CBCT) (Figure 1a). Since a greater amount of bone was needed to carry out the dental implant, she underwent bone grafting with custom manufactured SBoD. The operating technique required a horizontal and vertical augmentation: bone defect did not have a simple shape, so a customized graft was required. By 3D reconstruction a model of the patient's mandibular bone was generated first, and then the missing bone component was designed (Figures S1 and S2 in Supplementary Materials). The missing pieces were also tested on a stereolithographic model. The surgical operation required an engraving into the gum to reach the alveolar bone. Next, the custom-made pieces of SB were positioned in the area where an increase of the amount of bone was needed. When the right position for the bone graft was found, it was fixed with screws, to allow the tight anchoring of the graft to the patient receiving bone. Furthermore, in the procedure of soft tissue closure over the implant, good care was taken to release the tissue flaps proximally using an elevator to obtain a tension free flap.
- Case #2: The second patient, 57-year-old female, smoker, showed partial edentulia and lack of bone and teeth from 21 to 27 throughout the upper right dental arch, as diagnosed by CBCT. The patient's jaw was rebuilt based on CT and surgeon cut SB standard blocks on a sterile 3D model of the patient's anatomy (Figure 1b). A "periosteal elevation" was further performed, a procedure by which the periosteum together with the soft tissues is removed from the bone, to allow the positioning of the customized SB graft. The custom-made block grafts were implanted within the bone defect area. Screws in the bone stabilized the graft. After checking the stability of the system and having the screws firmly positioned, the incision was sutured; soft tissues covered the bone graft, and the two gum flaps were sutured.
- Case #3: The third patient, 59-year-old female, showed severe edentulia with only two teeth left on the upper arch, at diagnosis by CBCT (Figure 1c). This loss of teeth has led to bone reabsorption,

and, thus, the lack of bone portion was deep. She underwent surgery, after custom made SBoD blocks were obtained. A periosteum elevation procedure was performed, as previously described. Additionally, before placing the graft in the bone defect area, the surface of the bone was micro-drilled to induce bleeding intending to further enhance the regenerative processes (a.k.a. micro-channeling practice). Then, the bone graft was implanted and stabilized by screws. After checking the stability of the system and having the screws firmly positioned, the dentist deposited an autologous platelet concentrate (PRP) to promote tissue healing. Lastly, the bone graft was covered by soft tissues. and the two flaps of the gum were sutured.

- Case #4: The fourth patient, 57-year-old male, showed four different bone defects as diagnosis by CBCT (Figure 1d). The periosteum disconnection procedure was performed, as described in previous cases. Once the bone was reached, the surgeon customized by hand SB standard blocks, that were implanted and firmly stabilized by screws. As in previous cases, the wound was finally closed on all its levels till external gums.
- Case #5: The fifth patient, 65-year-old female, showed a meningioma tumor located at the back of the right eye, diagnosed by CT (Figure 1e). The tumor included temporal and sphenoid bone in the skull. The surgical operation involved the removal of the tumor as well as part of two bones, which were rebuilt with custom-made SBoD grafts (Figure S3 in Supplementary Materail). CT was used to design surgery, both in terms of tumor rescission and further bone reconstruction. Given the wide extension of the tumor mass, a significant portion of bone had to be removed, and custom-made SB was provided in pieces, which were assembled during surgery, bed-side, and soaked into blood before grafting, to accelerate the osteointegration process [35]. Once placed, the complete graft has been stabilized with two small titanium plates (KLS-Martin, Germany).
- Case #6: The sixth case, 65-year-old male, presented a clear lack of bone in the distal left radial epiphysis of the left hand, at diagnosis by CT. For a better design of bed-side hand customized SB standard blocks, a 3D model where the bone defect was visible at the apex of the radial bone was built (Figure 1f). The surgical operation required the insertion of the SB block inside the defect during stabilization.

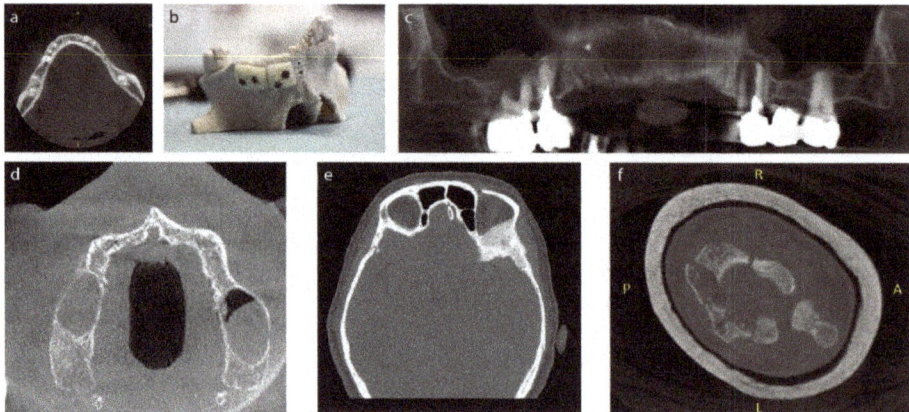

Figure 1. Initial conditions of the six investigated clinical cases. (**a**) Clinical case #1, patient with hypodontia in the lower dental arch; (**b**) Clinical case #2, sterile 3D real model of upper dental arch of partially edentulus patient, with bed-side hand cut SmartBone® blocks; (**c**) Clinical case #3, CBCT scan of upper arch of patient's severe edentulia; (**d**) Clinical case #4, CBCT scan of upper arch of patient's severe edentulia; (**e**) Clinical case #5, CT shows meningioma tumor located at the back of the right eye; (**f**) Clinical case #6, CT slice showing apex of the radial bone defect.

2.3. Computed Tomography (CT)

Table 1 shows radiological equipment and key settings used for image acquisition. For CBCT equipment, isotropic voxels are always intrinsically defined by the acquisition protocol, with dimensions ranging between 0.16 and 0.4 mm. For case #5 and #6, images were acquired with a multi slice computed tomography (MSCT), for which the pixel size is defined by the choice of the field of view combined with a standard 512 × 512 matrix, while the slice thickness is determined by the type of detector used. As part of a multi-planar and three-dimensional reconstruction from MSCT images, it is possible to reformat the voxels of the volume using reconstructions of partially overlapping tomographic sections. In any case, the spatial resolution will be lower than that commonly obtained with CBCT equipment.

The kilovolt and milliampere radiological output parameters (associated with energy and intensity of the X-ray beam) are common values for the indicated equipment, defined to obtain an adequate level of contrast and image noise. For each case, the images used to evaluate the temporal variations of bone volume were acquired on the same scanner.

Table 1. Type of radiological equipment, manufacturer, and exposure parameters used for image acquisition of the six analyzed cases.

Cases	Radiological Equipment	Manufacturer	FOW Diameter (mm)	Pixel Size (mm)	Slice Thickness	Exposure Parameters
Case 1	CBCT	Imaging Science Int. I CAT	96	0.2	0.2	120 kV, 5 mA
Case 2	CBCT	Imaging Science Int. I CAT	85	0.4	0.4	120 kV, 5 mA
Case 3	CBCT	de Gotzen Acteon Group	104	0.2	0.2	85 kV, 8 mA
Case 4	CBCT	Sirona	82	0.16	0.16	85 kV, 7 mA
Case 5	CT	Toshiba	256	0.5	2	120 kV, 50 mA
Case 6	CT	GE	148	0.3	0.625	100 kV, 100 mA

2.4. 3D Virtual Reconstruction: Model Building

The 3D bone model reconstruction was carried out using the Mimics Innovation Suite by Materialise (Materialise HQ, Technologielaan 15, 3001 Leuven, Belgium).

Patients' CT scans are mandatory to perform a 3D reconstruction: indeed, results accuracy mostly relies on how the CT is carried out. Artefacts can compromise the quality of the 3D reconstruction. It is advisable to check that all CT slices are in order and sequential, and show a correct orientation (right-anterior-back) so that the 3D image can be designed correctly with respect to the reference system. The software Mimics converts the clinical images according to specific instructions regarding the orientation of the individual slices, and displays the CT from different levels (as shown in Figure S4 in Supplementary Material).

To obtain a usable 3D model, it is necessary to segment images according to the most common methods of image discretization. Digital filters are applied to enhance the quality of the images by performing high degree noise reduction, with the final goal of making the model the most identical possible to the anatomy of the patients.

Binomial blur filters are traditionally used to remove noise from images, by attenuating high spatial frequencies. A curvature flow filter performs an edge-preserving smoothing on the images. The discrete Gaussian filter computes the convolution of the image with a Gaussian kernel. It is used to smooth and reduce the image detail, preserving the edges for the low variance. Gradient magnitude is mainly used to help in the determination of object contours and separation of homogenous regions. The mena filter is commonly used for simple image noise reduction. The median filter is useful to reduce speckle noise and salt and pepper noise [45].

It is necessary to define a mask, which is created by a digitization process that allows to convert tissue analogic signals so that they can be processed with numerical calculation devices, by considering the variation of the gray scale. A range of values is defined to represent a particular tissue: In our case, the adult compact bone range is around 500 to 2000 Hounsfield unit (HU) [46], while SmartBone® is in the range 100 to 400 HU. The gray value, defined in HU, precisely defines the tissue in each point. The HU is a value attributed to a voxel, which coincides to the average attenuation of the corresponding tissue volume. The choice of this range allows optimal tissue discrimination within the CT [47,48]. In some cases, this range value is modified to conceal the screws, to obtain a better view of SB and to have a better representation of the corresponding bone model.

Once the mask is created, it is possible to convert it into a 3D object. Next, the 3D model mesh quality is improved digitally by the software. If the model is highly consistent with the patient's anatomy no additional steps are required, otherwise, possible defects can be edited manually on the final model by the operator using 3-Matic, the CAD software of the Mimics Innovation Suite. It may be necessary to delete some artifacts that can be caused by poor CT quality or by the presence of metal implants or components that produce scattering. In those cases, a new definition of the slice contour on the slices of the CT scan is needed and Mimics software allow you to have many tools to correct those artefacts to obtain a consistent model.

2.5. Overlapping Models and Calculation of the Volumes

GOM Inspect (GOM GmbH, Braunschweig, Germany) is the software dedicated to the analysis of 3D measuring data for quality control, product development, and production. GOM software is used to evaluate 3D measuring data derived from GOM systems, 3D scanners, laser scanners, CTs and other sources, such as *STL (stereolithography file type, made basing on Standard Triangle Language)* models. The procedure of the overlapping of volumes is one among many possible methods to evaluate the volumetric bone growth that took place following the SB implant. Two 3D models are needed to perform the overlapping: The one built through pre-operation CT and the one constructed through post-operation CT.

Once models reproduce the patient's anatomy faithfully, it is possible to import the two geometric models into GOM Inspect to measure the differences between them. This image matching has to be done on images taken before the surgery *versus* those taken at least six months after when the patient is undergoing a control CT: Such timeframe allows seeing the beginning of the remodeling process supported by SB [29]. Moreover, this step overlap is necessary to get a comparison between the two models. The reference system of one model is converted into the reference system of the other model, to get a correct overlapping and avoid errors. It is very important to have a perfect alignment of the measuring model to the nominal model. Figure 2 shows an example of the pre-operative model imported as a mesh file (in gray) and the post-operative template imported as a CAD body file (in blue).

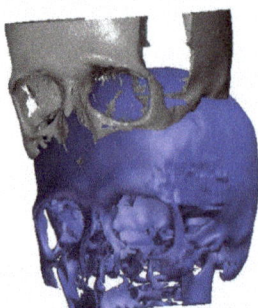

Figure 2. Example of the pre-operative model imported as a mesh file (in gray) and the post-operative template imported as a CAD body file (in blue).

It is crucial, in the overlapping procedure, to perform all possible alignment modes. Two types of alignment have been developed: 1) automatic pre-alignment and 2) alignments made by points. Pre-alignment is an automatic alignment created by the software through robust, effective algorithms. It works by recognizing three-dimensional features, such as edges or angles. Alignment by point consists of defining in the reference model a number of relevant anatomical points that are constant and also easily identifiable in the control model. The chosen points do not change in the two models enabling the chosen points to be perfectly aligned. After alignment, measurements are performed thanks to the GOM Inspects tools, which also provides the models' deviations and the measurements of increased bone volume (ΔV). That ΔV is the bone material regenerated from the SB graft.

The other method used to evaluate the volumetric bone growth is the Boolean subtraction between the two solid models. The software that carries out the subtraction is 3-Matic Medical (Materialise). With 3-Matic, the Boolean subtraction is performed on the 3D models obtained starting from two CT scans: one before the surgery and the other one always at least 6 months after the surgery. After an automatic alignment, the models obtained from the CT scan before surgery is subtracted from the model obtained from the CT scan after surgery. The software shows the remaining volume, which coincides with the bone regenerated (Figure 3).

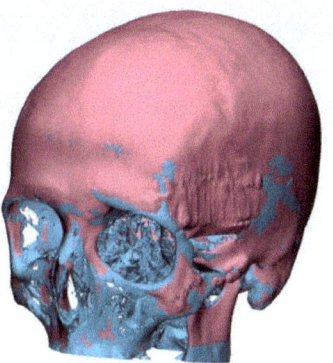

Figure 3. Example of the pre-operative model imported as a mesh file (in gray) and the post-operative template imported as a CAD body file (in blue).

3. Results

The cases included in the study were divided into two groups: The first group (1) included those cases in which the initial SB volume used during surgery was known, because they were custom-made implanted SB blocks (Table 2), hence, blocks designed and manufactured on demand specifically by the manufacturing company. The increase is considered with respect to the initial situation, i.e., the empty defect (considered as the 0 mm^3 reference); comparison is made between grafted SB (initial volume of SB) and final volumetric increase.

Table 2. Volumetric comparison on cases made with pre-customized SB blocks.

Cases	Region of Interest (ROI)	Final Volumetric Increase [mm^3]	Follow up Time	Initial Volume of SB [mm^3]
Case One	Dental	391	13 months	277
Case Three	Dental	605	6 months	781
Case Five	MCF	10,190	24 months	17831

The second group (2) included those other cases that did not have custom-made implants. Therefore, the surgeon had to cut and hand remodel standard blocks (Table 3). Here, again, the increase is considered with respect to the initial situation, i.e., the empty defect (considered as the 0 mm^3 reference); comparison between grafted SB (initial volume of SB not known) and the final volumetric increase was, hence, not possible.

Table 3. Volumetric increase on cases made with handy customized SB blocks during surgery.

Cases	Region of Interest (ROI)	Volumetric Increase [mm^3]	Follow up Time
Case Two	Dental	605	8 months
Case Four	Dental	1028	14 months
Case Six	Orthopedic	1794	6 months

These last cases resulted in a lack of exact bone grafted volume information, and, thus, it was not possible to make a direct and precise comparison between the resulting volume and the initially implanted volume. Nevertheless, these cases are relevant given the intent of this work to assess these types of situations, being frequent in current common clinical practice.

Table 2 shows the volumetric increase in all studied cases with respect to initial conditions. Group 1 collects three cases in which the initial volume of SB is known. Moreover, in one dental case, the resulting volume was greater than the initial volume of implanted SB. Importantly, after 7 to 9 months the new bone always represented a large part of the volume (80.8%), and SB was almost completely reabsorbed (0.5%). These data were consistent with previous results from the literature [29].

Group 2 shows instead that all patients had new bone generation because in the pre-surgery CT a lack of bone was evident, and in post-surgery CT the defect is corrected by the formation of new bone. This could be established because native bone and SB have different densities. Therefore, they can be distinguished, and such difference can be measured by HU. This difference in density was particularly noticeable in case #5, hence, presented in Figure 4a,b, where the red circle (the defective bone) had a smaller white part (the newly formed bone) in the same area. This deduction was straightforward: New bone was clearly visible after two years post-surgery. Further details for each case are here described:

- Case #1: The patient responded well to the implant: By comparing the CT before the operation and the CT 13 months after surgery, a volumetric increase of 114 mm^3 was calculated and no signs of inflammation. It was possible to proceed with the design of the dental implant, after checking that the body integrated the implant and the graft had allowed the regeneration of new bone. The project established dental implant positioning, which is important because they replaced the missing tooth roots. The surgery allowed the dentist to have the right plan specifications, for example, the distance between the teeth or the depth of the implant. One year later the patient still did not show any inflammation or foreign body reaction against implanted material so the implants could be fitted. They were implanted in the mandibular bone to create the base for the prosthesis crown that was fitted later on. The implants were ready to be attached to the abutment, which is the part connecting the implant to the crown. Moreover, it was evident that the graft maintained good stability for the implant, like natural bone. In Figure 5a, it is possible to observe the left mandible reconstruction. The anatomy of the new mandibular bone was highly similar to the healthy geometry (see the left part of the gray volume). This statement is supported by the fact that, if we divide the mandible with a sagittal plane in the center, we can compare the right part with the newly formed bone and check that both parts are symmetrically identical. On the other hand, in the gray part on the right, likely the bone was still regenerating because the natural geometry of the bone was not respected yet. In fact, symmetry, as regards the sagittal plane, has not occurred.
- Case #2: The patient responded very well to the implant: 8 months after the bone graft we calculated a volumetric increase of 142 mm^3, with respect to the empty defect and no signs of

inflammation. In the upper dental arch, it was possible to observe the formation of new bone, which did not appear in the first CT (Figure 5b). At that time after 8 months, it was necessary to re-operate to remove the five screws implanted to proceed with the insertion of the dental implants. Next, the abutment was fitted to the implant by means of a screw to allow dental implant anchoring. If we divided the jaw with a sagittal plane, we could observe that the geometry was completely restored after eight months, because the left and the right part were symmetrical. In this case, the patient was ready for the dental implant because the bone thickness needed for the implant had been fully restored.

- Case #3: In this case, 6 months after the bone graft implantation, we could already observe the formation of new bone, not present in the first CT, as well as bone resurfacing even in parts where SB was not implanted (Figure 5c). In the upper dental arch, it was possible to detect the presence of the three screws, which ensured the stability of the bone graft. The two grafts could no longer be seen as they have been replaced by one reconstructed bone. Not only bone cells generated bone within SB but also osteogenesis occurred outside the grafts. There was a marked horizontal bone increase, which led to the correct anatomical shape being restored.
- Case #4: Follow ups of the patient were performed at different times, 6, 9, and 14 months, respectively. After 6 months post-surgery, the grafts appear to have filled the lack of bone (image not shown), with four screws stabilizing the bone grafts. The second follow up, 9 months after surgery, was performed to check whether the patient had complications. The tissue appears healthy and free of inflammation, and the graft was fully integrated into the patient's bone. At this point, the dentist could remove the screws that ensured stability. After 14 months, SB was completely replaced by the patient's bone. In Figure 5d, it is possible to observe how the bone was regenerated in all four points where SB was implanted. In the two central parts, where the lack of bone was more significant, the growth of the new bone was greater than in the other two parts. Notably, the grafts grew symmetrically and restored the natural anatomy of the maxillary bone.
- Case #5: After 11 days post-surgery a CT was performed to check the complete removal of the tumor and that the SB was integrating without causing foreign body reaction or inflammation. After 2 years post-surgery, osteointegration was fully successful, with the reconstruction of the temporal and sphenoid bone. The bone was perfectly regenerated, and the patient's cranial anatomy was completely reconstructed (Figure 5e). When we compared the two regions of interest in the post-surgery CT, we observed that the second one included a greater amount of bone. The bone was grown not only within the SB plaque but it was also remodeled to restore the correct skull anatomy; as a result, the right and left sides were symmetrical.
- Case #6: The patient underwent a CT after 5 months post-surgery to check whether the insertion of the SB was functional (image not shown). In the post-surgery CT, the little SB block grafted was visible, which was allowing the generation of new bone. Figure 5f shows the radius and the ulna: the bone not only grew within the SB' but also around the graft, thus, completely filling the hole inside the epiphysis: The complete integration of the SB could be observed two years after surgery.

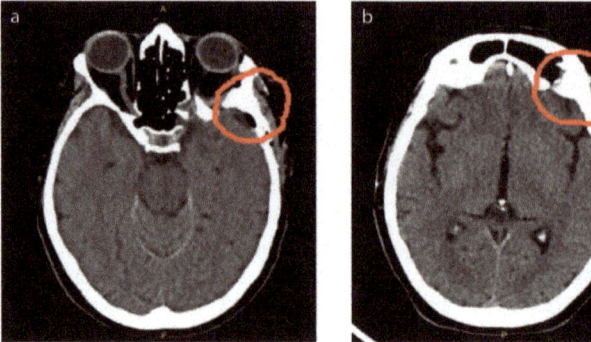

Figure 4. Clinical case #5; (**a**) CT slice immediately post-surgery, showing relatively low bone density, as highlighted in the graft are (red circle); (**b**) CT slice 2 years post-surgery, showing much higher signal, hence, higher bone density, due to new bone formation in the grafted region (red circle).

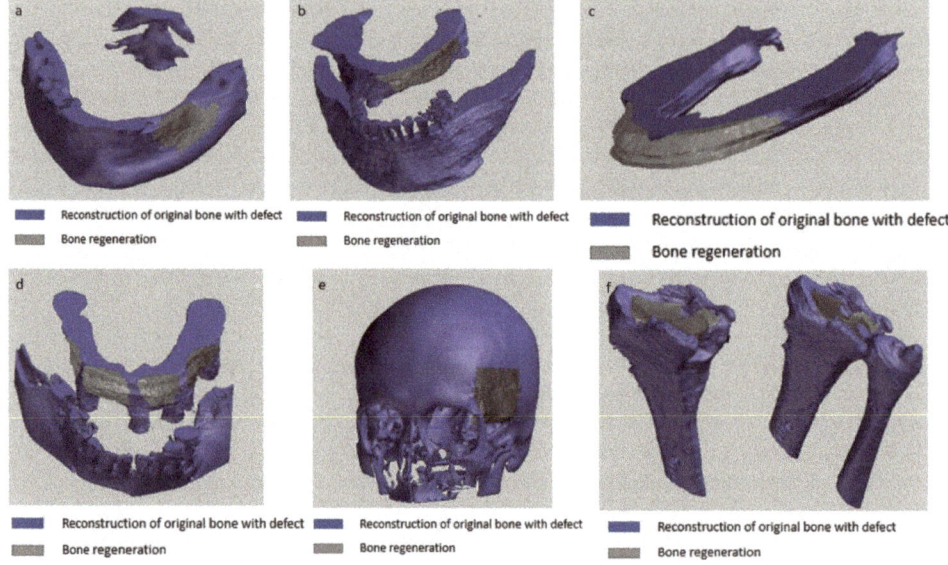

Figure 5. Follow-up images of the six investigated clinical cases; the gray area evidences the grafted volumes, indicated as bone regenerated volumes. (**a**) Clinical case #1, 13 months post-surgery reconstruction, volume stability is high and symmetry almost perfect. (**b**) Clinical case #2, 8 months post-surgery reconstruction, high volume stability of grafted SB. (**c**) Clinical case #3, 6 months post-surgery reconstruction, high volume stability and remodeling already in progress. (**d**) Clinical case #4, 14 months post-surgery reconstruction, excellent results on all SB grafted sites. (**e**) Clinical case #5, 24 months post-surgery reconstruction, complete graft integration and good symmetry. (**f**) Clinical case #6, 24 months post-surgery reconstruction, complete bone remodeling and restoration of functional anatomy.

4. Discussion

In the vast majority of cases, the quality of the new bone formation upon surgery is investigated through histology or densitometry, thus, implying a bone sampling from patient collected through a second operation. In our work, we have here proposed an innovative non-invasive method to establish a healthy bone volumetric increase after different time spans from the implant, which could be easily used in follow up analyses. Specifically, to achieve this goal, the unique radiographic properties of SB have been exploited and were investigated to create 3D templates that faithfully mirrored the anatomy of the individual patient. The trickiest aspect of the applied method was to find the right way to make pre- and post- 3D models overlay accurately, because if the superimposition is precise, the volumetric increase should have respected the real anatomy. The overlay depends on the correct alignment of the 3D templates, and the pre-model reference system should change into the post-model reference one. We tested two different methods to evaluate the volumetric bone growth that took place following the SB implant. Both model-measuring methods used, by means of GOM and by Boolean subtraction with 3-matic, showed equivalent results and depended on the accurate creation of the models from the CT images. Hence, we decided to merge them. Indeed, the peculiarity of the final method is to create templates faithfully respecting the patient's anatomy by the two above mentioned alignments to obtain the best accurate overlapping, which could help us in the understanding the correct volumetric increase for all cases analyzed in the study.

As reasonably expected, the quality of the CT played a primary role in this radiological approach: A good quality yield provided a better resolution and a greater discretization of tissues as it allowed to calculate 3D models identical to the bone anatomical region and, consequently, to reach a more accurate calculation of the possible volumetric increase. Importantly, it has to be taken into account that the SB has low density allowing an optimal CT quality to be recognized.

The main technical aspects related to the acquisition and processing of CT images to obtain quantitative information on the skeletal system have recently been reviewed in Troy et al. [49], providing recommendations finalized to maximize the repeatability and objectivity of measurements. It is particularly important to perform the scans on the same equipment, standardizing the X-ray tube settings, the field of view and the slice thickness. To properly evaluate bone mineral density and distinguish components of integral, cortical, and trabecular bone, a calibration phantom with known hydroxyapatite density standards should be scanned together with the anatomical district of interest. This kind of phantom can reduce the effects of many error sources, such as change in acquisition settings, resolution, or those due to the scanner itself. It is also important to consider that voxel density values are less stable for CBCT equipment than MSCT, with noticeable variations even within the same scan for materials with homogeneous composition [50]. For these reasons, the quantitative method used in this study was limited to the assessments of compact bone volume, after appropriate segmentation, without further investigations about bone densities and composition. The determination of the threshold used for the extraction of bone volumes was not particularly critical given the high degree of separation with respect to the soft tissue densities, for all the considered equipment [49,50].

The developed novel radiological approach not only was successfully tested in a set of different cases related to different anatomical districts confirming its robustness but also allowed drawing conclusions on SB performances. In each analyzed case, good results were recorded: The geometry of the volumetric increase was similar or identical to the lack of bone in the injured area, and, importantly, the amount was expected, considering both post-surgery timing and defect shape. Independent experienced users judged the overlapping of the images to define the acceptable score: This explains minor displacements differences, by a few millimeters, between first and second alignment.

As expected, the volumetric increase was not the same in all patients because of both different investigated anatomical sites and different post-surgery times. Additionally, bone resorption also differed among patient as it depends on age and on other possible pathologies as well as on the size of the region where SB was grafted. Thus, although it was not possible to estimate the growth of SB at a given time, the results showed that this scaffold allowed the formation of new bone in all the examined cases, coherent with literature evidences. We also demonstrated a volumetric increase in each patient. Moreover, there is a clear morphological pattern on the evolution of the standard X-Ray imaging series over time which shows the substitution of the grafted material with a more homogeneous signal in the area of graft implant. The progressive remodeling together with an increase of the mineral signal cannot be dependent on the active remodeling of the graft *per se* given it is a decellularized matrix.

Therefore, the increase in the density over time must be dependent on novel mineral matrix apposition likely induced by the graft as previously shown in vitro [30]. This neo-apposition is quantified in the measures reported using CT scan. Indeed, clinically, partial increase of bone regeneration was already evident from CT scans performed 6 to 7 months post-surgery, likely due to the regeneration process ongoing, while obtained bone gain allows obtaining complete anatomy in a two-years timeframe averagely. Furthermore, bone growth was not only limited to the site where SB was inserted, but new bone was also growing in the areas adjoining the implant, suggesting that bone growth continued until the natural anatomy of the site was fully restored, further confirming SB mechanism of action.

Supplementary Materials: The following are available online at http://www.mdpi.com/2076-3417/9/7/1469/s1, Figure S1: Clinical case #1, patient with hypodontia in the lower dental arch, highlighted in red, Figure S2: Clinical case #1, patient with hypodontia in the lower dental arch; 3D render model of mandibular bone with the design of the custom made SmartBone®on Demand™ graft, Figure S3: Case #5, custom-made SBoD grafts built bed-side, prior to implantation, to reconstruct the temporal and sphenoid bones of the skull which had been previously removed due to the tumor, Figure S4: Exemplificative clinical images converted and displayed by Mimics software, according to specific instructions regarding the orientation of the individual slices.

Author Contributions: Conceptualization, C.F.G. and G.P.; methodology, C.F.G, A.T., O.R., A.B. (Alda Borrè); software, C.F.G., L.P., A.T., O.R.; validation, C.F.G., A.T., O.R., A.B. (Alda Borrè); formal analysis, G.P., R.F., A.B. (Alda Borrè); investigation, R.F., A.B. (Alda Borrè), A.B. (Alessandro Bistolfi); resources, G.P.; data curation, R.F., A.C., M.C.; writing—original draft preparation, all; writing—review and editing, G.P., A.C., M.C.; supervision G.P. and R.F.

Funding: This research received no external funding.

Conflicts of Interest: Giuseppe Perale is among shareholders of I.B.I. sa, the Swiss Company owning intellectual property rights on SmartBone®, manufacturing and commercializing it, including its custom-made line SmartBone® on Demand™, that was here investigated. Ing. Carlo Grottoli and Alberto Cingolani work for the same company. Riccardo Ferracini is an external clinical advisor to the same company. Ing. Lucrezia Pilone was involved as a guest master student, from Politecnico di Torino (Italy), by the same company at the time of this study.

Ethical Use of Clinical Data: All procedures were performed in strict accordance with the recommendations of the Declaration of Helsinki as revised in Fortaleza (2013) for investigations with human subjects, and followed good clinical practice and ISO14155 prescriptions. Study protocol was approved by the United Ethical Committee of the "Città della Scienza e della Salute", Turin, Italy (approval n. 0004336). Informed consents have been recorded from all involved patients.

References

1. Planell, J.A. *Bone Repair Biomaterials*; Woodhead Publishing Limited: Shaston, UK, 2009; ISBN 9781845693763.
2. Sheikh, Z.; Sima, C.; Glogauer, M. Bone replacement materials and techniques used for achieving vertical alveolar bone augmentation. *Materials* **2015**, *8*, 2953–2993. [CrossRef]
3. Winkler, T.; Sass, F.A.; Duda, G.N.; Schmidt-Bleek, K. A review of biomaterials in bone defect healing, remaining shortcomings and future opportunities for bone tissue engineering. *Bone Joint Res.* **2018**, *7*, 232–243. [CrossRef] [PubMed]
4. Klouda, L.; Bouten, C.; Schenke-Layland, K. The Future of Tissue Engineering. *Curr. Opin. Biomed. Eng.* **2018**, *6*, iii–v. [CrossRef]
5. Stevens, B.; Yang, Y.; Mohandas, A.; Stucker, B.; Nguyen, K.T. A review of materials, fabrication methods, and strategies used to enhance bone regeneration in engineered bone tissues. *J. Biomed. Mater. Res. Part B Appl. Biomater.* **2008**, *85*, 573–582. [CrossRef] [PubMed]
6. Sarkar, S.K.; Lee, B.T. Hard tissue regeneration using bone substitutes: An update on innovations in materials. *Korean J. Intern. Med.* **2015**, *30*, 279–293. [CrossRef] [PubMed]
7. Ferracini, R.; Martínez Herreros, I.; Russo, A.; Casalini, T.; Rossi, F.; Perale, G. Scaffolds as Structural Tools for Bone-Targeted Drug Delivery. *Pharmaceutics* **2018**, *10*, 122. [CrossRef] [PubMed]
8. Roseti, L.; Parisi, V.; Petretta, M.; Cavallo, C.; Desando, G.; Bartolotti, I.; Grigolo, B. Scaffolds for Bone Tissue Engineering: State of the art and new perspectives. *Mater. Sci. Eng. C* **2017**, *78*, 1246–1262. [CrossRef]
9. Otsuki, B.; Takemoto, M.; Fujibayashi, S.; Neo, M.; Kokubo, T.; Nakamura, T. Pore throat size and connectivity determine bone and tissue ingrowth into porous implants: Three-dimensional micro-CT based structural analyses of porous bioactive titanium implants. *Biomaterials* **2006**, *27*, 5892–5900. [CrossRef]

10. Gupte, M.J.; Swanson, W.B.; Hu, J.; Jin, X.; Ma, H.; Zhang, Z.; Liu, Z.; Feng, K.; Feng, G.; Xiao, G.; et al. Pore size directs bone marrow stromal cell fate and tissue regeneration in nanofibrous macroporous scaffolds by mediating vascularization. *Acta Biomater.* **2018**, *82*, 1–11. [CrossRef]
11. Cingolani, A.; Grottoli, C.F.; Esposito, R.; Villa, T.; Rossi, F.; Perale, G. Improving Bovine Bone Mechanical Characteristics for the Development of Xenohybrid Bone Grafts. *Curr. Pharm. Biotechnol.* **2018**, *19*, 1005–1013. [CrossRef]
12. Bracey, D.; Seyler, T.; Jinnah, A.; Lively, M.; Willey, J.; Smith, T.; Van Dyke, M.; Whitlock, P. A Decellularized Porcine Xenograft-Derived Bone Scaffold for Clinical Use as a Bone Graft Substitute: A Critical Evaluation of Processing and Structure. *J. Funct. Biomater.* **2018**, *9*, 45. [CrossRef]
13. Guarnieri, R.; Belleggia, F.; DeVillier, P.; Testarelli, L. Histologic and Histomorphometric Analysis of Bone Regeneration with Bovine Grafting Material after 24 Months of Healing. A Case Report. *J. Funct. Biomater.* **2018**, *9*, 48. [CrossRef]
14. Bohner, M. Resorbable biomaterials as bone graft substitutes. *Mater. Today* **2010**, *13*, 24–30. [CrossRef]
15. Bignon, A.; Chouteau, J.; Chevalier, J.; Fantozzi, G.; Carret, J.P.; Chavassieux, P.; Boivin, G.; Melin, M.; Hartmann, D. Effect of micro- and macroporosity of bone substitutes on their mechanical properties and cellular response. *J. Mater. Sci. Mater. Med.* **2003**, *14*, 1089–1097. [CrossRef]
16. Hannink, G.; Arts, J.J.C. Bioresorbability, porosity and mechanical strength of bone substitutes: What is optimal for bone regeneration? *Injury* **2011**, *42*, S22–S25. [CrossRef]
17. Yuan, N.; Rezzadeh, K.S.; Lee, J.C. Biomimetic Scaffolds for Osteogenesis. *Recept Clin. Investig.* **2015**, 1–6. [CrossRef]
18. Salamanca, E.; Hsu, C.-C.; Huang, H.-M.; Teng, N.-C.; Lin, C.-T.; Pan, Y.-H.; Chang, W.-J. Bone regeneration using a porcine bone substitute collagen composite in vitro and in vivo. *Sci. Rep.* **2018**, *8*, 984. [CrossRef]
19. Chircov, C.; Grumezescu, A.M.; Bejenaru, L.E. Hyaluronic acid-based scaffolds for tissue engineering. *Rom. J. Morphol. Embryol.* **2018**, *59*, 71–76. [CrossRef]
20. Freed, L.E.; Vunjak-Novakovic, G.; Biron, R.J.; Eagles, D.B.; Lesnoy, D.C.; Barlow, S.K.; Langer, R. Biodegradable Polymer Scaffolds for Tissue Engineering. *Nat. Biotechnol.* **1994**, *12*, 1119–1124. [CrossRef]
21. Kroeze, R.J.; Helder, M.N.; Govaert, L.E.; Smit, T.H. Biodegradable polymers in bone tissue engineering. *Materials* **2009**, *2*, 833–856. [CrossRef]
22. Cingolani, A.; Casalini, T.; Caimi, S.; Klaue, A.; Sponchioni, M.; Rossi, F.; Perale, G. A Methodologic Approach for the Selection of Bio-Resorbable Polymers in the Development of Medical Devices: The Case of Poly(l-lactide-co-ε-caprolactone). *Polymers* **2018**, *10*, 851. [CrossRef]
23. Pertici, G.; Rossi, F.; Casalini, T.; Perale, G. Composite Polymer-Coated Mineral Grafts for Bone Regeneration: Material Characterisation and Model Study. *Ann. Oral Maxilofac. Surg.* **2014**, *2*, 1–7. [CrossRef]
24. Feng, P.; Wu, P.; Gao, C.; Yang, Y.; Guo, W.; Yang, W.; Shuai, C. A Multimaterial Scaffold With Tunable Properties: Toward Bone Tissue Repair. *Adv. Sci.* **2018**, *5*, 1–15. [CrossRef]
25. Sheikh, Z.; Najeeb, S.; Khurshid, Z.; Verma, V.; Rashid, H.; Glogauer, M. Biodegradable materials for bone repair and tissue engineering applications. *Materials* **2015**, *8*, 5744–5794. [CrossRef]
26. Fernandez de Grado, G.; Keller, L.; Idoux-Gillet, Y.; Wagner, Q.; Musset, A.-M.; Benkirane-Jessel, N.; Bornert, F.; Offner, D. Bone substitutes: A review of their characteristics, clinical use, and perspectives for large bone defects management. *J. Tissue Eng.* **2018**, *9*, 204173141877681. [CrossRef]
27. Haugen, H.J.; Lyngstadaas, S.P.; Rossi, F.; Perale, G. Bone grafts: Which is the ideal biomaterial? *J. Clin. Periodontol.* **2019**. [CrossRef]
28. Pertici, G.; Carinci, F.; Carusi, G.; Epistatus, D.; Villa, T.; Crivelli, F.; Rossi, F.; Perale, G. Composite Polymer-Coated Mineral Scaffolds for Bone Regeneration: From Material Characterization To Human Studies. *J. Biol. Regul. Homeost. Agents* **2015**, *29*, 136–148.
29. D'Alessandro, D.; Perale, G.; Milazzo, M.; Moscato, S.; Stefanini, C.; Pertici, G.; Danti, S. Bovine bone matrix/poly(L-lactic-co-ε-caprolactone)/gelatin hybrid scaffold (SmartBone®) for maxillary sinus augmentation: A histologic study on bone regeneration. *Int. J. Pharm.* **2017**, *523*, 534–544. [CrossRef]
30. Roato, I.; Belisario, D.C.; Compagno, M.; Verderio, L.; Sighinolfi, A.; Mussano, F.; Genova, T.; Veneziano, F.; Pertici, G.; Perale, G.; et al. Adipose-Derived Stromal Vascular Fraction/Xenohybrid Bone Scaffold: An Alternative Source for Bone Regeneration. *Stem Cells Int.* **2018**, *2018*, 1–11. [CrossRef]

31. Stacchi, C.; Lombardi, T.; Ottonelli, R.; Berton, F.; Perinetti, G.; Traini, T. New bone formation after transcrestal sinus floor elevation was influenced by sinus cavity dimensions: A prospective histologic and histomorphometric study. *Clin. Oral Implant. Res.* **2018**, 465–479. [CrossRef]
32. Spinato, S.; Galindo-Moreno, P.; Bernardello, F.; Zaffe, D. Minimum Abutment Height to Eliminate Bone Loss: Influence of Implant Neck Design and Platform Switching. *Int. J. Oral Maxillofac. Implant.* **2018**, *33*, 405–411. [CrossRef]
33. Secondo, F.; Grottoli, C.F.; Zollino, I.; Perale, G.; Lauritano, D. Positioning of a Contextual Implant along with a Sinus Lift Anchored with a Block of Heterologous Bone. *Oral Implantol.* **2017**, *4*, 457–467. [CrossRef]
34. Esposito, M.; Hirsch, J.-M.; Lekholm, U.; Thomsen, P. Biological factors contributing to failures of osseointegrated oral implants. *Eur. J. Oral Sci.* **1998**, *106*, 527–551. [CrossRef]
35. Grecchi, F.; Perale, G.; Candotto, V.; Busato, A.; Pascali, M.; Carinci, F. Reconstruction of the zygomatic bone with smartbone®: Case report. *J. Biol. Regul. Homeost. Agents* **2015**, *29*, 42–47.
36. Roato, I.; Belisario, D.C.; Compagno, M.; Lena, A.; Bistolfi, A.; Maccari, L.; Mussano, F.; Genova, T.; Godio, L.; Perale, G.; et al. Concentrated adipose tissue infusion for the treatment of knee osteoarthritis: Clinical and histological observations. *Int. Orthop.* **2018**. [CrossRef]
37. Taylor, D.; Hazenberg, J.G.; Lee, T.C. Living with cracks: Damage and repair in human bone. *Nat. Mater.* **2007**, *6*, 263–268. [CrossRef]
38. Huiskes, R.; Rulmerman, R.; Van Lenthe, G.H.; Janssen, J.D. Effects of mechanical forces on maintenance and adaptation of form in trabecular bone. *Nature* **2000**, *405*, 704–706. [CrossRef]
39. Jo, S.H.; Kim, Y.K.; Choi, Y.H. Histological evaluation of the healing process of various bone graft materials after engraftment into the human body. *Materials* **2018**, *11*, 714. [CrossRef]
40. An, H.Y.; Martin, K.L. *Handbook of Histology Methods for Bone and Cartilage*; Springer Science+Business Media: New york, NY, USA, 2003.
41. Mayer, Y.; Ginesin, O.; Khutaba, A.; Machtei, E.E.; Zigdon Giladi, H. Biocompatibility and osteoconductivity of PLCL coated and noncoated xenografts: An in vitro and preclinical trial. *Clin. Implant. Dent. Relat. Res.* **2018**, *20*, 294–299. [CrossRef]
42. Beaman, F.D.; Bancroft, L.W.; Peterson, J.J.; Kransdorf, M.J.; Menke, D.M.; James, K. Imaging Characteristics of Bone Graft Materials. *Radiographics* **2006**, 373–389. [CrossRef]
43. Bolland, B.J.R.F.; Kanczler, J.M.; Dunlop, D.G.; Oreffo, R.O.C. Development of in vivo µCT evaluation of neovascularisation in tissue engineered bone constructs. *Bone* **2008**, *43*, 195–202. [CrossRef]
44. Pertici, G. Bone Implant Matrix and Method of Preparing the Same. EP Patent EP2358407A1, 24 August 2011.
45. Senthilraja, S.; Suresh, P.; Suganthi, M. Noise Reduction in Computed Tomography Image Using WB – Filter. *Int. J. Sci. Eng. Res.* **2014**, *5*, 243–247.
46. Fat, D.L.; Kennedy, J.; Galvin, R.; O'Brien, F.; Grath, F.M.; Mullett, H. The Hounsfield value for cortical bone geometry in the proximal humerus-an in vitro study. *Skelet. Radiol.* **2012**, *41*, 557–568. [CrossRef]
47. Schreiber, J.J.; Anderson, P.A.; Hsu, W.K. Use of computed tomography for assessing bone mineral density. *Neurosurg. Focus* **2014**, *37*, E4. [CrossRef]
48. Langton, C.M.; Njeh, C.F. *The Physical Measurement of Bone*; Institute of Physics Publishing Bristol and Philadelphia: Bristol, UK, 2003; ISBN 9781420033342.
49. Troy, K.L.; Edwards, W.B. Practical considerations for obtaining high quality quantitative computed tomography data of the skeletal system. *Bone* **2018**, *110*, 58–65. [CrossRef]
50. Molteni, R. Prospects and challenges of rendering tissue density in Hounsfield units for cone beam computed tomography. *Oral Surg. Oral Med. Oral Pathol. Oral Radiol.* **2013**, *116*, 105–119. [CrossRef]

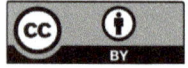 © 2019 by the authors. Licensee MDPI, Basel, Switzerland. This article is an open access article distributed under the terms and conditions of the Creative Commons Attribution (CC BY) license (http://creativecommons.org/licenses/by/4.0/).

Article

Influence of Implant Dimensions and Position on Implant Stability: A Prospective Clinical Study in Maxilla Using Resonance Frequency Analysis

Antonio Nappo [1], Carlo Rengo [1], Giuseppe Pantaleo [2], Gianrico Spagnuolo [2,*] and Marco Ferrari [1]

[1] Department of Prosthodontics and Dental Materials, University of Siena, 53100 Siena, Italy; dr.nappo@libero.it (A.N.); carlorengo@alice.it (C.R.); ferrarm@gmail.com (M.F.)
[2] Department of Neurosciences, Reproductive and Odontostomatological Sciences, University of Naples "Federico II", 80138 Naples, Italy; giuseppepantaleo88@gmail.com
* Correspondence: gspagnuo@unina.it; Tel.: +39-0817462080

Received: 6 February 2019; Accepted: 25 February 2019; Published: 27 February 2019

Abstract: Implant stability is relevant for the correct osseointegration and long-term success of dental implant treatments. The aim of this study has been to evaluate the influence of implant dimensions and position on primary and secondary stability of implants placed in maxilla using resonance frequency analysis. Thirty-one healthy patients who underwent dental implant placement were enrolled for the study. A total of 70 OsseoSpeed TX (Astra Tech Implant System—Dentsply Implants; Mölndal, Sweden) implants were placed. All implants have been placed according to a conventional two-stage surgical procedure according to the manufacturer instructions. Bone quality and implant stability quotient were recorded. Mean implant stability quotient (ISQ) at baseline (ISQ1) was statistically significant lower compared to 3-months post-implant placement (ISQ2) ($p < 0.05$). Initial implant stability was significantly higher with 4 mm diameter implants with respect to 3.5 mm. No differences were observed within maxilla regions. Implant length, diameter and maxillary regions have an influence on primary stability.

Keywords: dental implants; osseointegration; resonance frequency analysis

1. Introduction

In the literature many authors have proposed advantageous long-term results for implant-supported single-unit crowns, as well as, implant-supported short-span fixed dental prostheses (FDP) [1,2]. Implant success depends on tissue biological response and on several other factors such as smoking habit, periodontal status and surgical technique [3–6]. Primary and secondary stability are determining factors for successful implant osseointegration [7] and the absence of micro-movements is a necessary condition [8–10]. A combination of multiple variables could influence primary implant stability such as:

- The quality and quantity of bone at the recipient site;
- The surgical technique used in order to place the implant;
- The macro-/microscopic morphology of the implant [11–16].

Secondary stability is the progressive increase in stability as a consequence of the dynamic interrelationship between new bone formation and remodelling occurring at the bone-implant interfacial zone [17]. In the literature it is demonstrated that the implant success depends on the quality and quantity of the bone as most important factors [18–20]. Bone resorption and healing delay are the result of implant failure due to weak bone quantity and quality. Jaffin et al. showed a 35% failure rate in type 4 bone. In their study, the major risk factors for implant failure were weak bone quantity and quality [21]. Moreover, Bischof and co-workers demonstrated that the primary stability of the implant depends only on jaw and the bone type and not on other factors such as diameter, length and deepening of the implant [22].

Therefore, the aim of the present study was to evaluate the influence of implant dimensions (length and diameter) and position (anterior and posterior maxilla) on the primary and secondary stability of implants placed in the upper arch.

2. Materials and Methods

2.1. Study Design

The study was designed as a prospective clinical trial.

2.2. Patient Selection

Patients consecutively treated at the Department of Oral Surgery of the University of Siena and University "Federico II" of Napoli, Italy, were enrolled for the study, the recruitment period of included patients was 12 months. All patients agreed to participate in the study and signed informed consent. Thirty-one patients (mean age: 57; range from 31 to 77) have been enrolled in the study, 17 females (mean age: 56; range from 31 to 73) and 14 males (mean age: 59; range from 31 to 77). The study was conducted according to the principles of the Declaration of Helsinki on experimentation involving human subjects.

The inclusion criteria were as follows:

- Patients were aged 18 years or older;
- Absence of medical history or conditions that could contraindicate surgery;
- 4 to 6 months waiting time were necessary for healing after tooth extraction;
- Presence of sufficient residual alveolar bone volume to achieve primary implant stability without concomitant or previous bone augmentation;
- Full-mouth plaque score (FMPS) < 25% at baseline;
- Full-mouth bleeding score (FMBS) < 25% at baseline;

Exclusion criteria were:

- Tobacco smoking;
- Pregnancy and lactation;
- Bisphosphonates use;
- Untreated periodontal conditions;
- Absence at least of 2 mm of keratinized tissue;
- Lower arches.

2.3. Clinical Procedure

Dental implants ("OsseoSpeed TX", Astra Tech Implant System—Dentsply Implants; Mölndal, Sweden) were placed following a two-stage protocol according to the manufacturer's instructions. These kinds of implant have two main features: an exclusive implant surface with a fluoride-treated nanostructure that stimulates early bone formation and provides a firmer bone-implant connection; micro-threads on the neck of the implant that ensure optimal load distribution and optimal stress values. Implants were placed exclusively in the upper jaw. For definition purposes, implants placed in the "anterior" maxilla were meant to replace central and lateral incisors and canines; whereas in the "posterior" maxilla implants were placed to replace premolars and molars. Implants were usually positioned with the implant shoulder at the level of the alveolar bone crest and then covered with the mucosal flap. All the implants were placed in native bone and without bone regeneration. The torque was measured through the implant motor. The implants, placed with handpiece, had all torque up to 35 ncm. The second-phase surgery was carried out at 3 months. Different implant lengths (9, 11 and 13 mm) and diameters (3.5 and 4 mm) were used. The diameter of the last tool used was based on the diameter of the implants, it was 2.7 for diameter 3.5 and 3.2 for diameter 4. A beta-lactam antibiotic (Amoxicillin) was given to all patients for 5 days post-surgically. The postoperative therapy required good oral hygiene, rinsing with mouth wash containing 0.2% chlorhexidine solution twice a day for four post-operative weeks from the surgery. Sutures were removed at seven days at the surgery. All implants were evaluated with peri-apical x-rays immediately after insertion and after 3 months. Definitive crowns were delivered at 4–6 months post-surgery. All prosthesis were manufactured in order to facilitate oral hygiene procedures. No implant failures were recorded. The bone quality was clinically evaluated using the index of Lekholm and Zarb, in agreement with the radiographic evaluations and the drilling resistance perceived by the clinician operator [23]. Implants distribution according to bone quality is showed in Table 1. Implant stability measurements through resonance frequency analysis (RFA) were performed by a single operator immediately after implant placement in terms of the implant stability quotient (ISQ1) and after 3 months (ISQ2). The ISQ was obtained installing a "Smartpeg" transducer (Integration Diagnostics AB, Göteborg, Sweden) into the fixture and approaching it perpendicularly with the handpiece probe of the Osstell (Integration Diagnostics AB, Göteborg, Sweden) device.

Table 1. Implants distribution according to bone quality assessment.

Bone Quality	I	II	III	IV	Total
N	2	36	29	3	70
%	2.9	51.4	41.4	4.3	100%

2.4. Statistical Analysis

Descriptive statistics (e.g., means and standard deviation (SD)) were used to present the outcomes. The primary outcome was based on the ISQ. Analysis of variance and Tukey's multiple comparison tests and paired t-test were performed. A value of $p > 0.05$ was considered as level of statistical significance.

3. Results

Mean ISQ at implant placement (ISQ1) was 75.3 ± 5.5 whereas after 3 months (ISQ2) it was statistically significantly higher ($p < 0.05$), with a mean of 79.6 ± 5.8 (Figure 1). Descriptive statistics of ISQ values distribution within implant diameter and length, maxilla regions, sex and age are reported in Figures 2–4. Tukey's multiple comparison test of ISQ1 and ISQ2 values for all before mentioned parameters are shown in Tables 2–4.

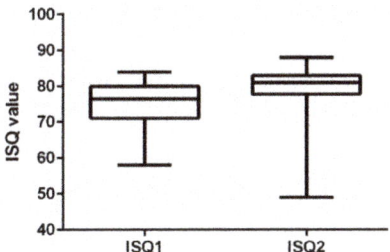

Figure 1. Paired t test for implant stability quotient (ISQ) values at implant placement (ISQ1) and after 3 months (ISQ2).

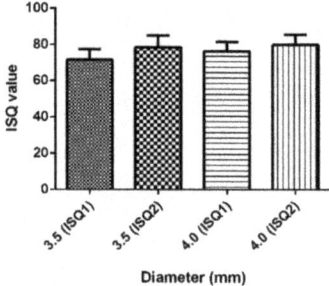

Figure 2. ISQ 1 and 2 values distribution within different implant diameters (3.5 and 4 mm).

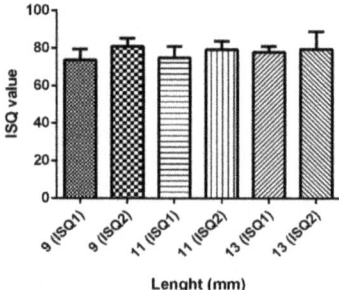

Figure 3. ISQ 1 and 2 values distribution within different implant lengths (9, 11 and 13 mm).

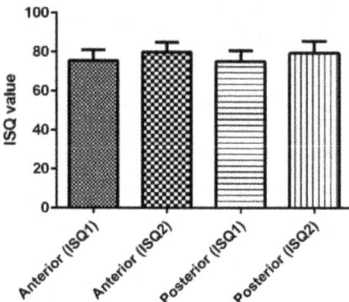

Figure 4. ISQ 1 and 2 values distribution within different maxilla regions (frontal and posterior).

Table 2. Tukey's multiple comparison test of ISQ1 and ISQ2 values for 3.5- and 4-mm diameter implants. Numbers are means and values in brackets are standard deviations. Lowercase letters indicate statistically significant differences among the diameter within the ISQ 1 or 2 values. Uppercase letters indicate statistically significant differences between the ISQ 1 or 2 values within the diameter.

Implant Diameter (mm)	ISQ1	ISQ2
3.5	71.38 (5.79) aA	78.46 (6.43) aB
4	76.23 (5.16) bA	79.89 (5.73) aB

Table 3. Tukey's multiple comparison test of ISQ1 and ISQ2 values for 9-, 11- and 13-mm implants. Numbers are means and values in brackets are standard deviations. Lowercase letters indicate statistically significant differences among the length within the ISQ 1 or 2 values. Uppercase letters indicate statistically significant differences between the ISQ 1 or 2 values within the length. * and ** indicate statistically significant differences between ISQ1 and 2 values across the lengths.

Implant Length (mm)	ISQ1	ISQ2
9	73.5 (5.91) aA *	80.93 (4.28) aB **
11	74.95 (5.95) aA **	79.25 (4.49) aB *
13	77.88 (3.13) abA	79.44 (9.31) aA

Table 4. Tukey's multiple comparison test of ISQ1 and ISQ2 values for different maxilla regions (frontal and posterior). Numbers are means and values in brackets are standard deviations. Uppercase letters indicate statistically significant differences between the ISQ 1 or 2 values within the maxillary region. * indicates statistically significant differences between ISQ 1 and 2 values across the maxillary regions.

Maxilla Region	ISQ1	ISQ2
Frontal	75.59 (5.57)	80.05 (4.97) *
Posterior	75.21 (5.62) A *	79.44 (6.24) B

3.1. Differences in Implant Stability Quotient (ISQ) Values According to Implant Diameter

At implant placement ISQ values were statistically significantly higher for 4 mm diameter implants (76.23 ± 5.16) compared with 3.5 mm diameter implants (71.38 ± 5.79) (Table 2).

3.2. Differences in ISQ Values According to Implant Length

At implant placement, ISQ values progressively increased with implant length, even if no statistically significant differences were observed within the groups (9, 11 and 13 mm). After 3 months, ISQ values were statistically significantly higher than baseline (ISQ1), but exclusively for 9- and 11-mm length implants. Implants with 13 mm length showed no differences between ISQ1 and ISQ2 values (Table 3).

3.3. Differences in ISQ Values According to Maxilla Regions

Both ISQ values at baseline and after 3 months post-implantation were found to be comparable for implants placed in anterior or posterior maxilla, although implants placed in posterior maxilla showed a significant increase of ISQ values after 3 months compared to baseline. No statistically significantly differences were observed within frontal and posterior maxilla at implant placement and after 3 months. ISQ values after 3 months compared to implant placement were statistically significantly higher exclusively for implants placed in the posterior maxilla (Table 4).

4. Discussion

This study has evaluated the influence of implant dimensions (length and diameter) on the primary and secondary stability of implants placed in the upper arch.

The results of the present study suggest that the ISQ values significantly increase during the three months of follow-up. The findings also include significant differences between some parameters analysed (implant diameter, implant length and maxilla regions).

Bone density seems to strongly influence implant stability and long-term success, as demonstrated by the higher implant survival rates in the mandible compared to the maxilla, especially the posterior maxilla [24]. Bone density can be objectively measured with different methods, including microCT [25] that may define the bone quality, even if the concept of "bone quality" is not clearly defined in literature.

Currently the most accepted method to assess the bone quality is the one proposed by Lekholm and Zarb [23], which give a scale from 1 to 4 based on the amount of cortical and trabecular bone evaluated in preoperative radiographs and the tactile sensation of resistance experienced by the clinician during the drilling procedure of implant site preparation. This method, however, is rather subjective [23]. Depending on the bone quality, surgeons may adapt the surgical protocol in order to increase implant primary stability. Adapted surgical protocols includes the preparation of undersized implant size, the use of osteotomes for bone condensation, the use of different specific drills such as countersink or screw tap drills [26–28].

Implant stability can be measured clinically with different more objective quantitative methods, such as the insertion torque, or electronic devices such as the Periotest (Medizintechnik Gulden, Germany) and the Osstell (Integration Diagnostics, Sweden). The insertion torque provides a reliable assessment of the implant stability, but it can be evaluated only at the implant insertion time and cannot be repeated in the follow-up. A recent systematic review concluded that there is no correlation between ISQ and insertion torque values [29]. The Periotest device produces vibrations on the implant and gives a value (PTV) from 8 to 50, while the Osstell device profits from RFA and gives a value (ISQ) from 1 to 100.

Among these two devices the first one raised some criticism since it seems to have a lower sensitivity and is more susceptible to the operator [30].

Implant stability quotient values recorded at the time of implant installation do not reflect the nature of the bone/implant interface and hence the degree of mechanical anchorage. Primary stability may not only be influenced by bone volumetric density and/or bone trabecular connectivity but also by the thickness and density of the cortical layer of the alveolar bone crest. Concerning the bone quality, the outcomes of the present study are in agreement with those presented by Degidi and co-workers, who reported that bone quality does not appear to be crucial for gaining high ISQ values [31], and the low association between bone quality and ISQ values has been demonstrated in clinical studies [32,33]. Moreover, Barewal [34] observed the correlation between the RFA and the Lekholm and Zarb classification and showed a difference only between bone types 1 and 4. By contrast, Östman [35] demonstrated a close correlation between bone quality and RFA values. Huang [36] demonstrated a direct correspondence between bone quality around implants and calculated a decreasing frequency trend. Moreover, Friberg [27] revealed a correlation between bone quality and implant stability measuring the cutting torque and RFA values during implant placement. Furthermore, it has been reported that this is due to the fact that cortical bone is 10 to 20 times stiffer than trabecular bone [37].

5. Conclusions

In conclusion, in this study no statistically significant differences in ISQ values were found in terms of different maxillary areas and, therefore, between different bone quality.

Within the limitations of this study, we conclude that some parameters such as implant length and diameter may influence only the primary stability. However, additional controlled and comparative studies are needed to confirm or refute these findings.

Author Contributions: All the authors contributed to this study. A.N., C.R., M.F.: conceptualization, funding acquisition, project administration, supervision, writing of review and editing; C.R., G.P.: investigation, writing of the original draft; A.N., G.S., M.F.: investigation.

Funding: This research received no external funding.

Conflicts of Interest: The authors declare no conflict of interest.

References

1. Pjetursson, B.E.; Lang, N.P. Prosthetic treatment planning on the basis of scientific evidence. *J. Oral Rehabil.* **2008**, *35*, 72–79. [CrossRef] [PubMed]
2. Aglietta, M.; Iorio Siciliano, V.; Zwahlen, M.; Bragger, U.; Pjetursson, B.E.; Lang, N.P.; Salvi, G.E. A systematic review of the survival and complication rates of implant supported fixed dental prostheses with cantilever extensions after an observation period of at least 5 years. *Clin. Oral Implant. Res.* **2009**, *20*, 441–451. [CrossRef] [PubMed]
3. Falco, A.; Berardini, M.; Trisi, P. Correlation Between Implant Geometry, Implant Surface, Insertion Torque, and Primary Stability: In Vitro Biomechanical Analysis. *Int. J. Oral Maxillofac. Implant.* **2018**, *33*, 824–830. [CrossRef] [PubMed]
4. Barikani, H.; Rashtak, S.; Akbari, S.; Fard, M.K.; Rokn, A. The effect of shape, length and diameter of implants on primary stability based on resonance frequency analysis. *Dent. Res. J. (Isfahan)* **2014**, *11*, 87–91.
5. Chen, M.H.; Lyons, K.M.; Tawse-Smith, A.; Ma, S. Clinical Significance of the Use of Resonance Frequency Analysis in Assessing Implant Stability: A Systematic Review. *Int. J. Prosthodont.* **2019**, *32*, 51–58. [CrossRef] [PubMed]
6. Trindade, R.; Albrektsson, T.; Wennerberg, A. Current concepts for the biological basis of dental implants: Foreign body equilibrium and osseointegration dynamics. *Oral Maxillofac. Surg. Clin. North. Am.* **2015**, *27*, 175–183. [CrossRef] [PubMed]
7. Lioubavina-Hack, N.; Lang, N.P.; Karring, T. Significance of primary stability for osseointegration of dental implants. *Clin. Oral Implant. Res.* **2006**, *17*, 244–250. [CrossRef] [PubMed]
8. Salama, H.; Rose, L.; Salama, M.; Betts, N. Immediate loading of bilaterally splinted titanium root-form implants in fixed prosthodontics—A technique reexamined; two case reports. *Int. J. Periodontics Restor. Dent.* **1995**, *15*, 344–361.
9. Zafar, M.S.; Farooq, I.; Awais, M.; Najeeb, S.; Khurshid, Z.; Zohaib, S. Bioactive Surface Coatings for Enhancing Osseointegration of Dental Implants. In *Biomedical, Therapeutic and Clinical Applications of Bioactive Glasses*; Woodhead Publishing: Cambridge, UK, 2019.
10. Esposito, M.; Grusovin, M.G.; Willings, M.; Coulthard, P.; Worthington, H.V. Interventions for replacing missing teeth: Different times for loading dental implants. *Cochrane Database Syst. Rev.* **2013**, *28*, CD003878. [CrossRef] [PubMed]
11. Marquezan, M.; Osório, A.; Sant'Anna, E.; Souza, M.M.; Maia, L. Does bone mineral density influence the primary stability of dental implants? A systematic review. *Clin. Oral Implant. Res.* **2012**, *23*, 767–774. [CrossRef] [PubMed]
12. Trisi, P.; Todisco, M.; Consolo, U.; Travaglini, D. High versus low implant insertion torque: A histologic, histomorphometric, and biomechanical study in the sheep mandible. *Int. J. Oral Maxillofac. Implant.* **2011**, *26*, 837–849.
13. Tabassum, A.; Meijer, G.J.; Wolke, J.G.; Jansen, J.A. Influence of surgical technique and surface roughness on the primary stability of an implant in artificial bone with different cortical thickness: A laboratory study. *Clin. Oral Implant. Res.* **2010**, *21*, 213–220. [CrossRef] [PubMed]
14. Sciasci, P.; Casalle, N.; Vaz, L.G. Evaluation of primary stability in modified implants: Analysis by resonance frequency and insertion torque. *Clin. Implant. Dent. Relat Res.* **2018**, *20*, 274–279. [CrossRef] [PubMed]
15. Norton, M.R. The Influence of Low Insertion Torque on Primary Stability, Implant Survival, and Maintenance of Marginal Bone Levels: A Closed-Cohort Prospective Study. *Int. J. Oral Maxillofac. Implant.* **2017**, *32*, 849–857. [CrossRef] [PubMed]
16. Novellino, M.M.; Sesma, N.; Zanardi, P.R.; Laganá, D.C. Resonance frequency analysis of dental implants placed at the posterior maxilla varying the surface treatment only: A randomized clinical trial. *Clin. Implant. Dent. Relat. Res.* **2017**, *19*, 770–775. [CrossRef] [PubMed]
17. Akoğlan, M.; Tatli, U.; Kurtoğlu, C.; Salimov, F.; Kürkçü, M. Effects of different loading protocols on the secondary stability and peri-implant bone density of the single implants in the posterior maxilla. *Clin. Implant. Dent. Relat. Res.* **2017**, *19*, 624–631. [CrossRef] [PubMed]
18. Chrcanovic, B.R.; Albrektsson, T.; Wennerberg, A. Bone Quality and Quantity and Dental Implant Failure: A Systematic Review and Meta-analysis. *Int. J. Prosthodont.* **2017**, *30*, 219–237. [CrossRef] [PubMed]
19. Kim, D.G.; Elias, K.L.; Jeong, Y.H.; Kwon, H.J.; Clements, M.; Brantley, W.A.; Lee, D.J.; Han, J.S. Differences between buccal and lingual bone quality and quantity of peri-implant regions. *J. Mech. Behav. Biomed. Mater.* **2016**, *60*, 48–55. [CrossRef] [PubMed]

20. Kim, D.G.; Kwon, H.J.; Jeong, Y.H.; Kosel, E.; Lee, D.J.; Han, J.S.; Kim, H.L.; Kim, D.J. Mechanical properties of bone tissues surrounding dental implant systems with different treatments and healing periods. *Clin. Oral Investig.* **2016**, *20*, 2211–2220. [CrossRef] [PubMed]
21. Jaffin, R.A.; Berman, C.L. The excessive loss of Branemark fixtures in type IV bone: A 5-year analysis. *J. Periodontol.* **1991**, *62*, 2–4. [CrossRef] [PubMed]
22. Bischof, M.; Nedeir, R.; Szmukler-Moncler, S.; Bernard, J.P.; Samson, J. Implant stability measurement of delayed and immediately loaded implants during healing. *Clin. Oral Implant. Res.* **2004**, *15*, 529–539. [CrossRef] [PubMed]
23. Lekholm, U.; Zarb, G.A. Patient selection and preparation. In *Tissue-Integrated Prostheses: Osseointegration in Clinical Dentistry*, 1st ed.; Brfinemark, P.I., Zarb, G.A., Alberktsson, T., Eds.; Quintessence International: Chicago, IL, USA, 1985; pp. 199–209.
24. Buser, D.; Mericske-Stern, R.; Bernard, J.P.; Behneke, A.; Behneke, N.; Hirt, H.P.; Belser, C.U.; Lang, N.P. Long-term evaluation of non-submerged ITI implants. Part 1: 8-year life table analysis of a prospective multi-center study with 2359 implants. *Clin. Oral Implant. Res.* **1997**, *8*, 161–172. [CrossRef]
25. Turkyilmaz, I.; McGlumphy, E.A. Influence of bone density on implant stability parameters and implant success: A retrospective clinical study. *BMC Oral Health* **2008**, *8*, 32. [CrossRef] [PubMed]
26. Alghamdi, H.; Anand, P.S.; Anil, S. Undersized implant site preparation to enhance primary implant stability in poor bone density: A prospective clinical study. *J. Oral Maxillofac. Surg.* **2011**, *69*, e506–e512. [CrossRef] [PubMed]
27. Nobrega, A.R.; Norton, A.; Silva, J.A.; Silva, J.P.; Branco, F.M.; Anitua, E. Osteotome versus conventional drilling technique for implant site preparation: A comparative study in the rabbit. *Int. J. Periodontics Restor. Dent.* **2012**, *32*, e109–e115.
28. Di Salle, A.; Spagnuolo, G.; Conte, R.; Procino, A.; Peluso, G.; Rengo, C. Effects of various prophylactic procedures on titanium surfaces and biofilm formation. *J. Periodontal Implant. Sci.* **2018**, *48*, 373–382. [CrossRef] [PubMed]
29. Lages, F.S.; Douglas-de Oliveira, D.W.; Costa, F.O. Relationship between implant stability measurements obtained by insertion torque and resonance frequency analysis: A systematic review. *Clin. Implant. Dent. Relat. Res.* **2018**, *20*, 26–33. [CrossRef] [PubMed]
30. Meredith, N. Assessment of implant stability as a prognostic determinant. *Int. J. Prosthodont* **1998**, *11*, 491–501. [PubMed]
31. Degidi, M.; Daprile, G.; Piattelli, A.; Carinci, F. Evaluation of factors influencing resonance frequency analysis values, at insertion surgery, of implants placed in sinus-augmented and nongrafted sites. *Clin. Implant. Dent. Relat Res.* **2007**, *9*, 144–149. [CrossRef] [PubMed]
32. Zix, J.; Kessler-Liechti, G.; Mericske-Stern, R. Stability measurement of 1-stage implants in the maxilla by means of resonance frequency analysis: A pilot study. *Int J. Oral Maxillofac Implant.* **2005**, *20*, 747–752.
33. Fu, M.W.; Fu, E.; Lin, F.G.; Chang, W.J.; Hsieh, Y.D.; Shen, E.C. Correlation Between Resonance Frequency Analysis and Bone Quality Assessments at Dental Implant Recipient Sites. *Int J. Oral Maxillofac Implant.* **2017**, *32*, 180–187. [CrossRef] [PubMed]
34. Barewal, R.M.; Oates, T.W.; Meredith, N.; Cochran, D.L. Resonance frequency measurement of implant stability in vivo on implants with a sandblasted and acid-etched surface. *Int J. Oral Maxillofac. Implant.* **2003**, *18*, 641–651.
35. Östman, P.O.; Hellman, M.; Wendelhag, I.; Sennerby, L. Resonance frequency analysis measurements of implants at placement surgery. *Int. J. Prosthodont* **2006**, *19*, 77–83. [PubMed]
36. Huang, H.M.; Lee, S.Y.; Yeh, C.Y.; Lin, C.T. Resonance frequency assessment of dental implant stability with various bone qualities: A numerical approach. *Clin. Oral Implant. Res.* **2000**, *13*, 65–74. [CrossRef]
37. Friberg, B.; Sennerby, L.; Roos, J.; Lekholm, U. Identification of bone quality in conjunction with insertion of titanium implants. A pilot study in jaw autopsy specimens. *Clin. Oral Implant. Res.* **1995**, *6*, 213–219. [CrossRef]

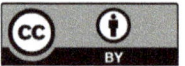

© 2019 by the authors. Licensee MDPI, Basel, Switzerland. This article is an open access article distributed under the terms and conditions of the Creative Commons Attribution (CC BY) license (http://creativecommons.org/licenses/by/4.0/).

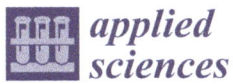

Article

Automatic Method for Bone Segmentation in Cone Beam Computed Tomography Data Set

Mantas Vaitiekūnas [1,*,†], Darius Jegelevičius [1,2,†], Andrius Sakalauskas [3,†] and Simonas Grybauskas [4,†]

1. Biomedical Engineering Institute, Kaunas University of Technology, 51423 Kaunas, Lithuania; darius.jegelevicius@ktu.lt
2. Department of Electronics Engineering, Kaunas University of Technology, 51367 Kaunas, Lithuania
3. JSC Telemed, 03154 Vilnius, Lithuania; sakalauskas.andrius@yahoo.com
4. Simonas Grybauskas' Orthognathic Surgery, 03229 Vilnius, Lithuania; simonas@drgrybauskas.com
* Correspondence: mantas.vaitiekunas@ktu.lt; Tel.: +370-626-63004
† These authors contributed equally to this work.

Received: 28 November 2019; Accepted: 20 December 2019; Published: 27 December 2019

Abstract: Due to technical aspects of Cone Beam Computed Tomography (CBCT), the automatic methods for bone segmentation are not widely used in the clinical practice of endodontics, orthodontics, oral and maxillofacial surgery. The aim of this study was to evaluate method's accuracy for bone segmentation in CBCT data sets. The sliding three dimensional (3D) window, histogram filter and Otsu's method were used to implement the automatic segmentation. The results of automatic segmentation were compared with the results of segmentation performed by an experienced oral and maxillofacial surgeon. Twenty patients and their forty CBCT data sets were used in this study (20 preoperative and 20 postoperative). Intraclass Correlation Coefficients (ICC) were calculated to prove the reliability of surgeon segmentations. ICC was 0.958 with 95% confidence interval [0.896 ... 0.983] in preoperative data sets and 0.931 with 95% confidence interval [0.836 ... 0.972] in postoperative data sets. Three basic metrics were used in order to evaluate the accuracy of the automatic method—Dice Similarity Coefficient (DSC), Root Mean Square (RMS), Average Distance Error (ADE) of surfaces mismatch and additional metric in order to evaluate computation time of segmentation was used. The mean value of preoperative DSC was 0.921, postoperative—0.911, the mean value of preoperative RMS was 0.559 mm, postoperative—0.647 mm, the ADE value of preoperative cases was 0.043 mm, postoperative—0.057 mm, the mean computational time to perform the segmentation was 46 s. The automatic method showed clinically acceptable accuracy results and thus can be used as a new tool for automatic bone segmentation in CBCT data. It can be applied in oral and maxillofacial surgery for performance of 3D Virtual Surgical Plan (VSP) or for postoperative follow-up.

Keywords: cone beam computed tomography; automatic segmentation; sliding window; 3D virtual surgical plan; Otsu's method

1. Introduction

Three dimensional (3D) segmentation of bones from Cone Beam Computed Tomography (CBCT) is very important for the orthodontics, endodontics, oral and maxillofacial surgeons. Accuracy of segmentation ensures a correct diagnosis, an accurate 3D Virtual Surgical Plan (VSP) and a successful postoperative follow-up of the patients with Cranio-maxillofacial (CMF) deformities [1,2]. Application of CBCT imaging modality in oral and maxillofacial surgery is increased due to its lower radiation dose and shorter acquisition time compared with the conventional multislice CT (MSCT). However, images of CBCT most often are noisier and have beam hardening artifacts.

Properties of CBCT also affect the ability to correctly display Hounsfield units (HU) of head tissues (immediately after surgery when edema of soft tissues is present) as opposed to traditional CT [3,4]. These disadvantages also influence image quality and accuracy of bone segmentation [5]. Due to these reasons, 3D VSP and evaluation of postoperative follow-up must be performed using segmentation by highly experienced experts. Such a procedure of bone segmentation becomes time-consuming [6].

Wang et al. published three studies dedicated to fully automatic bone segmentation using CBCT images [6–8]. In 2013 [6] and 2014 [7] studies, the principle of the automatic method was a patch-based sparse representation. Patient-specific atlas (probability map) using a sparse label fusion strategy from conventional CT atlases was used as a first estimation. Then a convex segmentation framework was used in order to get the final result. The introduced method led to an accurate segmentation but the basic limitation of this method was computation time (about 5 h [7]). Also, the variety of CBCT data sets (patients with metallic implants, metallic plates and different face deformities) was low in their studies. Data collection of CT to get more variety of the atlases is complicated in relation to the requirements of bioethics. In a 2016 study [8], the same authors also suggested a new automatic method that used the random forest. The multiclass classifier was used to create probability maps for each region of interest (mandible, maxilla and background). The results of the method were achieved almost the same as in the previous study [7] but also with some similar limitations: the limited amount of CBCT data and also computation time of segmentation (20 min). Gollmer and Buzug presented a fully automatic method for mandible segmentation. Segmentation was based on the idea of using a statistical shape model (SSM). They showed accurate results, however, they also—as did the previous authors—tested the algorithm with just six CBCT data sets [9]. Fan et al. [10] proposed an automatic method for mandible segmentation. Marker-based watershed transform method was used in their study. The authors performed accurate and fast enough (12-14 min per data set) segmentation on 20 CBCT data sets. The errors of segmentation were obtained mostly in these three basic areas—around the wisdom teeth, condyles and dental enamel. The reasons of segmentation errors were the different (bigger) or the same intensity of selected basic markers (mandible and background). Performance of manual editing in these areas was recommended. Eijnatten et al. [11] carried out a review of literature on different methods for bone segmentation. The authors discovered that global thresholding is the most used method for bone segmentation. However, a limitation of this method is that the manual post-processing is required.

This study presents a fully automatic 3D thresholding method which is based on local statistical information. In the previous pilot study [12], the automatic segmentation of ten CBCT data sets of preoperative patients was performed. We increased the amount and variety (postoperative cases) of data sets (n = 40) in the current study. Compared with the previous study, we included more anatomical areas of interest in order to better evaluate the accuracy of the presented method. Otsu's method [13], histogram filter and 3D sliding window [14] are used for the implementation of the segmentation method. The accuracy of the current method is evaluated using three metrics—Dice Similarity Coefficient (DSC) [15], Root Mean Square (RMS) [16,17], Average Distance Error (ADE). The computation time of the segmentation is also evaluated. The results of the automatic segmentation are compared with the segmentation results of an experienced oral and maxillofacial surgeon.

2. Materials and Methods

2.1. Data Acquisition

A retrospective study was performed by using 40 CBCT data sets from the database of the Simonas Grybauskas' Orthognathic Surgery clinic. Before the study, all CBCT data sets were anonymised in order to protect the patients' data. Half of them (n = 20) were preoperative (obtained one week before the surgery) and another half (n = 20) were postoperative (obtained about one week after surgery) scans of the same patients' group. All scans were done using the i-CAT FLX V17 machine. All patients undertook double jaws correction. CBCT data sets were acquired with a resolution of an isotropic voxel of 0.3 mm, 230 mm × 170 mm field of view (FOV), the time of exposure was 7 s, tube voltage 120 kV and tube current 5 mA. Preoperative and postoperative CBCT data sets were segmented by an experienced oral and maxillofacial surgeon using ITK-SNAP software (Version 3.4.0) selecting a global threshold value for each case individually. Mandible and lower parts of skull (including maxilla, zygomatic bone) were used to perform the segmentation. Therefore, mentioned anatomical regions were selected as the segmentation target assessing the importance of them to perform a surgery. The study framework is presented in Figure 1.

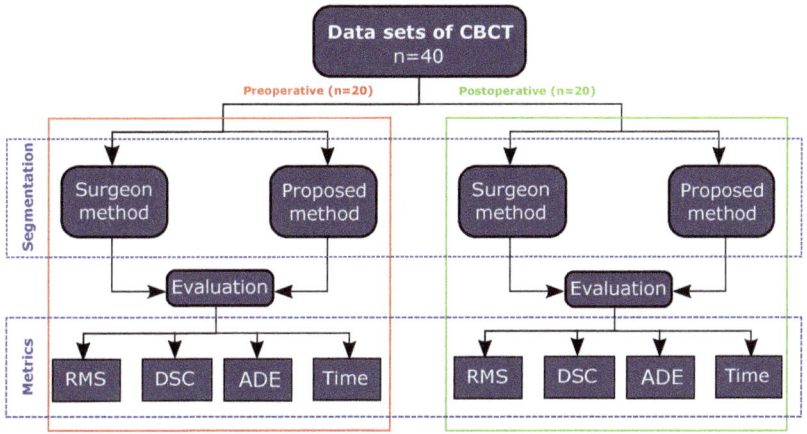

Figure 1. The framework of the current study. The study was performed using preoperative and postoperative Cone Beam Computed Tomography (CBCT) data sets. Four metrics (Root Mean Square (RMS), Dice Similarity Coefficient (DSC), Average Distance Error (ADE) and Time) were used to evaluate the proposed method.

2.2. Description of Proposed Method

The proposed method was based on the finding of an optimal threshold by using Otsu's method in a sliding 3D window. However, Otsu's method works most accurately when the analyzing histogram is bimodal. This means that the intensity values of voxels must be divided into two basic classes C_0 with intensity range $[1, \ldots, T]$ and C_1 with intensity range $[T + 1, \ldots, L]$ (where L is the upper limit of intensity in the volume), T representing the threshold optimally separating modes in bimodal histogram. The number of voxels with intensity threshold i is denoted by n_i. A probability of intensity threshold i in an image is

$$p_i = \frac{n_i}{N} \tag{1}$$

N—the total number of voxels. Then, the probabilities that a randomly selected voxels belong to one of the classes C_0 or C_1 are

$$C_0 : \omega_0(T) = \sum_{i=0}^{T} p_i \tag{2}$$

$$C_1 : \omega_1(T) = \sum_{i=T+1}^{L} p_i. \tag{3}$$

The average of classes is defined

$$C_0 : \mu_0 = \frac{\sum_{i=1}^{T} i \cdot p_i}{\omega_0(T)} \tag{4}$$

$$C_1 : \mu_1 = \frac{\sum\limits_{i=T+1}^{L} i \cdot p_i}{\omega_1(T)}. \tag{5}$$

The intensity average of the total image is defined by

$$\omega_0 \mu_0 + \omega_1 \mu_1 = \mu_T \tag{6}$$

$$\omega_0 + \omega_1 = 1. \tag{7}$$

Using discriminant analysis, Otsu's method defines both classes variance of the thresholded image

$$\sigma_B^2 = \omega_0(\mu_0 - \mu_T)^2 + \omega_1(\mu_1 - \mu_T)^2. \tag{8}$$

Then the optimal threshold value is calculated by

$$T^* = Arg \quad Max \quad \{\sigma_B^2(T)\} \tag{9}$$

$$1 \leq T < L. \tag{10}$$

The illustration of the proposed method is presented in Figure 2.

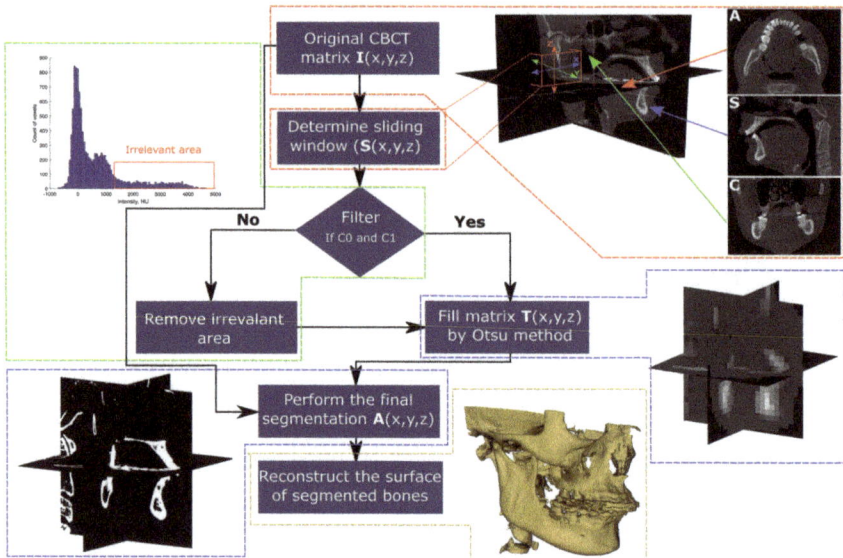

Figure 2. Implementation of segmentation by using the proposed automatic method.

The typical histogram of CBCT data set is not bimodal and Otsu's method does not work accurately in order to find optimal threshold value. The typical histogram of CBCT data set is presented in Figure 3.

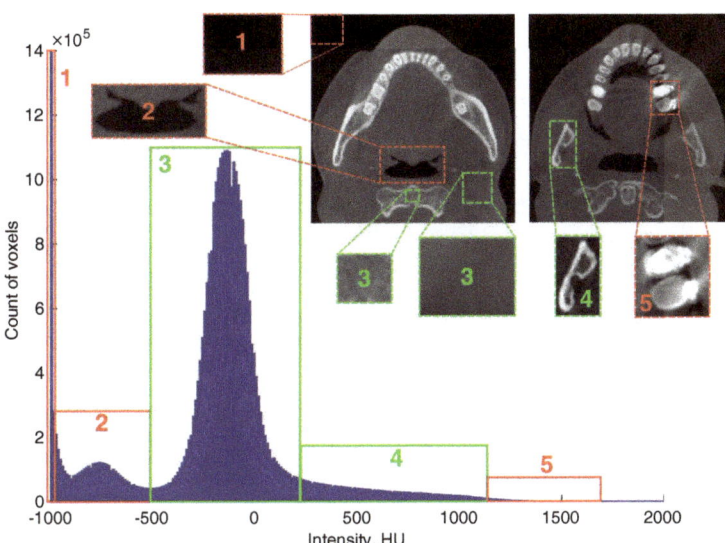

Figure 3. Typical histogram of CBCT data set. The basic areas: air (**1**), internal anatomical structures containing air (**2**), soft tissues/soft bone (**3**), bone (**4**) and metal artifacts/restorative materials (**5**).

In order to perform an accurate segmentation using Otsu's method, a histogram filter was involved. The purpose of the filter is to remove irrelevant areas and to make analysed histograms bimodal. The optimal threshold was found after filtration, that is, removal of the 1st, 2nd and 5th areas in the histogram (Figure 3). Intensity values for histogram filtering areas were defined by the results of studies published in References [18,19]. Misch et al. [18] determined that the intensity of cortical bone of mandible is 1250 HU and it cover about 8% of the volume of mandible, trabecular bone intensity of mandible is 850–1250 HU, 350–850 HU levels corresponds to trabecular bone intensity of maxilla, levels of 150–350 HU limit posterior maxilla and levels of 150 HU could be found in sinus areas where the bone is very soft. The study performed by Norton et al. [19] divided the intensity scale of bone into these ranges of HU: anterior mandible 850 HU, posterior mandible/anterior maxilla 500–850 HU, posterior maxilla 0–500 HU, tuberosity region 0 HU. Air intensity is −1000 HU and internal anatomical areas such as cavity of maxillary sinuses, nasal cavities, airways are between −950 HU and −500 HU. This analysis was used to set which areas of the histogram are useful for the segmentation and which areas should be filtered out. Then the filter was built to automatically remove areas in the sliding volume histogram with the intensities of more than 1250 HU and areas with the intensities less than −500 HU. An optimal threshold value using Otsu's method is found in the defined range [−500 HU ... 1250 HU]. The filter is involved before processing CBCT data set and it ensures that CBCT volumetric histogram is bimodal (Figure 4, C0—object, C1—background). Then the matrix of local thresholds ($T(x,y,z)$) is filled by the found T values and the final segmentation ($A(x,y,z)$) is performed by:

$$A(x,y,z) = \begin{cases} 0 \text{ if } I(x,y,z) < T(x,y,z) \\ 1 \text{ otherwise} \end{cases} \tag{11}$$

Here $A(x,y,z)$—3D final matrix of segmentation, $I(x,y,z)$—3D matrix of the original CBCT data set.

The local threshold value T is found in a volume of sliding window ($S(x,y,z)$), the segmentation object is the segment of bone (mandible and maxilla)—C0 and background is the segment of soft tissues (including soft bone)—C1 (Figure 4).

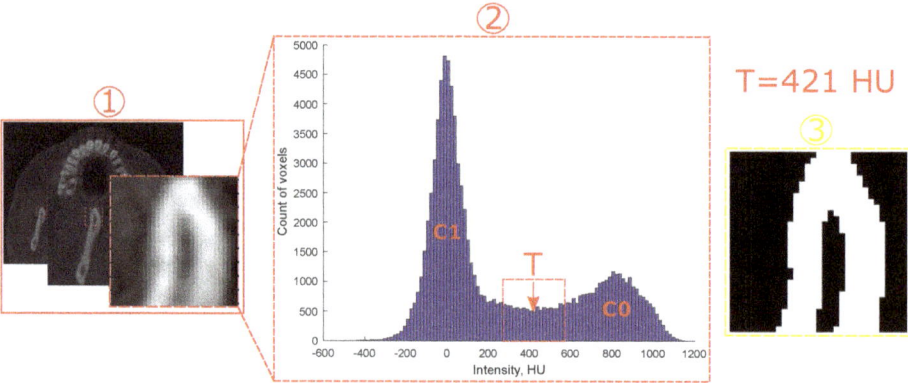

Figure 4. Analysing histogram (**2**) in selected sliding window volume (**1**) in order to find an optimal threshold **T** to segmented a bone (**3**).

2.3. Surface Reconstruction

Segmented bone ($A(x,y,z)$) is saved as a surface in the STereoLithography (STL) file format. The reconstruction of the bone surface from segmented voxels is performed by the volumetric reconstruction algorithm (Visualization and Computer Graphics (VCG) reconstruction filter) using MeshLab software (Visual Computing Lab of ISTI–CNR, University of Pisa) [20,21] (Figure 5).

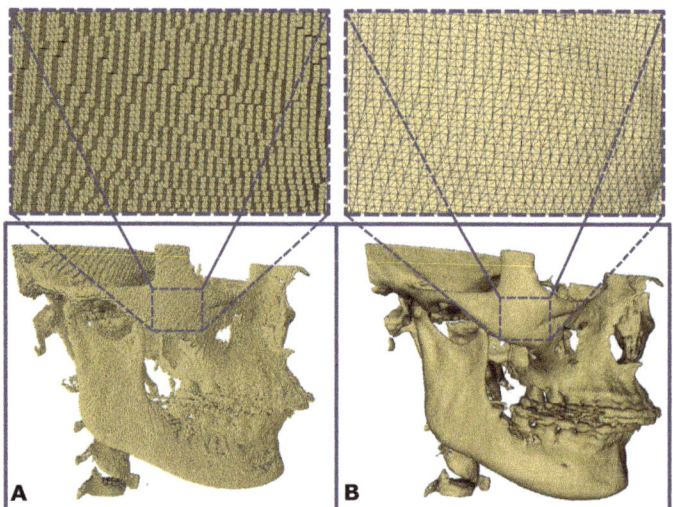

Figure 5. Reconstruction of segmented bone. (**A**) The surface of the bone after segmentation, (**B**) Reconstructed surface of the bone. At the top, are shown the small fragments of surfaces before and after reconstruction.

The basic parameters of the surface reconstruction ((1) voxel size, (2) the level of the subvolume reconstruction process, (3) geodesic weighting, number of Volume Laplacian iterations, (4) widening, (5) number of smoothing iterations) were used the same for all forty cases in order to have comparable results of reconstruction.

2.4. Evaluation of Method Accuracy

The results of the proposed algorithm were compared with the results of segmentation performed by an experienced surgeon. In order to evaluate the reliability of surgeon's segmentation, the segmentations were done twice with a 2 weeks interval. For the quantitative evaluation of the reliability, Intraclass Correlation Coefficient (ICC) by using a two-way mixed model, unit: single rater and the type of relationship: absolute agreement method [22] was calculated by:

$$ICC = \frac{MS_R - MS_E}{MS_R + (k-1)MS_E + \frac{k}{n}(MS_C - MS_E)}, \quad (12)$$

where MS_R = mean square for rows, k = number of raters/measurements; MS_E = mean square for error; MS_C = mean square for columns; n = number of subjects.

ICC was calculated separately for preoperative and postoperative cases and segmentation thresholds selected by the surgeon were used for this.

The evaluation of segmentation accuracy by using proposed method three basic metrics were used:

(1) Root mean square (RMS) of the intersurface distance used to evaluate reconstructed surface mismatch:

$$RMS = \frac{1}{\sqrt{n}} \cdot \sqrt{\sum_{x,y,z=1}^{n}(a_{x,y,z} - b_{x,y,z})^2}, \quad (13)$$

where $a_{x,y,z}$ represents the coordinates of reference surface point, $b_{x,y,z}$—the coordinates of surface point created with the proposed method;

(2) Dice similarity coefficient (DSC), used to evaluate volume discrepancy:

$$DSC = \frac{2|A \cap B|}{(|A| + |B|)}, \quad (14)$$

where A represents the volume of the reference model, B—volume of automatically segmented bone;

(3) Average intersurface distance error (ADE) was calculated by:

$$ADE = \frac{1}{N} \cdot \sum_{i=1}^{n}(a_{x,y,z} - b_{x,y,z}), \quad (15)$$

where $a_{x,y,z}$ represents the coordinates of 3D point of the reference model, $b_{x,y,z}$—the coordinates of 3D point of the automatically segmented model;

Positive and negative ADE values were calculated also.

Additional metric to evaluate the rapidity of segmentation the computation time of automatic segmentation was calculated. In this study, personal computer with parameters—processor—Intel(R) Core(TM) i7-4790 CPU @ 3.60 GHz, RAM—16 GB, system type—64-bit Windows 10 Operating System was used. The automatic method was implemented by using Matlab software.

3. Results

The reliability of segmentations performed by surgeon was evaluated by calculating ICC values for preoperative and postoperative CBCT data sets (Table 1).

Table 1. Results of Intraclass Correlation Coefficient (ICC) using single rater, absolute agreement and 2-way random effects model.

	Itraclass Correlation	95% Confidence Interval		F Test with True Value 0			
		Lower Bound	Upper Bound	Value	df1	df2	Sig
Single measures preoperative	0.958	0.896	0.983	49.03	19	19	0.000
Single measures postoperative	0.931	0.836	0.972	27.43	19	19	0.000

The results show that in preoperative data ICC = 0.958 with 95% confidence interval [0.896 ... 0.983] and in postoperative data ICC = 0.931 with 95% confidence interval [0.836 ... 0.972]. Calculated values of ICC show that the level of surgeon reliability is sufficient [22].

(1) The mean RMS value of intersurface distance in preoperative cases was 0.559 mm and in postoperative—0.647 mm. Calculated RMS values of intersurface distance for all cases are presented by a boxplot in Figure 6.

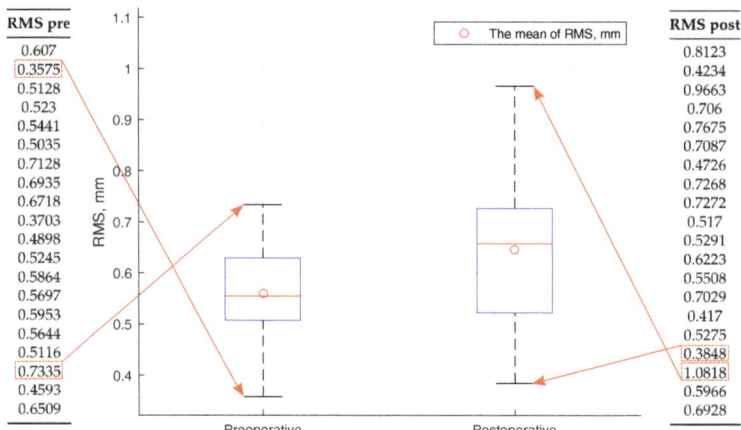

Figure 6. Distributions of RMS values of preoperative and postoperative segmentation data.

The interquartile range of boxplot is narrower for preoperative RMS values. The bigger distribution of RMS values is seen in postoperative cases. This could have been caused by a better quality of preoperative CBCT data sets.

(2) The mean value of DSC was 0.921 in preoperative cases. In postoperative cases, the mean value of DSC was 0.911. Calculated DSC values are similar and are very high—more than 0.9. The results of DSC in preoperative and postoperative segmentation data are presented by using the boxplot function in Figure 7.

The narrower range of interquartile is found in postoperative cases. Two DSC values are out of the DSC range in postoperative cases and are marked as outliers.

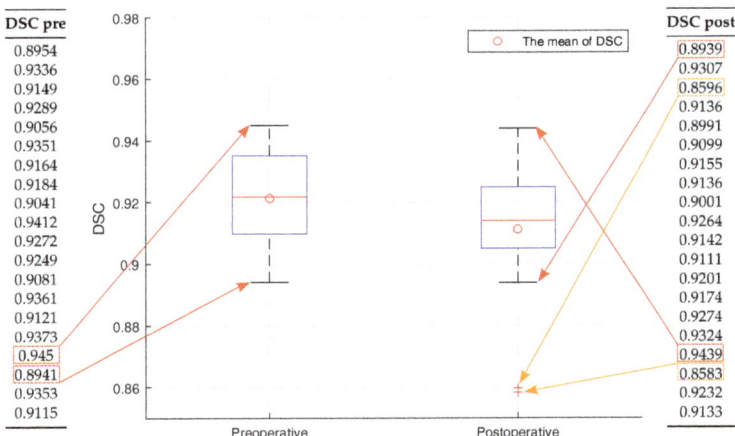

Figure 7. Distribution of DSC values of preoperative and postoperative segmentation data.

(3) The ADE values were calculated and divided into three groups: general average, positive average and negative average. The whole results are presented in Table 2.

The mean value of computational time to perform an automatic segmentation by using all CBCT data sets was 46 s. Compared with other studies, this computation time is very fast. The achieved results are compared with the results of other similar studies. The comparison is presented in Table 2.

Table 2. The comparison of different automatic methods by 4 metrics.

Metric	Wang et al. [6]	Wang et al. [7]	Wang et al. [8]	Fan et al. [10]	Proposed
RMS, mm	-	-	-	-	0.559 [a] | 0.647 [b]
DSC	0.91 [c] | 0.87 [d]	0.92 [c] | 0.87 [d]	0.94 [c] | 0.91 [d]	0.97	0.921 [a] | 0.911 [b]
ADE, mm	0.61	0.65	0.42	-	0.043 [1a] | 0.279 [2a] | −0.242 [3a] 0.057 [1b] | 0.293 [2b] | −0.282 [3b]
Time, s	-	18,000	1200	720–840	45 [a] | 47 [b]

a—preoperative, b —postoperative, c—region of interest maxilla, c—region of interest mandible, 1—average distance error, 2—possitive average distance error, 3—negative average distance error.

DSC is the most popular metric in order to prove the accuracy of segmentation. Achieved values of DSC were similar in comparison with other studies (values were near 0.9). ADE also is a frequent metric in order to evaluate the segmentation. In our study, ADE was calculated and divided into three groups. The results between ADE values in different groups (preoperative and postoperative) were compared. It was found that differences were similar (Table 2). In comparison with the other studies, in which the proposed method was used, ADE values were found lower. The proposed method showed a short computation time to an automatic segmentation performance. The comparison of segmentation results by using automatic and surgeon methods are shown in Figure 8.

The results of segmentation by using the proposed method showed that bones with low density were not fully segmented. However, areas of condyles and sinuses were segmented with fewer holes by using the proposed method, compared to the surgeon segmentation results (Figure 8).

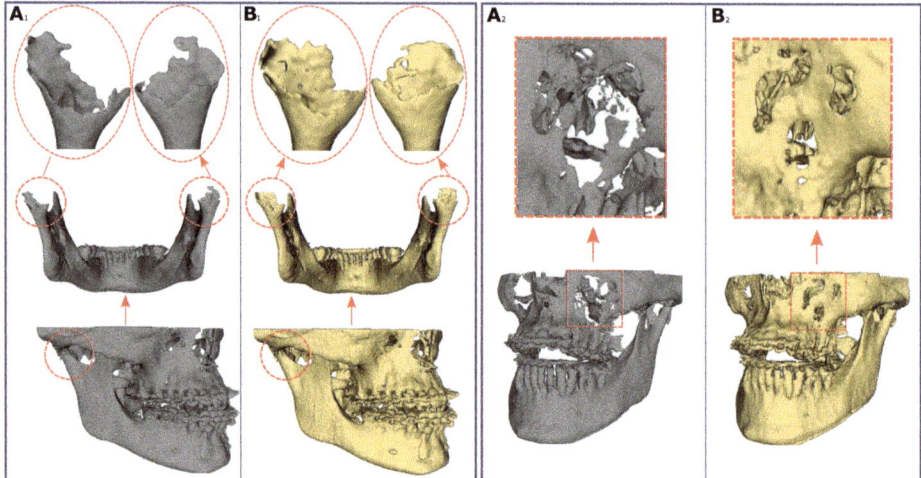

Figure 8. Evaluation of two random selected 3D models using different segmentation methods. (**A**) represents 3D models segmented using a global threshold method by the surgeon, (**B**)—segmented with proposed method (region of interest: **1**–condyles, **2**–sinuses).

4. Discussion

Automatic methods for bone segmentation are very important in order to get 3D surfaces. It helps surgeons in making correct diagnoses, in performing accurate and quicker VSP and in the evaluation of postoperative follow-up without the influence of surgeon's experience [23–27]. The aim of this study was to evaluate method's accuracy for bone segmentation in CBCT data sets. The method is based on the histogram filter, 3D sliding window and Otsu's thresholding. The results of automatic segmentation revealed sufficient accuracy of bone segmentation. For the evaluation of method accuracy, three kind of metrics were used: voxel-based–DSC [15,17,28], based on the intersurface distance evaluation–RMS and ADE [16,17]. Additional metric based on the time to perform segmentation–computation time was calculated. The mean DSC coefficient values of two groups (preoperative and postoperative) were bigger than 0.9, which proved the complete overlap and high accuracy of the automatic and surgeon segmented bone voxels. The mean RMS values of intersurface distance for preoperative (0.559 mm) and postoperative (0.647 mm) cases were about two times bigger than the voxel size (0.3 mm). Calculated ADE values showed small discrepancies of surfaces. It shows that segmentation result is good, either we succeeded to avoid superimposition step because both automatic and global segmentations were made by using the same source data sets. In this way, surface superimposition did not yield any additional errors. Compared with the other studies [7,8,10], the proposed method performed the segmentation very rapidly (46 s/case). The achieved results showed that the proposed automatic method worked accurately.

However, the proposed method had some limitations. CBCT images were not filtered for metal artefacts (brackets, metal plates and mini-implants) before or after segmentation. Due to this reason, metal artefacts were seen in 3D models. These artefacts hide important areas of bone. Therefore, assessment of the bone near these artefacts became complicated and inaccurate. Especially it is important when postoperative follow-ups are performed [29,30]. The other limitation of the proposed method is the difficulty to segment areas with low density (thin anatomical areas, e.g., alveolar part of the mandible, mandibular condyles or areas of maxillary sinuses) in CBCT images [31]. This is also valid for other threshold-based segmentation methods. Problematic areas could be segmented including more sensitive techniques [31–34].

Further studies may be concentrated to evaluate proposed method with higher amount and different kind of CT/CBCT data sets. The next direction of further study may be to increase accuracy of the segmentation for anatomical areas with low density. Fully automatic segmentation of selected anatomical areas especially condyles would be important tool to increase the evaluation of treatment or postoperative follow-up [35,36].

5. Conclusions

The presented study proposed a new automatic method for bone segmentation in a CBCT data set. The important feature of the proposed segmentation method is simple and rapid implementation. The results of segmentation were very accurate and reliable to use in the clinical practice of oral and maxillofacial surgery. The method does not require access to a computer with high computation power parameters. It can be integrated into the most popular software of 3D medical imaging processing using an ordinary computer.

Author Contributions: All authors contributed equally to this work. All authors have read and agreed to the published version of the manuscript

Funding: This research received no external funding.

Conflicts of Interest: The authors declare no conflict of interest.

Abbreviations

The following abbreviations are used in this manuscript:

CBCT	Cone Beam Computed Tomography
3D	Three dimensional
VSP	Virtual Surgical Plan
RMS	Root Mean Square
DSC	Dice Similarity Coefficient
ADE	Average Distance Error

References

1. Deeb, G.; Antonos, L.; Tack, S.; Carrico, C.; Laskin, D.; Deeb, J.G. Is Cone-Beam Computed Tomography Always Necessary for Dental Implant Placement? *J. Oral Maxillofac. Surg.* **2017**, *75*, 285–289. [CrossRef]
2. Fourie, Z.; Damstra, J.; Schepers, R.H.; Gerrits, P.O.; Ren, Y. Segmentation process significantly influences the accuracy of 3D surface models derived from cone beam computed tomography. *Eur. J. Radiol.* **2012**, *81*, 524–530. [CrossRef]
3. Pauwels, R.; Jacobs, R.; Singer, S.R.; Mupparapu, M. CBCT-based bone quality assessment: Are Hounsfield units applicable? *Dentomaxillofac. Radio* **2015**, *44*, 20140238. [CrossRef]
4. Pauwels, R.; Nackaerts, O.; Bellaiche, N.; Stamatakis, H.; Tsiklakis, K.; Walker, A.; Bosmans, H.; Bogaerts, R.; Jacobs, R.; Horner, K. Variability of dental cone beam CT grey values for density estimations. *Br. J. Radiol.* **2013**, *86*, 20120135. [CrossRef]
5. Katsumata, A.; Hirukawa, A.; Noujeim, M.; Okumura, S.; Naitoh, M.; Fujishita, M.; Ariji, E.; Langlais, R.P. Image artifact in dental cone-beam CT. *Oral. Surg. Oral Med. Oral Pathol. Oral Radiol. Endod.* **2006**, *101*, 652–657. [CrossRef]
6. Wang, L.; Chen, K.C.; Shi, F.; Liao, S.; Li, G.; Gao, Y.; Shen, S.G.; Yan, J.; Lee, P.K.; Chow, B.; et al. Automated segmentation of CBCT image using spiral CT atlases and convex optimization. *Med. Image Comput. Comput. Assist. Interv.* **2013**, *16*, 251–258.
7. Wang, L.; Chen, K.C.; Gao, Y.; Shi, F.; Liao, S.; Li, G.; Shen, S.G.; Yan, J.; Lee, P.K.; Chow, B.; et al. Automated bone segmentation from dental CBCT images using patch-based sparse representation and convex optimization. *Med. Phys.* **2014**, *41*, 043503. [CrossRef] [PubMed]
8. Wang, L.; Gao, Y.; Shi, F.; Li, G.; Chen, K.C.; Tang, Z.; Xia, J.J.; Shen, D. Automated segmentation of dental CBCT image with prior-guided sequential random forests. *Med. Phys.* **2016**, *43*, 336–346. [CrossRef] [PubMed]

9. Gollmer, S.T.; Buzug, T.M. Fully automatic shape constrained mandible segmentation from cone-beam CT data. In Proceedings of the 9th IEEE International Symposium on Biomedical Imaging (ISBI), Barcelona, Spain, 2–5 May 2012; pp. 1272–1275.
10. Fan, Y.; Beare, R.; Matthews, H.; Schneider, P.; Kilpatrick, N.; Clement, J.; Claes, P.; Penington, A.; Adamson, C. Marker-based watershed transform method for fully automatic mandibular segmentation from cBct images. *Dentomaxillofac. Radiol.* **2019**, *48*, 20180261. [CrossRef] [PubMed]
11. van Eijnatten, M.; van Dijk, R.; Dobbe, J.; Streekstra, G.; Koivisto, J.; Wolff, J. CT image segmentation methods for bone used in medical additive manufacturing. *Med. Eng. Phys.* **2018**, *51*, 6–16. [CrossRef]
12. Vaitiekunas, M.; Jegelevicius, D.; Sakalauskas, A.; Grybauskas, S. Method for automatic 3D bone segmentation in CBCT data. In Proceedings of the Joint Conference of the European Medical and Biological Engineering Conference (EMBEC) and the Nordic-Baltic Conference on Biomedical Engineering and Medical Physics (NBC), Tampere, Finland, 11–15 June 2017; pp. 1–4.
13. Otsu, N. A Threshold Selection Method from Gray-Level Histograms. *IEEE Trans. Syst. Man Cybern.* **1979**, *9*, 62–66. [CrossRef]
14. Yang, P.; Clapworthy, G.; Dong, F.; Codreanu, V.; Williams, D.; Liu, B.; Roerdink, J.B.; Deng, Z. GSWO: A programming model for GPU-enabled parallelization of sliding window operations in image processing. *Signal Process. Image Commun.* **2016**, *47*, 332–345. [CrossRef]
15. Dice, L.R. Measures of the Amount of Ecologic Association Between Species. *Ecology* **1945**, *26*, 297–302. [CrossRef]
16. Park, G.H.; Son, K.B.D.; Lee, K.B. Feasibility of using an intraoral scanner for a complete-arch digital scan. *J. Prosthet. Dent.* **2019**, *121*, 803–810. [CrossRef] [PubMed]
17. Hosseini, M.P.; Nazem-Zadeh, M.R.; Pompili, D.; Jafari-Khouzani, K.; Elisevich, K.; Soltanian-Zadeh, H. Comparative performance evaluation of automated segmentation methods of hippocampus from magnetic resonance images of temporal lobe epilepsy patients. *Med. Phys.* **2016**, *43*, 538–553. [CrossRef]
18. Misch, C.E. Density of bone: effect on treatment plans, surgical approach, healing, and progressive boen loading. *Int. J. Oral Implantol.* **1990**, *6*, 23–31.
19. Norton, M.R.; Gamble, C. Bone classification: an objective scale of bone density using the computerized tomography scan. *Clin. Oral Implants Res.* **2001**, *12*, 79–84. [CrossRef]
20. Meshlab Software. Available online: www.meshlab.net (accessed on 5 May 2019).
21. Curless, B.; Levoy, M. A volumetric method for building complex models from range images. In Proceedings of the 23rd Annual Conference on Computer Graphics and Interactive Techniques—SIGGRAPH '96, New York, NY, USA, 11–15 June 1996; pp. 303–312.
22. Koo, T.K.; Li, M.Y. A Guideline of Selecting and Reporting Intraclass Correlation Coefficients for Reliability Research. *J. Chiropr. Med.* **2016**, *15*, 155–163. [CrossRef]
23. Wallner, J.; Hochegger, K.; Chen, X.; Mischak, I.; Reinbacher, K.; Pau, M.; Zrnc, T.; Schwenzer-Zimmerer, K.; Zemann, W.; Schmalstieg, D.; et al. Clinical evaluation of semi-automatic open-source algorithmic software segmentation of the mandibular bone: Practical feasibility and assessment of a new course of action. *PLoS ONE* **2018**, *13*, e0196378. [CrossRef]
24. Lebre, M.A.; Vacavant, A.; Grand-Brochier, M.; Rositi, H.; Abergel, A.; Chabrot, P.; Magnin, B. Automatic segmentation methods for liver and hepatic vessels from CT and MRI volumes, applied to the Couinaud scheme. *Comput. Biol. Med.* **2019**, *110*, 42–51. [CrossRef]
25. Sakinis, T.; Milletari, F.; Roth, H.; Korfiatis, P.; Kostandy, P.; Philbrick, K.; Akkus, Z.; Xu, Z.; Xu, D.; Erickson, B.J. Interactive segmentation of medical images through fully convolutional neural networks. *arXiv* **2019**, arXiv:1903.08205.
26. Fripp, J.; Crozier, S.; Warfield, S.K.; Ourselin, S. Automatic segmentation of the bone and extraction of the bone-cartilage interface from magnetic resonance images of the knee. *Phys. Med. Biol.* **2007**, *52*, 1617–1631. [CrossRef] [PubMed]
27. Indraswari, R.; Arifin, A.Z.; Suciati, N.; Astuti, E.R.; Kurita, T. Automatic segmentation of mandibular cortical bone on cone-beam CT images based on histogram thresholding and polynomial fitting. *Int. J. Intell. Eng. Syst.* **2019**, *12*, 130–141. [CrossRef]
28. Taha, A.A.; Hanbury, A. Metrics for evaluating 3D medical image segmentation: Analysis, selection, and tool. *BMC Med. Imaging* **2015**, *15*, 29. [CrossRef] [PubMed]

29. Shokri, A.; Jamalpour, M.R.; Khavid, A.; Mohseni, Z.; Sadeghi, M. Effect of exposure parameters of cone beam computed tomography on metal artifact reduction around the dental implants in various bone densities. *BMC Med. Imaging* **2019**, *19*, 34. [CrossRef]
30. Scarfe, W.C.; Farman, A.G.; Sukovic, P. Clinical applications of cone-beam computed tomography in dental practice. *J. Can. Dent. Assoc.* **2006**, *72*, 75–80.
31. Chang, Y.B.; Xia, J.J.; Yuan, P.; Kuo, T.H.; Xiong, Z.; Gateno, J.; Zhou, X. 3D segmentation of maxilla in cone-beam computed tomography imaging using base invariant wavelet active shape model on customized two-manifold topology. *J. Xray Sci. Technol.* **2013**, *21*, 251–282. [CrossRef]
32. Xi, T.; Schreurs, R.; Heerink, W.J.; Bergé, S.J.; Maal, T.J. A novel region-growing based semi-automatic segmentation protocol for three-dimensional condylar reconstruction using cone beam computed tomography (CBCT). *PLoS ONE* **2014**, *9*, e111126. [CrossRef]
33. Descoteaux, M.; Audette, M.; Chinzei, K.; Siddiqi, K. Bone enhancement filtering: application to sinus bone segmentation and simulation of pituitary surgery. *Comput. Aided Surg.* **2006**, *11*, 247–255. [CrossRef]
34. Chuang, Y.J.; Doherty, B.M.; Adluru, N.; Chung, M.K.; Vorperian, H.K. A Novel Registration-Based Semiautomatic Mandible Segmentation Pipeline Using Computed Tomography Images to Study Mandibular Development. *J. Comput. Assist. Tomogr.* **2018**, *42*, 306–316. [CrossRef]
35. Engelbrecht, W.P.; Fourie, Z.; Damstra, J.; Gerrits, P.O.; Ren, Y. The influence of the segmentation process on 3D measurements from cone beam computed tomography-derived surface models. *Clin. Oral Investig.* **2013**, *17*, 1919–1927. [CrossRef] [PubMed]
36. Nicolielo, L.F.P.; Van Dessel, J.; Shaheen, E.; Letelier, C.; Codari, M.; Politis, C.; Lambrichts, I.; Jacobs, R. Validation of a novel imaging approach using multi-slice CT and cone-beam CT to follow-up on condylar remodeling after bimaxillary surgery. *Int. J. Oral Sci.* **2017**, *9*, 139–144. [CrossRef] [PubMed]

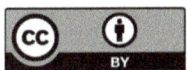

© 2019 by the authors. Licensee MDPI, Basel, Switzerland. This article is an open access article distributed under the terms and conditions of the Creative Commons Attribution (CC BY) license (http://creativecommons.org/licenses/by/4.0/).

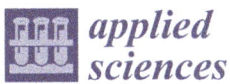

Article

Establishment of a Numerical Model to Design an Electro-Stimulating System for a Porcine Mandibular Critical Size Defect

Hendrikje Raben [1,*], Peer W. Kämmerer [2], Rainer Bader [3,4] and Ursula van Rienen [1,4]

1. Institute of General Electrical Engineering, University of Rostock, 18051 Rostock, Germany; ursula.van-rienen@uni-rostock.de
2. Department of Oral and Maxillofacial Surgery, University Medical Centre Mainz, 55131 Mainz, Germany; peer.kaemmerer@unimedizin-mainz.de
3. Department of Orthopaedics, University Medical Center Rostock, 18057 Rostock, Germany; rainer.bader@med.uni-rostock.de
4. Department Life, Light & Matter, University of Rostock, 18051 Rostock, Germany
* Correspondence: hendrikje.raben@uni-rostock.de

Received: 15 April 2019; Accepted: 18 May 2019; Published: 27 May 2019

Abstract: Electrical stimulation is a promising therapeutic approach for the regeneration of large bone defects. Innovative electrically stimulating implants for critical size defects in the lower jaw are under development and need to be optimized in silico and tested in vivo prior to application. In this context, numerical modelling and simulation are useful tools in the design process. In this study, a numerical model of an electrically stimulated minipig mandible was established to find optimal stimulation parameters that allow for a maximum area of beneficially stimulated tissue. Finite-element simulations were performed to determine the stimulation impact of the proposed implant design and to optimize the electric field distribution resulting from sinusoidal low-frequency ($f = 20\,\text{Hz}$) electric stimulation. Optimal stimulation parameters of the electrode length $h_{\text{el}} = 25$ mm and the stimulation potential $\varphi_{\text{stim}} = 0.5$ V were determined. These parameter sets shall be applied in future in vivo validation studies. Furthermore, our results suggest that changing tissue properties during the course of the healing process might make a feedback-controlled stimulation system necessary.

Keywords: finite-element simulation; electric stimulation; bone regeneration; computational modelling; electrically active implants; bioelectromagnetism; critical size defect; maxillofacial; minipig

1. Introduction

Electrical stimulation of bone has received a lot of attention in recent decades. It can be employed to improve bone healing in the case of fractures [1–5], non-unions [6,7], or other bone defects [8–10] such as those resulting after tumor resection. A further benefit could be stimulation of osseous healing capacities especially in compromised situations such as irradiated sites or patients with systemic intake of antiresorptive drugs [11,12]. The reason for the therapeutic effect of electrical stimulation is seen in the imitation of the electric fields that occur naturally in bone as a bioelectric tissue. The bioelectricity of bone has been an object of study for a long time. One example is in long bones showing the accumulation of charges when exposed to mechanical stress or strain: On the concave side negative charges accumulate and bone formation can be observed, whereas positive charges and bone resorption occur on the convex side [13]. These effects are attributed to streaming potentials [14–16] and piezoelectricity [17–19]. Also, some studies hypothesize strong interdependencies between both phenomena [20,21].

Taking advantage of bone's bioelectric properties, electrical stimulation for bone regeneration was attempted as early as in the 1950s with Yasuda [22] as the "pioneer" in the field of bone bioelectricity and stimulation. Since then, accelerated bone regeneration due to electrical stimulation has been widely investigated in numerous in vitro, in vivo, in silico, and clinical studies [23,24].

The naturally occurring electric fields in loaded bone contribute to a complicated signaling network involved in bone modelling and remodeling that has not yet been fully understood. However, cell experiments showed that stimulation of osteoblasts with low-frequency electromagnetic fields induces enhanced collagen synthesis [25]. Brighton et al. observed significantly enhanced DNA production following electric stimulation of bone cells [26]. Further in vitro studies could prove effects of electric stimulation on processes such as proliferation, differentiation, and migration of bone mesenchymal stem cells [27] and osteoblasts [28].

There are many ways of applying certain types of stimulating signals, for example constant, pulsed or alternating currents or fields (electric, magnetic, electromagnetic). These signals may be coupled to the tissue directly, capacitively, or inductively [29,30]. The diverse stimulation parameters applied in different studies are mainly used empirically or phenomenologically. This is because the complex physiological processes of bone remodeling are still not fully decoded. In clinical practice, low-frequency stimulation with sinusoidal electromagnetic fields between 5 and 70 V/m at $f = 20\,\text{Hz}$ empirically led to improved healing results [31]. Consequently, it is assumed that electric field strengths above 70 V/m might lead to harmful tissue damage due to overstimulation, whereas field strength below 5 V/m would show no supportive effect on bone regeneration. The method established by Kraus and Lechner [31] has been further developed. Mittelmeier et al. proposed the "bipolar induction screw system" (BISS) [32] that became an established method and that has been applied mainly to patients with loosened hip endoprostheses or femoral head necrosis. These findings were also supported by recent in vitro studies: Cell experiments applying an AC sinusoidal signal ($f = 20\,\text{Hz}$) on human osteoblasts showed voltage-dependent enhanced differentiation of the cells [33]. Using the BISS system, electromagnetic fields in combination with additional alternating electric fields at 20 Hz and 700 mV potential difference between the electrodes of the screw showed a positive impact on bone cell viability and differentiation [34].

As for the development of electro-stimulating implants for bone regeneration, numerical simulation is a useful tool in the design process. It allows testing of possible stimulation setups and the exclusion of unfeasible designs already at an early stage. In this context, electro-stimulating implants for a hip revision system were developed and numerically optimized [35–38]. Furthermore, electrically stimulating dental implants were designed and examined in vivo [39] and in silico [40].

However, large bone voids such as critical size defects in the mandible (lower jaw) have not been considered so far. Such defects extend over several centimeters and thus do not heal spontaneously without plastic reconstruction. Critical size defects occur mainly after partial resection of the mandible due to tumors, and are of great clinical relevance with over 3100 surgeries per year in Germany alone [41]. These defects are conventionally treated with a combination of bone replacement material and an osteosynthesis plate to keep the material in position with the help of screws. Unfortunately, this approach is frequently accompanied with complications that may make a revision surgery necessary. These complications include fracture of the plate, loosening of the fixation screws, or dehiscence [42–44]. To avoid such a second surgery with its additional risks for the patient, our aim is to use electrical stimulation as an approach to achieve faster bone healing and better fixation of bone and implant.

Although we already proposed preliminary numerical models of an electrically stimulated human mandible [45,46], the current work for the first time examines an electrical stimulation system for the regeneration of critical size defects in mandibular bone suitable for practical application in validation experiments. Specifically, in the current study we focus on a numerical model of a porcine, i.e., minipig mandible. This was chosen because of planned in vivo experiments with minipigs that will follow this numerical study. Compared to the human mandible, minipigs provide a similar geometry of the lower jaw. For the minipig mandible, a critical size defect is stated to be 2 cm [47].

The aim of the present study is to develop and numerically examine electro-stimulating devices that directly stimulate the tissue in the defect region. In this way, no external primary coil—in contrast to the BISS method [28,32]—is necessary. This would increase the patient's comfort and ensure patient compliance. In this context, this work introduces the procedure to numerically simulate and optimize an electro-stimulating device for a critical size defect in the lower jaw of a minipig. The conducted finite-element simulation studies constitute an important first step in preparation for in vivo experiments. These experiments will be described in the future.

In our current study, we hypothesize that the proposed design of a bipolar electro-stimulating device allows for a suitable region of beneficially stimulated tissue in the lower jaw of a minipig with a critical size defect. To support this hypothesis, the stimulation impact is estimated with the help of a finite-element simulation model. In addition, we assume that the resulting numerical model enables us to determine optimal stimulation parameters such as electrode length and stimulation potential for a given stimulation frequency of $f = 20\,\text{Hz}$ to achieve a maximum beneficially stimulated area. To optimize the electro-stimulating implant with respect to best possible electric field distribution within the defect region, the finite-element method was used. Prior to simulation, a 3D model of a minipig mandible with a critical size defect, surrounding soft tissue, and an electro-stimulating implant was created. The implant parameters, i.e., the length of the electrodes and the applied voltage were optimized. In addition, we assessed the impact of varying the electric conductivity assigned to the defect and concluded important requirements for the application and further development of future electro-stimulating implants.

2. Materials and Methods

Here, we introduce the steps that need to be performed to establish a bioelectric numerical model of electrically stimulated biological tissue. These steps include

- setting up the anatomical and technical model, i.e., segmenting computer tomographic (CT) data and computer-aided design (CAD) modelling based on the segmentation.
- setting up the physical model, i.e., the anatomical and technical models are assigned their dielectric properties.
- setting up the corresponding boundary value problem, i.e., the needed equations for simulating the electric field distribution.
- solving the boundary value problem.

The 3D models and the simulation models created in this study are available at [48]. For the Materialise 3-matic project files (Materialise, Leuven, Belgium. http://www.materialise.com) and the COMSOL Multiphysics® (COMSOL Inc., Stockholm, Sweden. https://www.comsol.com/) models the corresponding licenses are needed. Please note that the CT data and segmentation project files are excluded from public availability.

We would like to emphasize here that all modelling steps have been undertaken with respect to the planned in vivo experiments.

2.1. Anatomical and Technical Model Generation

The geometrical model that is subject to the finite-element studies is shown in Figure 1b and was built up from the results of two modelling steps: firstly the anatomical modelling, i.e., creating the model of the defective minipig mandible and its surrounding tissue; secondly, the technical modelling, where technical components such as the electro-stimulating implant or osteosynthesis plates and screws are created.

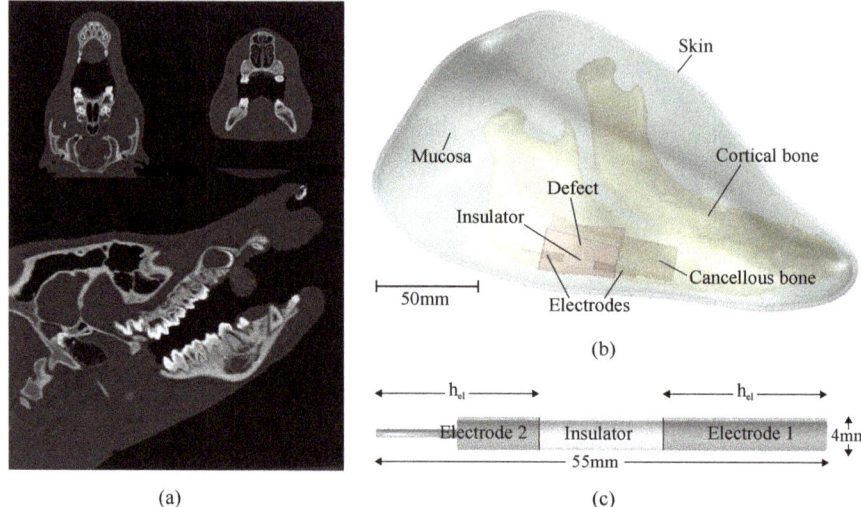

Figure 1. (**a**) Computer tomographic pictures of the head of a minipig. To reduce unnecessary computational costs in the later simulations the upper part of the head has been removed in the modelling process. (**b**) CAD model of a defective minipig mandible and its surrounding tissues, equipped with an electro-stimulating implant. The critical size defect (region of interest) is highlighted in red. (**c**) Bipolar electro-stimulating implant consisting of stimulating electrode ("Electrode 1"), insulator and counter-electrode ("Electrode 2"). The parameters h_{el} and φ_{stim} are to be optimized.

The anatomical modelling of the regarded model object, i.e., the minipig mandible, was done based on CT data of a 17-month-old male Göttingen minipig, see Figure 1a. The CT data comprised 442 slices with 512 × 512 pixels each and a pixel spacing of ca. 0.39 mm. The slice thickness was 1 mm and the spacing between the slices was 0.5 mm. By segmenting the data, i.e., assigning certain thresholds of gray values to the respective biological tissue (cortical bone, teeth, and soft tissue) a first rough anatomical model was created. For this, we used the image processing software Materialise Mimics® version 19 (Materialise, Leuven, Belgium. http://www.materialise.com).

One part of the anatomical model is the mandible (cortical bone) from which the teeth were subtracted. This was done to avoid unnecessary small details in the geometry that might lead to problems during the simulation. This is valid since the field amplitude can be easily estimated to be well below the stimulation threshold in the neighborhood of the teeth. The resulting coarse anatomical model (stereolithography (STL) file) was imported into the CAD software Materialise 3-matic® version 11 (Materialise, Leuven, Belgium. http://www.materialise.com) to be further processed. The modifications included manually filling larger holes in the geometry object that resulted from subtracting the teeth, wrapping (i.e., automatically filling smaller holes and creating a "watertight" model), smoothing of the surface, and removing other geometrical artefacts such as spikes, double or intersecting triangles, and sharp triangles. The latter modifications were performed automatically using 3-matic's "Fix Wizard". In addition, manually performed local smoothing of the surface ensured removal of further unwanted and unrealistic geometric features (little bumps and unevenness of the surface). Finally, the number of triangles describing the STL object were reduced, while preserving the mesh quality.

The soft tissue domain was created analogously: Firstly, the coarse STL file resulting after segmentation was imported into Materialise 3-matic® and the ears and the upper part of the minipig head were removed. Again, here the fields can be assessed to be negligible with respect to the stimulation threshold. Secondly, wrapping, smoothing, and repairing analogously to the bone geometry was performed. To create a skin domain, the *hollow* operation was used to create a shell with a uniform thickness of 2.28 mm [49]. Soft tissue and skin object were uniformly remeshed with a desired edge length of 3 mm. After importing the bone geometry, all domains, i.e., bone, soft tissue, and skin, were then combined into one final model object by creating a non-manifold assembly.

Due to the limited CT scan resolution, the cancellous bone region was not modelled based on segmentation. Instead, we modelled it as a generically shaped object (see Figure 1b) directly inside the geometry preprocessor of the simulation software COMSOL Multiphysics® version 5.3a (COMSOL; COMSOL Inc., Stockholm, Sweden. https://www.comsol.com). Apart from that, the cancellous bone layer was neglected in bone parts far away from the so-called region of interest (ROI). The ROI is defined as the volume inside the defect domain, highlighted in red in Figure 1b.

Due to technical reasons, the geometry file of the anatomical model (consisting of the mandible and the surrounding soft tissue) and the cancellous bone firstly had to be imported into COMSOL, secondly exported as a COMSOL-internal geometry file type *.mphbin*, and could only then be reimported and further modified inside the simulation software. The critical size defect in the angular region of the mandible, measuring 35 mm in width and ca. 20 mm in height, was modelled within COMSOL by subtracting a cuboid from the cortical bone geometry. The defect is supposed to be filled with cancellous bone from another part of the body and will be equipped with growth factors in the in vivo experiment. Finally, so-called virtual operations were used to simplify the topological structure of the geometry, namely forming composite domains and composite faces. This allows for an easier and more regular finite-element mesh generation.

In the current study, the technical modelling of the implant design and positioning was performed directly in the geometry module of COMSOL. The technical model only comprises the electro-stimulating implant, whereas a reconstruction plate is not modelled geometrically to reduce the problem size. Instead, a boundary condition (see Section 2.4) mimics the stabilizing Ti6Al4V mesh tray around the defect domain that is supposed to hold the filling material in place. It will be 3D printed for the in vivo experiments.

The proposed cylindrical electro-stimulating implant is 55 mm long and designed in a bipolar manner, see the parametrized implant geometry in Figure 1c: Two electrodes (stimulating electrode "Electrode 1" and counter-electrode "Electrode 2") of length h_{el} are separated by an insulator of length 55 mm—$2h_{el}$. This geometry was chosen due to comparably easy manufacturing and very regular field distribution around the electrodes. Because the mandible's thickness is only around 5 mm in its posterior region, here the last 10 mm of the electrode are realized as a thin fixation pin of 1 mm in diameter. The diameter of the remaining implant is 4 mm and it is positioned approximately in the center of the defect.

The electrode length h_{el} is a fundamental parameter influencing the electric field distribution and hence the regeneration success. Therefore, this parameter will be optimized to aim for the most beneficial electric field distribution (see Section 2.5).

2.2. Generation of the Physical Model

The physical modelling step regards assigning the physical tissue and material properties and distribution to the anatomical and technical model. In this study, it is necessary to assign the dielectric tissue and material properties, i.e., electric conductivity σ and relative permittivity ε_r, to the respective model domains to simulate the electric field distribution resulting from electric stimulation of the mandible. These quantities are highly frequency-dependent and their values at the stimulation frequency of $f = 20$ Hz have been taken from the literature [50,51] in the case of the biological tissues (a practical online tool can be found at [52]). As described earlier, the model takes into account two types of bone: cortical bone representing the mandible and cancellous bone inside the mandible and filling the defect domain.

As for the electro-stimulating implant, the assigned biocompatible material commonly used in orthopedics and maxillofacial surgery are Ti6Al4V for the electrodes and PEEK (polyether ether ketone) for the insulator. The dielectric properties of these materials have been taken from technical data sheets [53,54]. The assigned dielectric tissue and material properties are summarized in Table 1.

Table 1. Dielectric properties (electric conductivity σ and relative permittivity ε_r) of the tissues and materials used in the simulation at $f = 20$ Hz.

Tissue/Material	σ (S/m)	ε_r
Cortical bone [50]	0.02	25,100
Cancellous bone [50]	0.079	4,020,200
Soft tissue (buccal mucosa) [51]	0.01	3×10^6
Skin [50]	2×10^{-4}	1140
Ti6Al4V [53]	5.6×10^5	1
PEEK [54]	10^{-12}	3.2

In this study, the individual tissues and materials are modelled macroscopically. Furthermore, they are simplified to be linear, isotropic, and locally homogeneous. In that case, the constitutive relations $\mathbf{J} = \sigma \mathbf{E}$ and $\mathbf{D} = \varepsilon_0 \varepsilon_r \mathbf{E}$ apply, with the current density $\mathbf{J}$, the electric field strength $\mathbf{E}$, the electric flux density $\mathbf{D}$, and the dielectric constant of vacuum ε_0. Still, it must be noted that bone is in general a highly anisotropic tissue with a hierarchic microscopic substructure [55]. Nonetheless, to employ a homogenization approach is feasible in our case. This holds especially true since only macroscopic dielectric tissue properties are available in the literature [50].

2.3. Modelling of the Electrode–Tissue Interface

In the numerical model, the electrochemical processes at the electrode–electrolyte interface between the electro-stimulating implant and the conductive tissue need to be taken into account, because part of the applied potential drops over this interface layer. These processes include the capacitive charging of the electrical double layer (non-Faradaic processes) as well as transfer of charges through the interface (Faradaic processes), as they determine the ratio of flowing current and the associated voltage drop. The electrical double layer results from the redistribution of ions in the surrounding electrolyte when interacting with the charged electrode surface. Its pseudocapacitive behavior is empirically modelled by a so-called constant phase element (CPE) [56]. This means that a constant phase difference between voltage and current exists, but generally with a larger value than the $-90°$ that would apply to a pure capacitance. The CPE is described by the equation

$$Z_{\text{CPE}} = K \left(j \frac{\omega}{\omega_0} \right)^{-\beta}, \qquad (1)$$

with K being the ratio of the amplitudes of voltage and current, j the imaginary unit, ω the angular frequency $\omega = 2\pi f$, and $\omega_0 = 1\, \text{s}^{-1}$ a normalization frequency to account for proper units of Ω for Z_{CPE}. The parameter $\beta = 0, \ldots, 1$ reflects the frequency dependence of the CPE and how much it deviates from a pure capacitance ($\beta = 1$).

The electrode–tissue interface is modelled via an equivalent circuit model that is commonly used to model simple systems: a parallel connection of the impedance of a constant phase element Z_{CPE} and a charge transfer resistance R_{CT} [56], see Figure 2. The impedance of the tissue Z_{Tissue} is defined by its dielectric properties σ and ε_r (ref. Section 2.2).

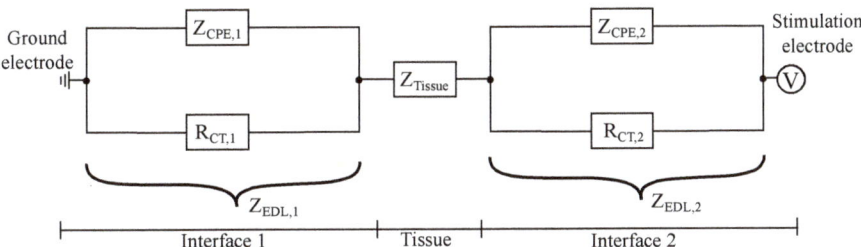

Figure 2. Equivalent circuit model for the electrode–tissue interface.

Thus, each of the two electrode–tissue interfaces of the bipolar electrode is described by one double layer impedance $Z_{EDL,i}$ ($i = 1, 2$), with

$$\frac{1}{Z_{EDL,i}} = \frac{1}{Z_{CPE,i}} + \frac{1}{R_{CT,i}} \tag{2}$$

$$= \left(\frac{A_{meas}}{A_{el,i}} K \left(j \frac{\omega}{\omega_0} \right)^{-\beta} \right)^{-1} + \left(\frac{A_{meas}}{A_{el,i}} R_{CT} \right)^{-1}. \tag{3}$$

In Equation (3), the contributions to the impedance have been scaled with respect to the surface of the measurement electrode used in electrochemical impedance spectroscopy (EIS) measurements with $A_{meas} = 314\,\text{mm}^2$ [57] and the surface of the stimulation electrode $A_{el,i}$ used in the simulations.

The parameters (β, K, R_{CT}) to model the electrode–tissue interface have been derived via EIS measurements of polished titanium specimens [57]. Their values from [57] are $\beta = 0.95$, $K = (Y_0[1/F])^{-\beta}\,\Omega = (38.95 \times 10^{-6})^{-0.95}\,\Omega = 15453\,\Omega$, $R_{CT} = 137.7\,\text{k}\Omega$. Please note that in EIS measurements, using the capacitance parameter Y_0 instead of the parameter K (used by Richardot and McAdams [56]) is more common.

The charge transfer resistance R_{CT} is generally non-linear, but as we use rather small stimulation voltages we may assume its measured value to be also valid in our simulations. As the interface behavior mainly depends on the surface structure and not so much on the material itself, it can be well assumed that the values measured for titanium also give a good approximation for the titanium alloy Ti6Al4V employed in the current study.

2.4. Electro-Quasistatic Boundary Value Problem

In general, the macroscopic behavior of electromagnetic fields is described by Maxwell's equations. Assuming negligible magnetic inductive effects and propagation in the low-frequency regime ($f = 20\,\text{Hz}$) as is commonly valid for bioelectric phenomena, Maxwell's equations can be simplified and the so-called electro-quasistatic approximation can be applied. In this case, the time-harmonic electric field is uniquely defined by the complex scalar potential $\underline{\varphi}$ with $\underline{\mathbf{E}} = -\nabla \underline{\varphi}$. Assuming no impressed currents, this leads to

$$\nabla \cdot \left([j\omega\varepsilon_0 \varepsilon_r(\mathbf{r}, \omega) + \sigma(\mathbf{r}, \omega)] \nabla \underline{\varphi}(\mathbf{r}) \right) = 0, \tag{4}$$

with the imaginary unit j, the angular frequency ω, the permittivity of free space ε_0, the relative permittivity $\varepsilon_r(\mathbf{r}, \omega)$, and the electric conductivity $\sigma(\mathbf{r}, \omega)$. Details on the derivation can be retraced in, e.g., [58–60].

We apply terminals with Dirichlet boundary conditions at the electrodes, with ground potential ($\varphi = 0\,\text{V}$) at the surface of the posterior electrode and the stimulation potential to be optimized $\varphi_{stim} \neq 0\,\text{V}$ at the surface of the anterior electrode (Figure 3). Homogeneous Neumann boundary conditions are applied to the surface of the skin domain representing the insulating air.

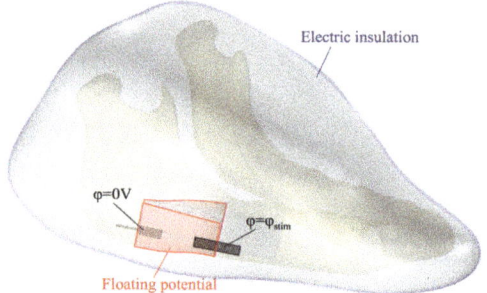

Figure 3. Boundary conditions applied in the simulation model: We assigned Dirichlet boundary conditions to the surfaces of both electrodes (black), homogeneous Neumann boundary conditions to the surface of the skin (blue), and a floating potential boundary condition to the surface enclosing the defect (red).

The mesh tray introduced in Section 2.1 serves as an additional stabilization for the bone but also has an impact on the resulting electric field distribution. To reduce the complexity of the model and computation time, the mesh tray has not been modelled explicitly, but only been regarded as a floating potential boundary condition at the lateral and lower boarder of the defect region (Figure 3). The floating potential boundary condition

$$\underline{\varphi} = \underline{\varphi}_0, \quad \int_{\partial\Omega} -\mathbf{n} \cdot \mathbf{J}\, dS = I_0 = 0\,\mathrm{A} \tag{5}$$

applies a constant potential φ_0 on the chosen surfaces, implying that the tangential electric field is zero and the electric field is perpendicular to the boundary. The value of the resulting potential depends on the integral source current I_0. In our study, we regard $I_0 = 0\,\mathrm{A}$, implying that the boundary will act as an unconnected perfect conductor. As the conductivity of the mesh tray is several orders of magnitude higher than that of the surrounding tissue, this is a valid approximation. Comparative simulations in a simplified model setup showed that the error in the electric field norm compared to a fully modelled mesh tray is less than 3% but the reduction in CPU time is 45%.

Considering the mentioned boundary conditions summarized in Figure 3, Equation (4) is solved for the complex electric potential $\underline{\varphi}(\mathbf{r})$. From this quantity, the complex amplitude of the electric field strength $\underline{\mathbf{E}} = -\nabla\underline{\varphi}$ can be derived. Finally, the electric field norm $|\underline{\mathbf{E}}|$ is computed that is used to rate the stimulation impact.

2.5. Optimization of the Stimulation Parameters

The stimulation parameters, i.e., the electrode length h_{el} and the stimulation voltage φ_{stim} need to be optimized to achieve the best possible electric stimulation in the ROI. In this context, a goal function is defined concerning the volume of beneficially stimulated tissue in the ROI. Here, *beneficially stimulated* means that in the considered region the following applies:

$$5\,\mathrm{V/m} \leq |\underline{\mathbf{E}}| \leq 70\,\mathrm{V/m}, \tag{6}$$

whereas overstimulation would correspond to $|\underline{\mathbf{E}}| > 70\,\mathrm{V/m}$ and understimulation would imply $|\underline{\mathbf{E}}| < 5\,\mathrm{V/m}$.

For optimizing the stimulation parameters for a most beneficial electric field distribution, the objective is a maximum volume of beneficially stimulated tissue in the ROI. At the same time, the volume of overstimulated and understimulated tissue is to be minimized. In the *Optimization module* of COMSOL these goals are expressed in terms of integral objective functions

$$s_{\text{ben}} \cdot \int 1 - \text{if}(|\mathbf{E}| \geq 5\,\text{V/m}\,\&\&\,|\mathbf{E}| \leq 70\,\text{V/m})\,dV, \tag{7}$$

$$s_{\text{over}} \cdot \int \text{if}(|\mathbf{E}| > 70\,\text{V/m})\,dV, \tag{8}$$

$$s_{\text{under}} \cdot \int \text{if}(|\mathbf{E}| < 5\,\text{V/m})\,dV. \tag{9}$$

Simply put, the objective functions represent the volume of beneficially stimulated (7), overstimulated (8), or understimulated (9) tissue and are only computed inside the ROI. The sum of the goal functions (7)–(9) is to be minimized to achieve the best possible stimulation impact. The goal functions are scaled with scale factors $s_{\text{ben}} = s_{\text{under}} = 4 \times 10^{-5}$, $s_{\text{over}} = 2 \times 10^{-4}$ so that the goal functions are in the order of one. This ensures stability of COMSOL's optimization methods. Because overstimulation is especially harmful as it might lead to tissue damage, goal function (8) is weighed with a higher factor than the other goal functions.

We consider the goal functions only in the ROI because at the current application of electro-stimulation we are not interested in an optimal fixation of the electrodes inside the residual bone. In this case, one would also consider the cortical and cancellous bone domains. Instead, we are only interested in how the electric field evolves inside a large volume of tissue to be regenerated.

The control variable is the stimulation amplitude φ_{stim} only, since optimizing both h_{el} and φ_{stim} simultaneously was unfortunately not possible due to the rather complicated model geometry. Instead, the electrode length h_{el} was varied parametrically for an exemplary stimulation amplitude of 1 V. The parameter was varied between $h_{\text{el}} = 10.5\,\text{mm}$ and $h_{\text{el}} = 27\,\text{mm}$ in increments of a few mm which is admissible for the manufacturing tolerances to be expected. The "optimal" electrode length yielded $h_{\text{el}} = 25\,\text{mm}$ (see Section 3.2). This value was then further used during the optimization of the stimulation amplitude φ_{stim}.

The stimulation potential applied to the electrodes has been optimized using the *Optimization* module of COMSOL. For this purpose, the Nelder–Mead–Simplex optimization algorithm [61,62] was used. We specified an optimality tolerance of 0.001, representing the relative accuracy in the final values of the scaled control variables. Scaling of the control variables, i.e., dividing the variables by their associated scale, ensures stability of the optimization method if the scaled control variables are in the order of unity. The derivative-free Nelder–Mead algorithm explores the design space around the current iterate by evaluating the objective function. Transformations are applied on the point of the simplex with the worst objective function value. If no further improvement of the objective function is achieved with relative increments of the scaled control variables greater or equal to the tolerance, the optimization iteration stops. In our study, the stimulation amplitude was optimized within lower and upper bounds of the control variable $\varphi_{\text{stim}} = 0.2 \ldots 4\,\text{V}$ with an initial value of $\varphi_{\text{stim}} = 0.2\,\text{V}$. We defined a scaling factor of 2 V to ensure that this control variable is in the order of 1, enabling the optimization algorithm to work properly.

2.6. Finite-Element Simulation

The finite-element simulations were conducted with COMSOL Multiphysics® version 5.4, using the *Electric Currents* and *Electrical Circuit* interfaces of the *ACDC* module in order to solve the electro-quasistatic approximation of Maxwell's equations (Equation (4)). The electrode–tissue interface was modelled via an *Electrical Circuit* interface at each electrode. The coupling between electrical circuit and the terminal boundary condition is achieved via a so-called *External-I-Terminal* that applies a voltage relative to ground to the circuit node, i.e., the surface of the electrodes. For the optimization of the stimulation amplitude we used the *Optimization* Module of COMSOL.

As for the finite-element discretization, second-order Laplace elements were used on a tetrahedral mesh to approximate the dependent variable in the model, i.e., the electric potential φ. The finite-element mesh consisted of ca. 1.24 million tetrahedral elements resulting in ca. 1.68 million degrees of freedom solved for. Based on a mesh convergence study we ensured that further refining the mesh would only change the electric energy in the whole computational domain by less than 0.04% with respect to the finest mesh resolution used. Additionally, we made sure that the mesh quality, especially in the ROI, is quite high, i.e., close to 1.

The computations were performed using the frequency domain solver of COMSOL that uses the iterative solver BiCGStab (biconjugate gradient stabilized method) with a relative tolerance of tol= 1×10^{-3} and a factor $\rho = 400$ in COMSOL's error estimate. This ensures that the desired tolerance would be achieved even in ill-conditioned problems. The computations were performed on a Windows workstation with 24 × 3.00 GHz CPU and 256 GB RAM. The computation time for one simulation run was about three minutes on the chosen mesh. 22 simulation runs were necessary to reach the desired optimality tolerance in the optimization study.

3. Results

3.1. Electric Field Distribution

Figure 4a shows the simulated electric field norm $|\underline{E}|$ and the electric field lines in a vertical slice of the mandible bone right through the defect region and electrodes. The field plot is shown for the optimized stimulation parameters $h_{el} = 25$ mm and $\varphi_{stim} = 0.523$ V (details in Section 3.2). Please note that the color legend only reaches from 5–70 V/m to emphasize the thresholds for beneficial bone stimulation. The field evolves rod-shaped around the electrodes where it achieves the desired values between 5 and 70 V/m, but also quickly diminishes with increasing distance to the electrodes, as the conductivity of the tissue is comparably high.

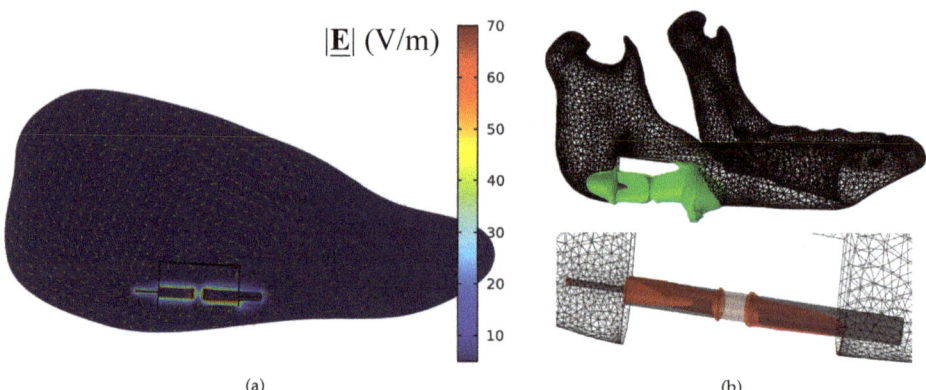

Figure 4. (a) Simulated electric field norm $|\underline{E}|$ in a slice through the electrically stimulated minipig mandible ($h_{el} = 25$ mm and $\varphi_{stim} = 0.523$ V). Scale is bounded for field strengths between 5 and 70 V/m and the arrow length is normalized. (b) Region with beneficially (top, green) and overstimulated (bottom, red) tissue around the electro-stimulating implant. The depicted mesh on the mandible bone corresponds to the finite-element discretization used in the simulations.

Figure 4b depicts the volumes of beneficially stimulated and overstimulated tissue in the defect. It can be seen that the beneficial stimulation volume reaches at least 6 mm into the tissue. As the field is not limited by the mesh tray at the sides outside of the defect, here the beneficial stimulation volume extends even further into the soft tissue. However, at a distance of roughly 10 mm away from the electrode, the electric field norm has decreased below 2 V/m. The region with overstimulation ($|\mathbf{E}| > 70$ V/m) is restricted to a small area directly around the electrodes.

3.2. Optimized Electrode Parameters

Figure 5 shows the volume percentage of beneficially, over-, and understimulated tissue in the defect domain in dependence on the electrode length h_{el} for an exemplary stimulating voltage of $\varphi_{stim} = 1$ V.

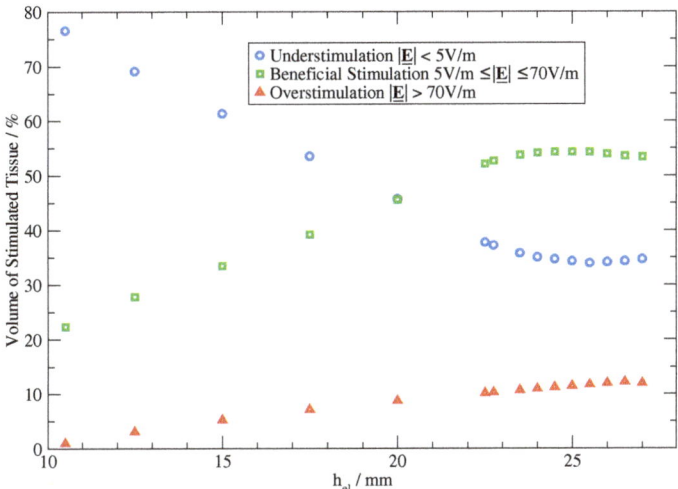

Figure 5. Volume of under-, beneficially, and overstimulated tissue in the ROI at a stimulation amplitude of $\varphi_{stim} = 1$ V as a function of the electrode length h_{el}.

It can be observed that the electrode length has a strong impact on the volume of stimulated tissue. Over the whole range of h_{el} the stimulated volumes vary by factors of ca. 2.2 (understimulation), 2.4 (beneficial stimulation), and 12 (overstimulation). Generally, with increasing electrode length the volume of beneficially stimulated tissue (5 V/m $\leq |\mathbf{E}| \leq$ 70 V/m) increases linearly, reaching a plateau at around 23 mm–27 mm. At $h_{el} = 25$ mm the volume of beneficially stimulated tissue reaches a maximum with 54% of the defect volume being stimulated. Smaller and larger electrode lengths lead to slightly reduced volumes of beneficially stimulated tissue. The volume of understimulated tissue ($|\mathbf{E}| < 5$ V/m) generally shows an inverse behavior: It decreases from ca. 77% to ca. 35% with increasing electrode length. The volume of overstimulated tissue ($|\mathbf{E}| > 70$ V/m) in the considered domain is generally about one order of magnitude smaller than the volumes for beneficial and understimulation. It increases from ca. 1% to ca. 12% with increasing electrode length.

Based on the optimum electrode length $h_{el} = 25$ mm, the stimulation potential applied to the electrode was also optimized numerically. For the optimal stimulation amplitude, we obtain $\varphi_{stim,opt} = 0.523$ V. With this parameter setting, approximately 49% of the tissue in the defect is stimulated beneficially, 49% is understimulated and 2% is overstimulated.

3.3. Impact of Varying Tissue Conductivity

Furthermore, the electrical conductivity of the defect domain, which is not exactly known, was varied parametrically between the extreme values of cancellous bone and cortical bone. This was done on the assumption that during the healing process the formerly soft cancellous bone develops and begins to resemble more structured and dense cortical bone [63]. Recent studies proposed the electrical properties of bone as a biomarker for bone fracture healing [64], e.g., increasing bone resistance as an indicator for bone fracture healing [65]. Hence, we may assume that the electrical conductivity in the defect domain—formerly being cancellous bone—decreases and approaches that of cortical bone during bone remodeling. The simulations show that decreasing the conductivity from $\sigma_{\text{defect}} = 0.079\,\text{S/m}$ (cancellous bone) to $\sigma_{\text{defect}} = 0.02\,\text{S/m}$ (cortical bone) results in a volume of beneficially stimulated tissue that is increased by ca. 21%, as can be seen in Figure 6.

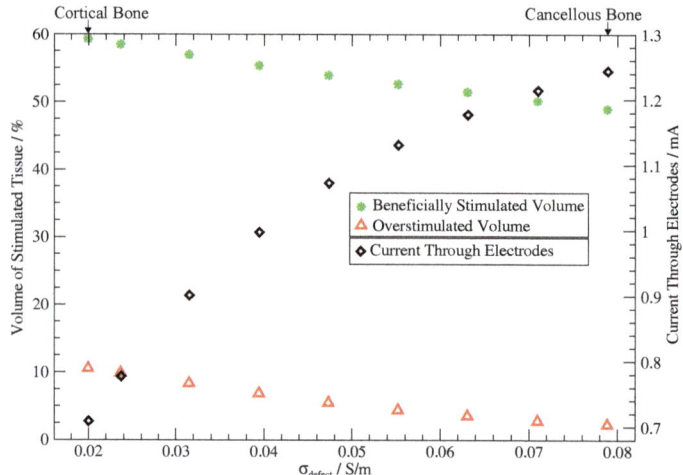

Figure 6. Impact of changing the electrical conductivity σ_{defect} in the defect domain on the volume of stimulated tissue and the current flowing through the electrodes.

However, there is also an increase in the volume of overstimulated tissue: from 2.3 to 10.6%. Hence, a reduction of the stimulation amplitude might be recommendable in the course of the physical treatment to avoid tissue damage. The current flowing through the electrodes is ca. 1.244 mA in the original, optimized setting (cancellous bone). With decreasing defect conductivity, it decreases to ca. 0.71 mA (cortical bone), thus leading to a reduced power consumption of the implant.

4. Discussion

In this study, a finite-element simulation model of a minipig mandible with an electro-stimulating implant without contact to the oral cavity could be built. This model enabled us to determine optimized stimulation parameters for the electro-stimulating setup. Furthermore, we could draw conclusions on the impact of changing material properties during bone healing.

The simulation results lead to a recommendation for the stimulation parameters to be used in the in vivo experiments following this study. Applying the optimized parameters $h_{\text{el}} = 25$ mm and $\varphi_{\text{stim,opt}} = 0.523$ V, nearly one half of the defect volume is being stimulated beneficially (Figure 6, case for $\sigma_{\text{defect}} = 0.078\,\text{S/m}$). By specifying strict weighting of the objective function for overstimulation, in the optimized setting only 2% of the tissue receives unfavorable electric field strengths greater than 70 V/m. It is favorable that the simulated volume of overstimulated tissue is generally much smaller than the volume of beneficially stimulated tissue. Otherwise, the related tissue damage would undo the healing impact of the electric stimulation in certain regions of the defect. However, we observed that the desired field threshold between 5 and 70 V/m is not only achieved in the bone, but also in the soft tissue (Figure 4b). The consequences of this need to be carefully studied in the in vivo experiments as the impact of such fields on soft tissue is not exactly known.

Forcing the optimization to avoid overstimulation, a relatively low optimal stimulation amplitude of ca. $\varphi_{\text{stim,opt}} = 0.5$ V results. This is also favorable in terms of ensuring long lifetime of the battery being used in the planned animal experiments. Furthermore, Liboff et al. [66] observed profound electrolysis at stimulation potentials higher than 1 V. Therefore, in the planned electro-stimulating devices voltages as high as this should be avoided. In this context, comparative numerical test studies with higher stimulation amplitudes of $\varphi_{\text{stim}} = 1$ V and $\varphi_{\text{stim}} = 2$ V showed that the volume of beneficially stimulated tissue could be increased by 11.0% and 15.6% respectively, but these lead to a 5-fold or 11-fold increase respectively in the overstimulated volume. This brings us to the conclusion that the stimulation voltage should be monitored carefully and kept low to avoid possible tissue damage during application.

To sum up, the optimized stimulation parameters $h_{\text{el}} = 25$ mm and $\varphi_{\text{stim,opt}} = 0.5$ V allow for an energy-efficient beneficial electrical stimulation of roughly one half of the defect volume with only very small regions of overstimulated tissue.

The computed currents of 1.244 mA flowing between electrode and tissue may be perceptible according to [67] (reproduced in [68]); however, this value is far from the threshold for muscular reactions (5 mA [67]). Consequently, the electric currents present in the optimized stimulation setup may be acceptable for long-term stimulation. However, in the end only the in vivo experiments can reveal the actual impact.

Analyzing the consequences of changing conductivity in the defect domain allowed us to roughly estimate how the stimulation impact might change over the whole treatment time. For the in vivo experiments this might extend over 6–12 weeks. We draw the conclusion that a corresponding adjustment in the stimulation parameters is necessary to ensure proper stimulation throughout the entire therapy. Specifically, decreasing the conductivity in the defect domain (Figure 6) revealed that with the same amplitude of the signal driving the stimulation a higher percentage of the defect region could be stimulated beneficially. What this implies is that a lower stimulation potential would be sufficient to obtain the same volume of beneficially stimulated tissue, or that the healing stimulation would reach further into the tissue, enabling a better growth of new tissue into the volume. However, substantially increased overstimulation could also be observed in this case. Therefore, the ideal stimulation unit would be feedback—controlled and able to adjust the stimulation signal during the treatment. As the flowing current decreases with the healing progress, the power consumption is reduced as well. This may allow for a longer lifetime of the battery.

For the future application in vivo—and later also in the clinic—a stimulation unit that will control and monitor the stimulation signal is under development. Regarding the design of the circuitry, the electrical impedance of the electrodes in the biological tissue is an important measure. For the optimized stimulation configuration the impedance is $Z = \frac{\varphi_{\text{stim,opt}}}{I} = \frac{0.523 \text{ V}}{1.244 \text{ mA}} = 420.4 \, \Omega$. Ex vivo experiments are planned to validate the numerical results. These experiments will include impedance measurements as well as measurements of the electric potential around the electrode in a porcine mandible.

Regarding the assumptions and limitations of the numerical study, there are different aspects to be noted. With respect to the dielectric tissue properties, we chose to include only the conductivity but not the permittivity. This has the advantage of simplifying the mathematical and numerical model and thus reducing computational demands. This decision is well justified since it is the conductivity which has the main impact when simulating electric stimulation of biological tissue [69]. A limitation of all such numerical studies on bioelectric effects is given by the fact that the dielectric properties of biological tissues available in the literature vary strongly among different species and also depend on the experimental conditions and the specific anatomic site [70–72]. Furthermore, the tissue properties depend on age [73] and health conditions of the subject: osteoporosis [74,75] will have an impact, for example. In addition, we assumed the defect to be filled purely with cancellous bone. In practice however, the cancellous bone material that is taken from another part of the body will be molded to fit into the defect, and equipped with growth factors. Hence, the cancellous bone will not be available in its original structure, thus having an unknown effect on its dielectric properties. Aside from that, we assumed each single sub-domain of the model that is representing one kind of tissue to be homogeneous and isotropic, neglecting the possible impact on the dielectric properties due to tissue heterogeneity and composition. To better capture the impact of the latter assumptions and the only vaguely known dielectric tissue properties, our future studies will include *Uncertainty Quantification* (UQ) methods in the numerical model. With this, the impact of the uncertain input parameters, especially the electric conductivity, on the obtained stimulation parameters could be identified. UQ methods are currently gaining in importance for this reason in numerical simulations of biological tissues [76–78]. In addition to the uncertainties in tissue parameters, geometrical uncertainties resulting from different jaw geometries or from manufacturing limitations of the implant could be estimated in terms of stochastic measures as well.

As the electric field decays rapidly with increasing distance to the electrodes (Figure 4a) and multiple simulations are necessary in UQ studies, future simulation models of the stimulation setup will be restricted to model only parts of the jaw geometry fully, e.g., only one half of it. This will reduce the degrees of freedom solved for and therefore reduce the computation time accordingly. Faster calculations would be especially favorable regarding UQ studies. In addition, upon success of the in vivo experiments, further numerical models including critical size defects in human mandibles will be established and analyzed.

In the current study, we neglected the complex hierarchic substructure of bone by assuming homogeneous, isotropic materials. Also, the physiological processes during bone remodeling have not been modelled. Future studies should include such microscopic details, as already quite simple studies in 2D showed notably increased electric field strengths as compared to the homogeneous case [79]. Therefore, so-called multi-scale models of electrical bone stimulation should be established. These would enable the inclusion of information from micro-scale simulations in the macro-scale model via appropriate scale-bridging techniques as presented, for instance, by Chopard et al. [80].

Author Contributions: Conceptualization, H.R., P.W.K., R.B., and U.v.R.; Formal analysis, H.R.; Funding acquisition, P.W.K., R.B. and U.v.R.; Investigation, H.R.; Methodology, P.W.K., R.B., and U.v.R.; Resources, U.v.R.; Supervision, P.W.K., R.B., and U.v.R.; Visualization, H.R.; Writing—original draft, H.R.; Writing—review & editing, H.R., P.W.K., R.B., and U.v.R.

Funding: This research was funded by a scholarship of the "Landesgraduiertenförderung Mecklenburg–Vorpommern" and is supported by the German Science Foundation (DFG) in the scope of the CRC 1270 "Electrically Active Implants" ELAINE.

Acknowledgments: The authors would like to thank Frank Krüger, Max Schröder (Institute of Communications Engineering, University of Rostock), and the Rostock University Library for providing the infrastructure to make the data publicly available. Further thanks to Dirk Timmermann and his team for extensive discussions on the technical realization of the proposed stimulation unit. Finally, we thank Jan Liese (Department of Oral, Maxillofacial and Plastic Surgery, University Medical Center Rostock) for providing the CT data of the minipig.

Conflicts of Interest: The authors declare no conflict of interest.

References

1. Bassett, C.A.; Pawluk, R.J.; Pilla, A.A. Acceleration of Fracture Repair by Electromagnetic Fields. A Surgically Noninvasive Method. *Ann. N. Y. Acad. Sci.* **1974**, *238*, 242–262. [CrossRef] [PubMed]
2. Ryaby, J.T. Clinical Effects of Electromagnetic and Electric Fields on Fracture Healing. *Clin. Orthop. Relat. Res.* **1998**, *355*, S205–S215. [CrossRef]
3. Brighton, C.T.; Hozack, W.J.; Brager, M.D.; Windsor, R.E.; Pollack, S.R.; Vreslovic, E.J.; Kotwick, J.E. Fracture Healing in the Rabbit Fibula when Subjected to Various Capacitively Coupled Electrical Fields. *J. Orthop. Res.* **1985**, *3*, 331–340. [CrossRef] [PubMed]
4. Kuzyk, P.R.; Schemitsch, E.H. The Science of Electrical Stimulation Therapy for Fracture Healing. *Indian J. Orthop.* **2009**, *43*, 127–131.
5. Daish, C.; Blanchard, R.; Fox, K.; Pivonka, P.; Pirogova, E. The Application of Pulsed Electromagnetic Fields (PEMFs) for Bone Fracture Repair: Past and Perspective Findings. *Ann. Biomed. Eng.* **2018**, *46*, 525–542. [CrossRef]
6. Aaron, R.K.; Ciombor, D.M.; Simon, B.J. Treatment of Nonunions With Electric and Electromagnetic Fields. *Clin. Orthop. Relat. Res.* **2004**, *419*, 21–29. [CrossRef]

7. Brighton, C.T.; Black, J.; Friedenberg, Z.B.; Esterhai, J.L.; Day, L.J.; Connolly, J.F. A Multicenter Study of the Treatment of Non-Union with Constant Direct Current. *J. Bone Jt. Surg. Am.* **1981**, *63*, 2–13. [CrossRef]
8. Shandler, H.S.; Weinstein, S.; Nathan, L.E. Facilitated Healing of Osseous Lesions in the Canine Mandible after Electrical Stimulation. *J. Oral Surg.* **1979**, *37*, 787–792.
9. Kohavi, D.; Pollack, S.R.; Brighton, C. Short-Term Effect of Guided Bone Regeneration and Electrical Stimulation on Bone Growth in a Surgically Modelled Resorbed Dog Mandibular Ridge. *Biomater. Artif. Cells Immobil. Biotechnol.* **1992**, *20*, 131–138.
10. Leppik, L.; Zhihua, H.; Mobini, S.; Parameswaran, V.T.; Eischen-Loges, M.; Slavici, A.; Helbing, J.; Pindur, L.; Oliveira, K.M.; Bhavsar, M.B.; et al. Combining Electrical Stimulation and Tissue Engineering to Treat Large Bone Defects in a Rat Model. *Sci. Rep.* **2018**, *8*, 6307. [CrossRef] [PubMed]
11. Schiegnitz, E.; Al-Nawas, B.; Kämmerer, P.W.; Grötz, K.A. Oral Rehabilitation with Dental Implants in Irradiated Patients: A Meta-Analysis on Implant Survival. *Clin. Oral Investig.* **2014**, *18*, 687–698. [CrossRef]
12. Khojasteh, A.; Dehghan, M.M.; Nazeman, P. Immediate Implant Placement Following 1-Year Treatment with Oral Versus Intravenous Bisphosphonates: A Histomorphometric Canine Study on Peri-Implant Bone. *Clin. Oral Investig.* **2019**, *23*, 1803–1809. [CrossRef] [PubMed]
13. Bassett, C.A.; Becker, R.O. Generation of Electric Potentials by Bone in Response to Mechanical Stress. *Science* **1962**, *137*, 1063–1064. [CrossRef] [PubMed]
14. Cerquiglini, S.; Cignitti, M.; Marchetti, M.; Salleo, A. On the Origin of Electrical Effects Produced by Stress in the Hard Tissues of Living Organisms. *Life Sci.* **1967**, *6*, 2651–2660. [CrossRef]
15. Pollack, S.R.; Petrov, N.; Salzstein, R.; Brankov, G.; Blagoeva, R. An Anatomical Model for Streaming Potentials in Osteons. *J. Biomech.* **1984**, *17*, 627–636. [CrossRef]
16. Riddle, R.C.; Donahue, H.J. From Streaming-Potentials to Shear Stress: 25 Years of Bone Cell Mechanotransduction. *J. Orthop. Res.* **2009**, *27*, 143–149. [CrossRef]
17. Fukada, E.; Yasuda, I. On the Piezoelectric Effect of Bone. *J. Phys. Soc. Jpn.* **1957**, *12*, 1158–1162. [CrossRef]
18. Anderson, J.C.; Eriksson, C. Piezoelectric Properties of Dry and Wet Bone. *Nature* **1970**, *227*, 491–492. [CrossRef]
19. Wieland, D.; Krywka, C.; Mick, E.; Willumeit-Römer, R.; Bader, R.; Kluess, D. Investigation of the Inverse Piezoelectric Effect of Trabecular Bone on a Micrometer Length Scale Using Synchrotron Radiation. *Acta Biomater.* **2015**, *25*, 339–346. [CrossRef]
20. Ahn, A.C.; Grodzinsky, A.J. Relevance of Collagen Piezoelectricity to "Wolff's Law": A Critical Review. *Med. Eng. Phys.* **2009**, *31*, 733–741. [CrossRef]
21. Min, S.; Lee, T.; Lee, S.H.; Hong, J. Theoretical Study of the Effect of Piezoelectric Bone Matrix on Transient Fluid Flow in the Osteonal Lacunocanaliculae. *J. Orthop. Res.* **2018**. [CrossRef]
22. Yasuda, I. The classic: Fundamental Aspects of Fracture Treatment by Iwao Yasuda, reprinted from J. Kyoto Med. Soc., 4:395–406, 1953. *Clin. Orthop. Relat. Res.* **1977**, *124*, 5–8.
23. Shuai, C.; Yang, W.; Peng, S.; Gao, C.; Guo, W.; Lai, Y.; Feng, P. Physical Stimulations and their Osteogenesis-Inducing Mechanisms. *Int. J. Bioprint.* **2018**, *4*. [CrossRef]
24. Massari, L.; Benazzo, F.; Falez, F.; Perugia, D.; Pietrogrande, L.; Setti, S.; Osti, R.; Vaienti, E.; Ruosi, C.; Cadossi, R. Biophysical Stimulation of Bone and Cartilage: State of the Art and Future Perspectives. *Int. Orthop.* **2019**, *43*, 539–551. [CrossRef] [PubMed]
25. Soda, A.; Ikehara, T.; Kinouchi, Y.; Yoshizaki, K. Effect of Exposure to an Extremely Low Frequency-Electromagnetic Field on the Cellular Collagen with Respect to Signaling Pathways in Osteoblast-like Cells. *J. Med. Investig.* **2008**, *55*, 267–278. [CrossRef]
26. Brighton, C.T.; Wang, W.; Seldes, R.; Zhang, G.; Pollack, S.R. Signal Transduction in Electrically Stimulated Bone Cells. *J. Bone Jt. Surg. Am.* **2001**, *83-A*, 1514–1523. [CrossRef]
27. Wang, X.; Gao, Y.; Shi, H.; Liu, N.; Zhang, W.; Li, H. Influence of the Intensity and Loading Time of Direct Current Electric Field on the Directional Migration of Rat Bone Marrow Mesenchymal Stem Cells. *Front. Med.* **2016**, *10*, 286–296. [CrossRef]
28. Grunert, P.; Jonitz-Heincke, A.; Su, Y.; Souffrant, R.; Hansmann, D.; Ewald, H.; Krüger, A.; Mittelmeier, W.; Bader, R. Establishment of a Novel in Vitro Test Setup for Electric and Magnetic Stimulation of Human Osteoblasts. *Cell Biochem. Biophys.* **2014**, *70*, 805–817. [CrossRef]
29. Black, J. *Electrical Stimulation: Its Role in Growth, Repair and Remodeling of the Musculoskeletal System*; Greenwood Press: Westport, CT, USA, 1986; pp. 85–101.

30. Griffin, M.; Bayat, A. Electrical Stimulation in Bone Healing: Critical Analysis by Evaluating Levels of Evidence. *Eplasty* **2011**, *11*, e34.
31. Kraus, W. Magnetic Field Therapy and Magnetically Induced Electrostimulation in Orthopedics. *Orthopaede* **1984**, *13*, 78–92.
32. Mittelmeier, W.; Lehner, S.; Kraus, W.; Matter, H.P.; Gerdesmeyer, L.; Steinhauser, E. BISS: Concept and Biomechanical Investigations of a New Screw System for Electromagnetically Induced Internal Osteostimulation. *Arch. Orthop. Trauma Surg.* **2004**, *124*, 86–91. [CrossRef]
33. Dauben, T.J.; Ziebart, J.; Bender, T.; Zaatreh, S.; Kreikemeyer, B.; Bader, R. A Novel In Vitro System for Comparative Analyses of Bone Cells and Bacteria under Electrical Stimulation. *BioMed Res. Int.* **2016**, *2016*, 5178640. [CrossRef]
34. Hiemer, B.; Ziebart, J.; Jonitz-Heincke, A.; Grunert, P.C.; Su, Y.; Hansmann, D.; Bader, R. Magnetically Induced Electrostimulation of Human Osteoblasts Results in Enhanced Cell Viability and Osteogenic Differentiation. *Int. J. Mol. Med.* **2016**, *38*, 57–64. [CrossRef]
35. Klüß, D.; Souffrant, R.; Bader, R.; van Rienen, U.; Ewald, H.; Mittelmeier, W. A New Concept of an Electrostimulative Acetabular Revision System with Patient Individual Additional Fixation. In *4th European Conference of the International Federation for Medical and Biological Engineering*; Vander Sloten, J., Verdonck, P., Nyssen, M., Haueisen, J., Eds.; Springer: Berlin/Heidelberg, Germany, 2009; pp. 1847–1850.
36. Klüß, D.; Souffrant, R.; Ewald, E.; van Rienen, U.; Bader, R.; Mittelmeier, W. Acetabuläre Hüftendoprothese mit einer Vorrichtung zur Elektrostimulation des Knochens. Patent DE202008015661 U1, 20 May 2009.
37. Potratz, C.; Kluess, D.; Ewald, H.; van Rienen, U. Multiobjective Optimization of an Electrostimulative Acetabular Revision System. *IEEE Trans. Biomed. Eng.* **2010**, *57*, 460–468. [CrossRef]
38. Su, Y.; Souffrant, R.; Kluess, D.; Ellenrieder, M.; Mittelmeier, W.; van Rienen, U.; Bader, R. Evaluation of Electric Field Distribution in Electromagnetic Stimulation of Human Femoral Head. *Bioelectromagnetics* **2014**, *35*, 547–558. [CrossRef]
39. Song, J.K.; Cho, T.H.; Pan, H.; Song, Y.M.; Kim, I.S.; Lee, T.H.; Hwang, S.J.; Kim, S.J. An Electronic Device for Accelerating Bone Formation in Tissues Surrounding a Dental Implant. *Bioelectromagnetics* **2009**, *30*, 374–384. [CrossRef]
40. Delenda, B.; Bader, R.; van Rienen, U. Modeling and Simulation of Platelet Reaction and Diffusion towards an Electro-Stimulating Dental Implant. In Proceedings of the 37th Annual International Conference of the IEEE Engineering in Medicine and Biology Society (EMBC), Milan, Italy, 25–29 August 2015; pp. 2584–2587. [CrossRef]
41. The Federal Health Monitoring System. Keyword "Operations and Procedures in Hospitals". Available online: http://www.gbe-bund.de/gbe10/pkg_isgbe5.prc_isgbe?p_uid=gast&p_aid=0&p_sprache=E (accessed on 15 February 2019).
42. Kämmerer, P.W.; Klein, M.O.; Moergel, M.; Gemmel, M.; Draenert, G.F. Local and Systemic Risk Factors Influencing the Long-Term Success of Angular Stable Alloplastic Reconstruction Plates of the Mandible. *J. Craniomaxillofac. Surg.* **2014**, *42*, e271–e276. [CrossRef]
43. Sadr-Eshkevari, P.; Rashad, A.; Vahdati, S.A.; Garajei, A.; Bohluli, B.; Maurer, P. Alloplastic Mandibular Reconstruction: A Systematic Review and Meta-Analysis of the Current Century Case Series. *Plast. Reconstr. Surg.* **2013**, *132*, 413e–427e. [CrossRef]
44. Maurer, P.; Eckert, A.W.; Kriwalsky, M.S.; Schubert, J. Scope and Limitations of Methods of Mandibular Reconstruction: A Long-Term Follow-Up. *Br. J. Oral Maxillofac. Surg.* **2010**, *48*, 100–104. [CrossRef]
45. Raben, H.; Schmidt, C.; Sridhar, K.; Kämmerer, P.W.; van Rienen, U. Numerical Design Studies on a Novel Electrostimulative Osteosynthesis System for the Mandible. *Curr. Dir. Biomed. Eng.* **2017**, *3*, 613–617. [CrossRef]
46. van Rienen, U.; Zimmermann, U.; Raben, H.; Kämmerer, P.W. Preliminary Numerical Study on Electrical Stimulation at Alloplastic Reconstruction Plates of the Mandible. *Sci. Comput. Electr. Eng.* **2018**. [CrossRef]
47. Ma, J.L.; Pan, J.L.; Tan, B.S.; Cui, F.Z. Determination of Critical Size Defect of Minipig Mandible. *J. Tissue Eng. Regener. Med.* **2009**, *3*, 615–622. [CrossRef]
48. Raben, H.; van Rienen, U.; Kämmerer, P.W.; Bader, R. Data for: Establishment of a Numerical Model to Design an Electro-Stimulating System for a Porcine Mandibular Critical Size Defect. Dataset, May 2019, University Library, University of Rostock. Available online: http://purl.uni-rostock.de/rosdok/id00002450 (accessed on 23 May 2019). [CrossRef]

49. Qvist, M.H.; Hoeck, U.; Kreilgaard, B.; Madsen, F.; Frokjaer, S. Evaluation of Göttingen Minipig Skin for Transdermal in vitro Permeation Studies. *Eur. J. Pharm. Sci.* **2000**, *11*, 59–68. [CrossRef]
50. Gabriel, S.; Lau, R.W.; Gabriel, C. The Dielectric Properties of Biological Tissues: II. Measurements in the Frequency Range 10 Hz to 20 GHz. *Phys. Med. Biol.* **1996**, *41*, 2251–2269. [CrossRef] [PubMed]
51. Lackovic, I.; Stare, Z. Low-Frequency Dielectric Properties of the Oral Mucosa. In *13th International Conference on Electrical Bioimpedance and the 8th Conference on Electrical Impedance Tomography*; Springer: Berlin/Heidelberg, Germany, 2007. [CrossRef]
52. Dielectric Properties IT'IS Foundation Web Page. Available online: https://itis.swiss/virtual-population/tissue-properties/database/dielectric-properties/ (accessed on 9 January 2019).
53. MatWeb Web Page on Titanium Ti-6Al-4V (Grade 5), Annealed. Available online: http://www.matweb.com/search/datasheet.aspx?MatGUID=a0655d261898456b958e5f825ae85390 (accessed on 21 March 2019).
54. Mitsubishi Chemical Advanced Materials Web Page, Product Data Sheets. Available online: https://media.mcam.com/fileadmin/quadrant/documents/QEPP/Global/English/Product_Data_Sheets_AEP/Ketron_1000_PEEK_PDS_GLOB_E_19092016.pdf?_ga=2.7651570.1148302848.1554475020-1676376043.1553176436 (accessed on 5 April 2019).
55. Rho, J.Y.; Kuhn-Spearing, L.; Zioupos, P. Mechanical Properties and the Hierarchical Structure of Bone. *Med. Eng. Phys.* **1998**, *20*, 92–102. [CrossRef]
56. Richardot, A.; McAdams, E.T. Harmonic Analysis of Low-Frequency Bioelectrode Behavior. *IEEE Trans. Med. Imag.* **2002**, *21*, 604–612. [CrossRef] [PubMed]
57. Lange, R.; Lüthen, F.; Beck, U.; Rychly, J.; Baumann, A.; Nebe, B. Cell-Extracellular Matrix Interaction and Physico-Chemical Characteristics of Titanium Surfaces Depend on the Roughness of the Material. *Biomol. Eng.* **2002**, *19*, 255–261. [CrossRef]
58. Plonsey, R.; Heppner, D.B. Considerations of Quasi-Stationarity in Electrophysiological Systems. *Bull. Math. Biophys.* **1967**, *29*, 657–664. [CrossRef]
59. van Rienen, U.; Flehr, J.; Schreiber, U.; Motrescu, V. *Modeling, Simulation, and Optimization of Integrated Circuits*; Volume 146 of International Series of Numerical Mathematics, Chapter Modeling and Simulation of Electro-Quasistatic Fields; Birkhäuser Verlag: Basel, Switzerland, 2003; pp. 17–31.
60. van Rienen, U.; Flehr, J.; Schreiber, U.; Schulze, S.; Gimsa, U.; Baumann, W.; Weiss, D.; Gimsa, J.; Benecke, R.; Pau, H.W. Electro-Quasistatic Simulations in Bio-Systems Engineering and Medical Engineering. *Adv. Radio Sci.* **2005**, *3*, 39–49. [CrossRef]
61. Nelder, J.A.; Mead, R. A Simplex Method for Function Minimization. *Comput. J.* **1965**, *7*, 308–313. [CrossRef]
62. Conn, A.R.; Scheinberg, K.; Vicente, L.N. *Introduction to Derivative-Free Optimization*; Number 8 in MPS-SIAM Series on Optimization; SIAM: Philadelphia, PA, USA, 2009.
63. Doblare, M.; Garcia, J.M.; Gomez, M.J. Modelling Bone Tissue Fracture and Healing: A Review. *Eng. Fract. Mech.* **2004**, *71*, 1809–1840. [CrossRef]
64. Gupta, K.; Gupta, P.; Singh, G.; Kumar, S.; Singh, R.; Srivastava, R. Changes in Electrical Properties of Bones as a Diagnostic Tool for Measurement of Fracture Healing. *Hard Tissue* **2013**, *2*, 3. [CrossRef]
65. Kumaravel, S.; Sundaram, S. Monitoring of Fracture Healing by Electrical Conduction: A New Diagnostic Procedure. *Indian J. Orthop.* **2012**, *46*, 384–390. [CrossRef]
66. Liboff, A.R.; Rinaldi, R.A.; Lavine, L.S.; Shamos, M.H. On Electrical Conduction in Living Bone. *Clin. Orthop.* **1975**, *106*, 330–335. [CrossRef] [PubMed]
67. IEC 2016. *IEC 60479-1: Effects of Current on Human Beings and Livestock*; International Electrotechnical Commission: Geneva, Switzerland, 2016.
68. Kono, M.; Takahashi, T.; Nakamura, H.; Miyaki, T.; Rekimoto, J. Design Guideline for Developing Safe Systems that Apply Electricity to the Human Body. *ACM Trans. Comput. Hum. Interact.* **2018**, *25*, 19. [CrossRef]
69. Schmidt, C.; Wagner, S.; Burger, M.; Rienen, U.V.; Wolters, C.H. Impact of Uncertain Head Tissue Conductivity in the Optimization of Transcranial Direct Current Stimulation for an Auditory Target. *J. Neural Eng.* **2015**, *12*, 046028. [CrossRef]
70. Gabriel, C.; Gabriel, S.; Corthout, E. The Dielectric Properties of Biological Tissues: I. Literature Survey. *Phys. Med. Biol.* **1996**, *41*, 2231–2249. [CrossRef]
71. McCann, H.; Pisano, G.; Beltrachini, L. Variation in Reported Human Head Tissue Electrical Conductivity Values. *bioRxiv* **2019**. [CrossRef]

72. Amin, B.; Elahi, M.A.; Shahzad, A.; Porter, E.; O'Halloran, M. A Review of the Dielectric Properties of the Bone for Low Frequency Medical Technologies. *Biomed. Phys. Eng. Express* **2019**, *5*, 022001. [CrossRef]
73. Wendel, K.; Väisänen, J.; Seemann, G.; Hyttinen, J.; Malmivuo, J. The Influence of Age and Skull Conductivity on Surface and Subdermal Bipolar EEG Leads. *Comput. Intell. Neurosci.* **2010**, *2010*, 397272. [CrossRef] [PubMed]
74. Amin, B.; Elahi, M.A.; Shahzad, A.; Parle, E.; McNamara, L.; O'Halloran, M. An Insight into Bone Dielectric Properties Variation: A Foundation for Electromagnetic Medical Devices. In Proceedings of the 2018 EMF-Med 1st World Conference on Biomedical Applications of Electromagnetic Fields (EMF-Med), Split, Croatia, 10–13 September 2018; pp. 1–2.
75. Amin, B.; Elahi, M.A.; Shahzad, A.; Porter, E.; McDermott, B.; O'Halloran, M. Dielectric Properties of Bones for the Monitoring of Osteoporosis. *Med. Biol. Eng. Comput.* **2019**, *57*, 1–13. [CrossRef] [PubMed]
76. Schmidt, C.; Zimmermann, U.; van Rienen, U. Modeling of an Optimized Electrostimulative Hip Revision System under Consideration of Uncertainty in the Conductivity of Bone Tissue. *IEEE J. Biomed. Health Inf.* **2015**, *19*, 1321–1330. [CrossRef] [PubMed]
77. Römer, U.; Schmidt, C.; Van Rienen, U.; Schöps, S. Low-Dimensional Stochastic Modeling of the Electrical Properties of Biological Tissues. *IEEE Trans. Magn.* **2017**, *53*, 1–4. [CrossRef]
78. Saturnino, G.B.; Thielscher, A.; Madsen, K.H.; Knösche, T.R.; Weise, K. A Principled Approach to Conductivity Uncertainty Analysis in Electric Field Calculations. *Neuroimage* **2018**. [CrossRef] [PubMed]
79. Zimmermann, U.; van Rienen, U. The Impact of Bone Microstructure on the Field Distribution of Electrostimulative Implants. In Proceedings of the 2015 37th Annual International Conference of the IEEE Engineering in Medicine and Biology Society (EMBC), Milan, Italy, 25–29 August 2015; pp. 3545–3548. [CrossRef]
80. Chopard, B.; Borgdorff, J.; Hoekstra, A.G. A Framework for Multi-Scale Modelling. *Philos. Trans. Ser. A Math. Phys. Eng. Sci.* **2014**, *372*. [CrossRef] [PubMed]

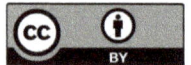

© 2019 by the authors. Licensee MDPI, Basel, Switzerland. This article is an open access article distributed under the terms and conditions of the Creative Commons Attribution (CC BY) license (http://creativecommons.org/licenses/by/4.0/).

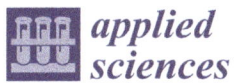 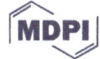

Article
Analysis of Damage Models for Cortical Bone

Jacobo Baldonedo [1], José R. Fernández [2,*], José A. López-Campos [1] and Abraham Segade [1]

[1] Departamento de Ingeniería Mecánica, Máquinas y Motores Térmicos y Fluídos, Escola de Enxeñería Industrial, Campus As Lagoas Marcosende s/n, 36310 Vigo, Spain
[2] Departamento de Matemática Aplicada I, Universidade de Vigo, ETSI Telecomunicación, Campus As Lagoas Marcosende s/n, 36310 Vigo, Spain
* Correspondence: jose.fernandez@uvigo.es; Tel.: +34-986-818-746

Received: 6 June 2019; Accepted: 1 July 2019; Published: 3 July 2019

Abstract: Bone tissue is a material with a complex structure and mechanical properties. Diseases or even normal repetitive loads may cause microfractures to appear in the bone structure, leading to a deterioration of its properties. A better understanding of this phenomenon will lead to better predictions of bone fracture or bone-implant performance. In this work, the model proposed by Frémond and Nedjar in 1996 (initially for concrete structures) is numerically analyzed and compared against a bone specific mechanical model proposed by García et al. in 2009. The objective is to evaluate both models implemented with a finite element method. This will allow us to determine if the modified Frémond–Nedjar model is adequate for this purpose. We show that, in one dimension, both models show similar results, reproducing the qualitative behaviour of bone subjected to typical engineering tests. In particular, the Frémond–Nedjar model with the introduced modifications shows good agreement with experimental data. Finally, some two-dimensional results are also provided for the Frémond–Nedjar model to show its behaviour in the simulation of a real tensile test.

Keywords: cortical bone; damage; finite elements; numerical results

1. Introduction

Damage models arise in order to describe how mechanical properties of materials degrade over time. This degradation can be caused both because of the loading it is subjected to, and due to external causes (such as crack formation due to thermal shock or chemical attack). These models have been deeply studied for structures, usually concrete structures, where the progressive wear of the materials can be critical to its integrity. In this field, works about damage exist since the decade of 1980 [1]. A later work from Frémond and Nedjar in 1996 [2] became a reference for new concrete damage models based on the continuum elastoplastic damage approach [3]. In this approach, the principle of virtual power is modified, including the damage in the term of the power of the internal forces. Also, damage is represented by a scalar field.

The study of engineering concepts in the field of biology and medicine is more recent, but it is growing fast. In the particular case of bone tissue, biological aspects such as bone remodelling were studied also since the decade of 1980 [4]. The model proposed by Weinans, Huiskes and Grootenboer in 1992 [5] started the possibility of simulating this effect numerically, and led to a large number of contributions in this field. The effect of damage described previously can be seen in bones too. In bone tissue, both loading and external causes (now related to illness such as osteoporosis) produce again a growing deterioration of its elastic properties [6]. The first studies of damage were focused on cumulative damage caused by cyclic loading [7,8]. This approach allows for fatigue estimations of the number of cycles that a probe can withstand, but it is not effective for its implementation in numerical simulations. In 1999, Fondrk, Bahniuk and Davy proposed a model that reproduced the tensile behaviour of cortical bone [9]; however, it is limited to one-dimensional simulations, obtaining bending results by applying beam theory assumptions. A recent work from and García et al. in 2009 [10] introduced rheological bone specific models that reproduced uniaxial and cyclic tests and could be extended to three dimensional simulations. Other works about bone damage can be seen in [11–14].

In this work, the Frémond–Nedjar model is compared against the García et al. model in order to assess its capabilities to reproduce bone tissue behaviour. Indeed, one of the main novelties of this work is its application in the simulation of the bone damage process. The selection and the interest of analysing the Frémond-Nejdar model relies on the fact that its formulated as a set of partial differential equations (in particular a subdifferential inclusion) that couples the damage evolution with the well known linear elasticity model. This allows for its numerical analysis and its implementation in a finite element simulation. Also, it is not restricted to one dimensional simulations, like the previously mentioned Fondrk, Bahniuk and Davy model.

Furthermore, since the formulation is similar to the Weinans–Huiskes–Grootenboer model of bone remodelling, it would allow for a direct coupling of these models, a future objective of the authors. Although an existing work presents a coupling between damage and a remodelling model [15], it is based on a simple remodelling rule and the numerical analysis is not performed.

The paper is structured as follows. In Section 2, the formulations of the studied models are presented, then, in Section 3, the implementation and results obtained are shown and discussed, followed by some conclusions in Section 4.

2. Damage Models

In this paper, as mentioned before, two damage models for numerical simulations are analyzed: the Frémond–Nedjar model, first developed for concrete structures, and the model proposed by García et al. (bone specific). The particular formulation of each model is described in the following subsections. Special emphasis is placed on the Frémond–Nedjar model, for which the numerical analysis of the algorithm proposed for its resolution is shown.

2.1. Frémond–Nedjar Model

The damage model proposed by Frémond and Nedjar in 1996 considers damage as an unknown of the problem (β) that varies between 1 (undamaged material) and 0 (completely damaged). This counter-intuitive definition accounts for the fact that the variable multiplies the mechanical properties of the material (the elastic modulus in the one-dimensional case) in such a way that, in a damaged material, they will be affected by this variable.

As mentioned before, this model was presented for concrete structures, so some modifications to include bone behaviour were necessary. Since bone tissue is a living material that can heal over time, the assumption that this variable cannot recover, $\dot{\beta} < 0$, is no longer true and it is removed from the initial formulation.

The mathematical formulation of this model with the modifications to account for bone properties is defined in what follows.

In [2] the damage source function ϕ was defined by

$$\phi(\varepsilon(u), \beta) = \lambda_d \left(\frac{1-\beta}{\beta}\right) - \lambda_u |\varepsilon(u)|^2 + \lambda_w,$$

where λ_d, λ_u and λ_w are constitutive parameters. The second term becomes unmanageable mathematically when strains are very large, but then the whole model becomes inadequate, so we truncate the term as follows. Given $q^* > 0$, a sufficiently large strain energy truncation constant, let Ψ_{q^*} be given by

$$\Psi_{q^*}(\tau) = \begin{cases} |\tau|^2 & \text{if } |\tau|^2 \leq q^*, \\ q^* & \text{otherwise,} \end{cases}$$

where $|\tau|^2 = \tau_{ij}\tau_{ij}$, and here and below, $i, j = 1, \ldots, d$ (d is the dimension of the problem), and a repeated index indicates summation. Therefore, we use the truncated damage source function:

$$\phi(\varepsilon(u), \beta) = \lambda_d \left(\frac{1-\beta}{\beta}\right) - \lambda_u \Psi_{q^*}(\varepsilon(u)) + \lambda_w. \tag{1}$$

Finally, the mechanical problem is written as follows.

Problem P. Find the displacement field $u = (u_i)_{i=1}^d : \overline{\Omega} \times [0, T] \to \mathbb{R}^d$ and the damage field $\beta : \overline{\Omega} \times [0, T] \to \mathbb{R}$ such that

$$\sigma = 2\beta \mu \varepsilon(u) + \beta \lambda \text{Div}(u)\mathcal{I} \quad \text{in} \quad \Omega \times (0, T), \tag{2}$$

$$-\text{Div}\, \sigma = f_0 \quad \text{in} \quad \Omega \times (0, T), \tag{3}$$

$$\dot{\beta} - \kappa^* \Delta \beta + \partial I_{[\beta_*, 1]}(\beta) \ni \phi(\varepsilon(u), \beta) \quad \text{in} \quad \Omega \times (0, T), \tag{4}$$

$$u = 0 \quad \text{on} \quad \Gamma_D \times (0, T), \tag{5}$$

$$\frac{\partial \beta}{\partial \nu} = 0 \quad \text{on} \quad \Gamma \times (0, T), \tag{6}$$

$$\sigma \nu = g \quad \text{on} \quad \Gamma_N \times (0, T), \tag{7}$$

$$\beta(x, 0) = \beta_0(x) \quad \text{in} \quad \Omega, \tag{8}$$

where Ω represents the bone, whose boundary Γ is assumed to be decomposed into two parts Γ_D and Γ_N such that $\Gamma = \Gamma_D \cup \Gamma_N$, with $\text{meas}(\Gamma_D) > 0$, $[0, T]$, for $T > 0$, denotes the time interval of interest, and let Div be the divergence of tensor-valued functions. λ and μ are the classical Lame's coefficients and $\kappa^* > 0$ is a damage diffusion coefficient. Moreover, β_0 is an initial condition for the damage field, f_0 and g represent volume and traction forces, respectively, and we include the subdifferential of the indicator function $I_{[\beta_*, 1]}$ into (4) to ensure that the damage function belongs to the interval $[\beta_*, 1]$. Here, $\beta_* > 0$ is a positive constant, assumed small, and it is introduced for mathematical reasons. In any case, when damage becomes zero, the material is dense with microcracks and modelling it as elastic ceases to make sense (see [16] for details). Finally, we note that damage function ϕ is given in (1), where constants λ_d, λ_u and λ_w are constitutive parameters.

Now, in order to obtain the variational formulation of Problem P, let $Y = L^2(\Omega)$, $H = [L^2(\Omega)]^d$ and $Q = [L^2(\Omega)]^{d \times d}$ and denote by $(\cdot, \cdot)_Y$, $(\cdot, \cdot)_H$ and $(\cdot, \cdot)_Q$ the respective scalar products in these spaces. Moreover, let us define the variational space V as follows,

$$V = \{v \in [H^1(\Omega)]^d ; v = 0 \quad \text{on} \quad \Gamma_D\},$$

with the scalar product $(\cdot, \cdot)_V$, and norm $\|\cdot\|_V$.

Finally, let us define the convex set of admissible damage functions,

$$K = \{\zeta \in H^1(\Omega) ; \beta_* \leq \zeta \leq 1 \text{ a.e. in } \Omega\}.$$

By using Green's formula and boundary conditions (5)–(7), we write the variational formulation of problem P.

Problem VP. Find the displacement field $u : [0, T] \to V$ and the damage field $\beta : [0, T] \to K$ such that $\beta(0) = \beta_0$ and, for a.e. $t \in (0, T)$, and for all $v \in V$ and $\zeta \in K$,

$$c(\beta(t); u(t), v) = (f(t), v)_V, \tag{9}$$

$$(\dot{\beta}(t), \zeta - \beta(t))_Y + \kappa^*(\nabla \beta(t), \nabla(\zeta - \beta(t)))_H \geq (\phi(\varepsilon(u(t)), \beta(t)), \zeta - \beta(t))_Y, \tag{10}$$

where the bilinear functional $c: K \times V \times V \to \mathbb{R}$ is defined as follows, for all $v, w \in V$ and $\zeta \in K$,

$$c(\zeta; v, w) = \int_\Omega \zeta \left(2\mu \varepsilon(v) : \varepsilon(w) + \lambda \mathrm{div}\, v\, \mathrm{div}\, w\right)\, dx.$$

The operator div represents now the divergence of vector-valued functions, the element $f(t) \in V'$ (as usual, V' denotes the dual space of V) is obtained from Riesz' theorem as

$$(f(t), w)_V = (f_0(t), w)_H + (g(t), w)_{[L^2(\Gamma_N)]^d} \quad \forall w \in V,$$

and we recall that damage function ϕ is defined in (1).

We now consider a fully discrete approximation of problem VP. To solve it numerically, a finite element scheme is used. This is done in two steps. First, we assume that the domain $\overline{\Omega}$ is polyhedral and we denote by $\mathcal{T}^h$ a regular triangulation in the sense of [17]. Thus, we construct the finite dimensional spaces $V^h \subset V$ and $E^h \subset H^1(\Omega)$ given by

$$V^h = \{v^h \in [C(\overline{\Omega})]^d \,;\, v^h_{|Tr} \in [P_1(Tr)]^d \quad \forall Tr \in \mathcal{T}^h, \quad v^h = 0 \text{ on } \Gamma_D\},$$
$$E^h = \{\xi^h \in C(\overline{\Omega}) \,;\, \xi^h_{|Tr} \in P_1(Tr) \quad \forall Tr \in \mathcal{T}^h\},$$

where $P_1(Tr)$ represents the space of polynomials of degree less or equal to one in the element Tr, i.e., the finite element spaces V^h and E^h are composed of continuous and piecewise affine functions. Here, $h > 0$ denotes the spatial discretization parameter. Moreover, let $K^h = K \cap E^h$ and assume that the discrete initial condition, denoted by β_0^h, is given by

$$\beta_0^h = \mathcal{P}^h \beta_0,$$

where $\mathcal{P}^h$ is the classical finite element interpolation operator over E^h (see, e.g., [17]).

Secondly, we consider a partition of the time interval $[0, T]$, denoted by $0 = t_0 < t_1 < \cdots < t_N = T$. In this case, we use a uniform partition with step size $k = T/N$ and nodes $t_n = nk$ for $n = 0, 1, \ldots, N$.

Therefore, using a combination of both implicit and explicit Euler schemes, the fully discrete approximations are considered as follows.

Problem VP^{hk}. Find the discrete displacement field $u^{hk} = \{u_n^{hk}\}_{n=0}^N \subset V^h$ and the discrete damage field $\beta^{hk} = \{\beta_n^{hk}\}_{n=0}^N \subset K^h$ such that $\beta_0^{hk} = \beta_0^h$ and, for all $v^h \in V^h$, $\zeta^h \in K^h$,

$$c(\beta_n^{hk}; u_n^{hk}, v^h) = (f_n, v^h)_V \quad n = 0, 1, \ldots, N, \tag{11}$$

$$(\beta_n^{hk}, \zeta^h - \beta_n^{hk})_Y + k\kappa^*(\nabla \beta_n^{hk}, \nabla(\zeta^h - \beta_n^{hk}))_H \geq (\beta_{n-1}^{hk}, \zeta^h - \beta_n^{hk})_Y$$
$$+ k\left(\phi(\varepsilon(u_{n-1}^{hk}), \beta_{n-1}^{hk}), \zeta^h - \beta_n^{hk}\right)_Y \quad n = 1, \ldots, N. \tag{12}$$

We remark that in problem VP^{hk} the "initial condition" u_0^{hk} for the displacement field must be calculated because it is not previously given. Thus, we take it as the solution to the corresponding discrete problem:

$$c(\beta_0^h; u_0^{hk}, v^h) = (f_0, v^h)_V \quad \forall v^h \in V^h.$$

We have the following theorem which states the linear convergence of these approximations under suitable additional regularity conditions.

Theorem 1. *Assume that problem VP has a unique solution (u, β) with the following regularity:*

$$u \in \mathcal{C}([0, T]; [H^2(\Omega)]^d) \cap \mathcal{C}^1([0, T]; V),$$
$$\beta \in H^2(0, T; Y) \cap H^1(0, T; H^1(\Omega)) \cap \mathcal{C}([0, T]; H^2(\Omega)),$$

and let (u^{hk}, β^{hk}) be the solution to Problem VP^{hk}. Then, it follows that the numerical approximation is linearly convergent; that is, there exists a positive constant C, independent of the discretization parameters h and k, such that

$$\max_{0 \leq n \leq N} \left\{ \|u_n - u_n^{hk}\|_V + \|\beta_n - \beta_n^{hk}\|_Y \right\} \leq C(h+k).$$

Proof. First, proceeding as in [16], we have the following estimates for the damage field, for all $\zeta^h = \{\zeta_j^h\}_{j=0}^n \subset K^h$,

$$\|\beta_n - \beta_n^{hk}\|_Y^2 + k \sum_{j=1}^n \|\nabla(\beta_n - \beta_n^{hk})\|_Y^2 \leq C \Big(\|\beta_0 - \beta_0^h\|_Y^2 + \|\beta_1 - \zeta_1^h\|_Y^2 + \|\beta_n - \zeta_n^h\|_Y^2$$
$$+ k \sum_{j=1}^n \|\beta_{j-1} - \beta_{j-1}^{hk}\|_Y^2 + k \sum_{j=1}^n \|u_j - u_j^{hk}\|_V^2 + k \sum_{j=1}^n \|\beta_j - \zeta_j^h\|_{H^1(\Omega)}^2 + k^2 + k \sum_{j=1}^n \|\delta\beta_j - \dot{\beta}_j\|_Y^2$$
$$+ k \sum_{j=1}^n \|\phi(\varepsilon(u_j), \beta_j) - \delta\beta_j + \kappa^* \Delta \beta_j\|_Y \|\beta_j - \zeta_j^h\|_Y + k^{-1} \sum_{j=1}^{n-1} \|\beta_{j+1} - \zeta_{j+1}^h - (\beta_j - \zeta_j^j)\|_Y^2 \Big),$$

where we used the notation $\delta\beta_j = (\beta_j - \beta_{j-1})/k$ and the regularity of the continuous solution β.

Now, we obtain the estimates for the displacement fields. Subtracting the variational Equation (9) at time t_n for $v = v^h \in V^h \subset V$ and the discrete variational Equation (11) we have

$$c(\beta_n; u_n, v^h) - c(\beta_n^{hk}; u_n^{hk}, v^h) \quad \forall v^h \in V^h,$$

so it follows that, for all $v^h \in V^h$,

$$c(\beta_n; u_n, u_n - u_n^{hk}) - c(\beta_n^{hk}; u_n^{hk}, u_n - u_n^{hk}) = c(\beta_n; u_n, u_n - v^h) - c(\beta_n^{hk}; u_n^{hk}, u_n - v^h).$$

Taking into account that

$$c(\beta_n; u_n, u_n - u_n^{hk}) - c(\beta_n^{hk}; u_n^{hk}, u_n - u_n^{hk}) = c(\beta_n^{hk}; u_n - u_n^{hk}, u_n - u_n^{hk}) + c(\beta_n - \beta_n^{hk}; u_n, u_n - u_n^{hk}),$$
$$c(\beta_n^{hk}; u_n - u_n^{hk}, u_n - u_n^{hk}) \geq C\|u_n - u_n^{hk}\|_V^2,$$

using the fact that $\beta_n^{hk} \in K^h$ (and so, $\beta_n^{hk} \geq \beta_*$) and the regularity $u \in \mathcal{C}([0,T]; [H^2(\Omega)]^d)$ we have

$$\|u_n - u_n^{hk}\|_V^2 \leq C \Big(\|\beta_n - \beta_n^{hk}\|_Y^2 + \|u_n - v^h\|_V^2 \Big) \quad \forall v^h \in V^h.$$

Therefore, combining the previous estimates of both damage and displacement fields we conclude that

$$\|\beta_n - \beta_n^{hk}\|_Y^2 + \|u_n - u_n^{hk}\|_V^2 \leq C \Big(\|\beta_0 - \beta_0^h\|_Y^2 + \|\beta_1 - \zeta_1^h\|_Y^2 + \|\beta_n - \zeta_n^h\|_Y^2 + k \sum_{j=1}^n \|\beta_{j-1} - \beta_{j-1}^{hk}\|_Y^2$$
$$+ k \sum_{j=1}^n \|u_j - u_j^{hk}\|_V^2 + k \sum_{j=1}^n \|\beta_j - \zeta_j^h\|_{H^1(\Omega)}^2 + k^2 + k \sum_{j=1}^n \|\delta\beta_j - \dot{\beta}_j\|_Y^2 + \|u_n - v^h\|_V^2$$
$$+ k \sum_{j=1}^n \|\phi(\varepsilon(u_j), \beta_j) - \delta\beta_j + \kappa^* \Delta \beta_j\|_Y \|\beta_j - \zeta_j^h\|_Y + k^{-1} \sum_{j=1}^{n-1} \|\beta_{j+1} - \zeta_{j+1}^h - (\beta_j - \zeta_j^j)\|_Y^2 \Big).$$

Finally, keeping in mind that

$$k^{-1} \sum_{j=1}^{n-1} \|\beta_{j+1} - \zeta_{j+1}^h - (\beta_j - \zeta_j^j)\|_Y^2 \leq Ch^2 \|\beta\|_{H^1(0,T;H^1(\Omega))}^2,$$

using the well-known approximation properties by finite elements (see [17]) and a discrete version of Gronwall's inequality, we obtain the desired linear convergence. □

The fully discrete scheme provided in problem VP^{hk} has been solved using a penalty-duality algorithm, related to Uzawa's algorithm, for the numerical resolution of the discrete variational inequality. The discrete displacements have been obtained solving the discrete linear variational equation with the classical conjugate gradient method. We note that a similar scheme has also been employed for the numerical approximation of dynamic contact problems (see, for example, [16]). Moreover, the resulting algorithm has been implemented within the well-known code MATLAB in a 3.3 GHz PC (with 16 Gb of RAM memory), and a typical 1D run with parameters $h = k = 10^2$ took about 1.54 s of CPU time.

In order to show the numerical convergence of the algorithm we solve Problem P with the following parameters:

$$T = 2, \quad \Omega = (0,1), \quad \Gamma_D = \{0\}, \quad \Gamma_N = \{1\}, \quad \mathbf{g} = \mathbf{0},$$
$$\lambda = 0, \quad \mu = 1.348 \times 10^{10}, \quad \kappa^* = 0.5, \quad \beta_* = 0.01,$$
$$q^* = 10^5, \quad \lambda_d = 17, \quad \lambda_u = 4.2 \times 10^5, \quad \lambda_w = 0,$$

with the initial condition:

$$\beta_0(x) = 1 \quad \text{for all} \quad x \in (0,1),$$

and the volumetric force:

$$f_0(x,t) = \begin{cases} 90 \times 10^6 \cdot t & \text{if } t < 1, \\ 90 \times 10^6 & \text{if } t \geq 1. \end{cases}$$

The numerical errors are given by

$$E^{hk} = \max_{0 \leq n \leq N} \left\{ \|u_n - u_n^{hk}\|_V + \|\beta_n - \beta_n^{hk}\|_Y \right\},$$

considering as "exact solution" (u_n, β_n) the one obtained for $h = 2^{-12}$ and $k = 10^{-5}$. The errors (multiplied by 100), obtained for different discretizations, are shown in Table 1 and depicted in Figure 1 against $h + k$. As shown, the linear convergence of the algorithm stated in Theorem 1 seems to be achieved.

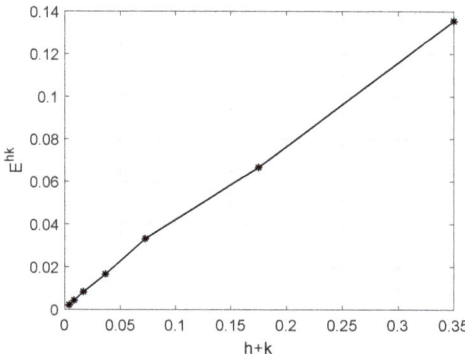

Figure 1. Asymptotic constant error.

Table 1. Numerical errors (×100) for some discretization parameters.

$h \downarrow k \rightarrow$	0.1	0.01	0.001	0.0001
2^{-2}	13.5490	13.5613	13.561268	13.561268
2^{-3}	6.6596	6.6679	6.667863	6.667863
2^{-4}	3.3080	3.3054	3.305386	3.305386
2^{-5}	1.6641	1.6457	1.645661	1.645661
2^{-6}	0.8460	0.8210	0.821036	0.821036
2^{-7}	0.4370	0.4099	0.409942	0.409942
2^{-8}	0.2328	0.2046	0.204565	0.204565
2^{-9}	0.1315	0.1017	0.101652	0.101653
2^{-10}	0.0822	0.0496	0.049597	0.049596

2.2. García et al. Model

The other model examined is the one proposed by García et al. [10,18]. It consists of a rheological model developed specifically for cortical bone, to reproduce the macroscopical phenomenon observed in this tissue. The model is written using several internal variables for damage and plastic strain, as well as laws to describe the evolution of these internal variables.

In [10], several models are presented. For the present study the rate independent model is chosen, since it allows for a more immediate comparison. The rheological model is composed of an elastic spring in series with the damageable part, which consists of a secondary spring, whose elasticity varies with damage, and a friction element that determines the plasticity threshold.

From this rheological model a free energy potential is obtained, which is convex and nonsmooth:

$$\Psi(\varepsilon, \varepsilon^p, D) = \begin{cases} \frac{1}{2} E_0 (\varepsilon - \varepsilon^p)^2 + \frac{1}{2} E_0 \frac{1-D}{D} \varepsilon^{p2} + I_{[0,1]}(D) & \text{if } D > 0, \\ \frac{1}{2} E_0 \varepsilon^2 + I_{\{0\}}(\varepsilon^p) & \text{if } D = 0, \end{cases} \quad (13)$$

and the state laws of the material can be derived from this potential. The details of this derivation can be found in [10], and we omit them for the sake of clarity in the presentation.

Regarding the García et al. model, the algorithm they developed to solve their model was used. Again, we refer to [10] for more details about its implementation. It is based on the combination of the classical finite element method with a Newton integration scheme and a projection operator. The latter one is used to satisfy the criterion defined for the internal variables.

3. Numerical Results and Discussion

3.1. Comparison in a One-Dimensional Problem

To compare the performance of the models presented in the previous section, a one-dimensional version of both was implemented. To test the models, a typical tensile test was reproduced, since there is experimental data in the literature to evaluate the performance [18]. The one-dimensional model represents a bone fixed on one end and with an increasing displacement imposed on the other end. Stress was computed in postprocessing once the deformation was obtained.

First, we solve the Frémond–Nedjar model with the following data:

$$T = 2, \quad \Omega = (0,1), \quad \Gamma_D = \{0,1\}, \quad \Gamma_N = \emptyset, \quad f_0 = 0,$$
$$g = 0, \quad \lambda = 0, \quad \mu = 1.348 \times 10^{10}, \quad \kappa^* = 0.5, \quad \beta_* = 0.01,$$
$$q^* = 10^5, \quad \lambda_d = 17, \quad \lambda_u = 4.2 \times 10^5, \quad \lambda_w = 0,$$

and the initial condition:

$$\beta_0(x) = 1 \quad \text{for all} \quad x \in (0,1).$$

That is, at initial time we assumed that the bone was completely healed. Moreover, since no mechanical forces were applied, the deformation is produced defining an imposed displacement at the right corner as,

$$u(1,t) = 5 \times 10^{-3} \cdot t \quad \text{for all} \quad t \in [0,2].$$

We note that the modifications needed to include this case into problem P were really straightforward, so the analysis performed in the previous section could be extended easily.

Using the discretization parameters $k = 0.01$ and $h = 0.05$ in Figure 2 (up) the stress–strain curve obtained with the Frémond–Nedjar model is shown. As it can be seen in the evolution of the damage variable (down), the mechanical properties of the bone degrade as the strain increases, leading to the "plastic" region which corresponds with the damage regime of the stress–strain curve.

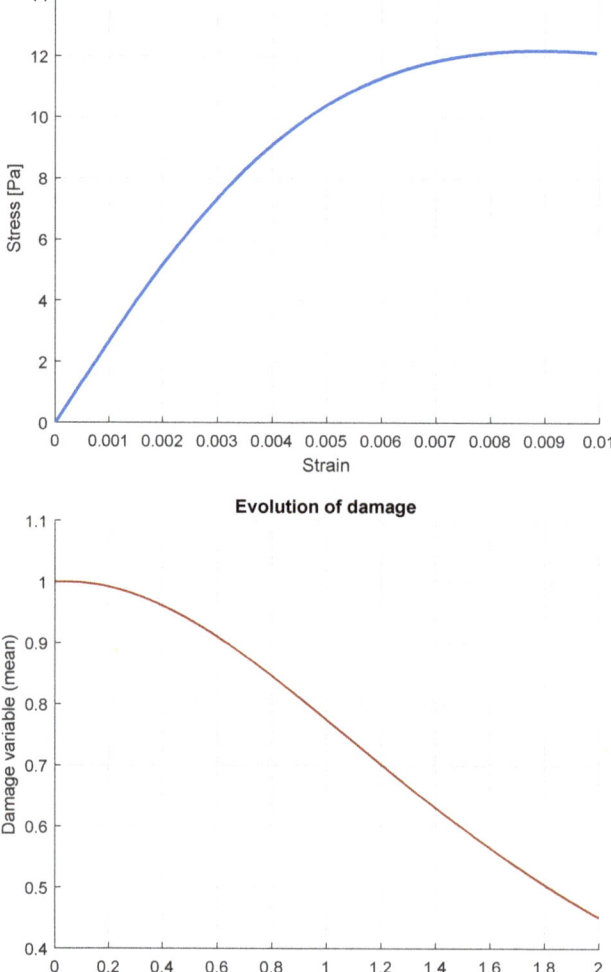

Figure 2. Stress–strain curve obtained with the Frémond–Nedjar model in a tensile test (**up**) and evolution of the damage variable in the tensile test (**down**).

Secondly, the García et al. model was solved, so in Figure 3 the shape of the stress–strain curve seen before is reproduced again with the rheological model.

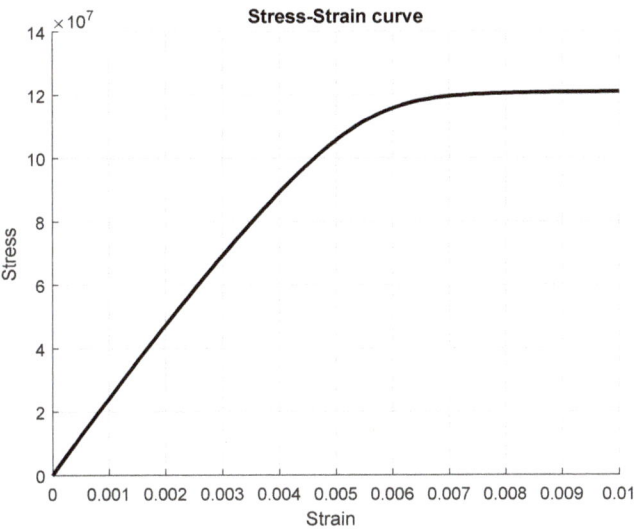

Figure 3. Stress–strain curve obtained with the García et al. model in a tensile test.

Finally, both models were compared with experimental data obtained from [18]. Figure 4 shows the stress–strain curves obtained from both models against the experimental data (black dots). Both models show good agreement with the experimental results, with small differences in the linear part of the curve and the beginning of the damage range. The Frémond–Nedjar model shows better agreement in the linear part, but the curvature of the damage range fits worse than the rheological model. However, these small differences were not significant, since mechanical properties vary greatly from bone to bone, making very accurate fittings not useful.

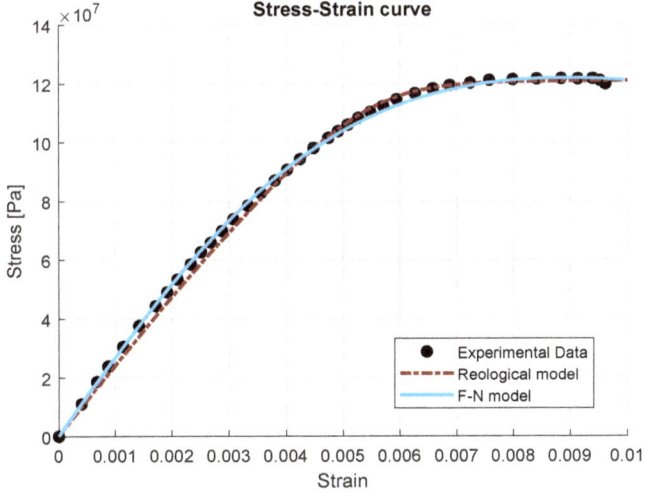

Figure 4. Comparative of both models with experimental data. Source of the experimental data: [18].

In any case, both models were capable of reproducing the qualitative characteristics of bone mechanics. In particular, the modified Frémond–Nedjar model shows its capability to be used to model bone tissue in spite of it being proposed to model concrete structures.

3.2. A Two-Dimensional Problem Solved Using Frémond–Nedjar Model

Now, we consider a two-dimensional case to simulate a more realistic setting. Thus, the bone occupied a two-dimensional domain Ω, which was assumed fixed on its left part Γ_D (the whole part clamped on the vertical direction and its lower point also in the horizontal one), and subjected to the action of a surface force on its right part Γ_N (see Figure 5).

The following data have been used in this example:

$T = 5$, $f_0 = 0$, $g = (5,0)$, $\lambda = 21.1 \times 10^{10}$, $\mu = 24.61 \times 10^{10}$, $\kappa^* = 1$, $\beta_* = 0.01$, $q^* = 10^5$, $\lambda_d = 0.01$, $\lambda_u = 15$, $\lambda_w = -0.0001$,

and the initial condition:

$$\beta_0(x,y) = 1 \quad \text{for all} \quad (x,y) \in \Omega.$$

That is, again at initial time we assumed that the bone was completely healed.

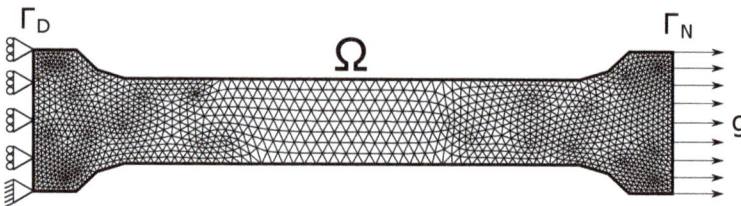

Figure 5. Physical settting and finite element mesh.

Using the time discretization parameter $k = 0.1$ and the finite element mesh shown in Figure 5, the damage field at final time is plotted over the deformed configuration in Figure 6. As expected, the most damaged areas concentrated in the middle of the bone due to the applied force and the clamping conditions.

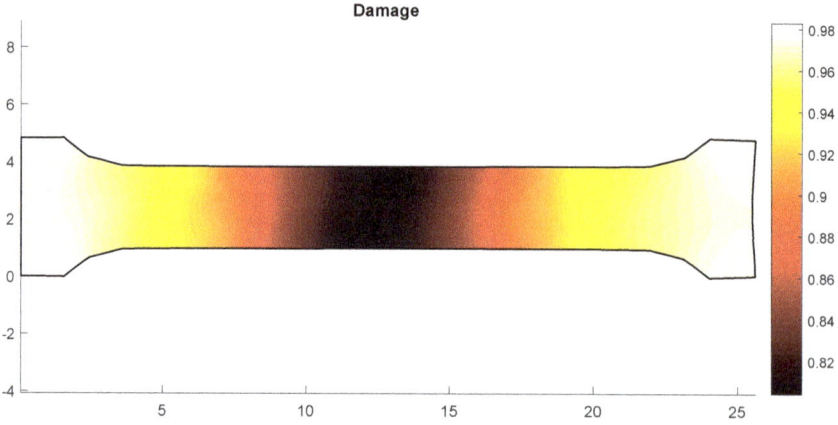

Figure 6. Damage field at final time over the deformed configuration.

Finally, in Figure 7 the stress field is shown at final time over the deformed configuration. We note that now the highest stressed areas concentrated in the middle part of the bone. The concentration of the damage and stress in the middle of the sample agree with the observed fracture of the real probes in uniaxial tests by on middle section.

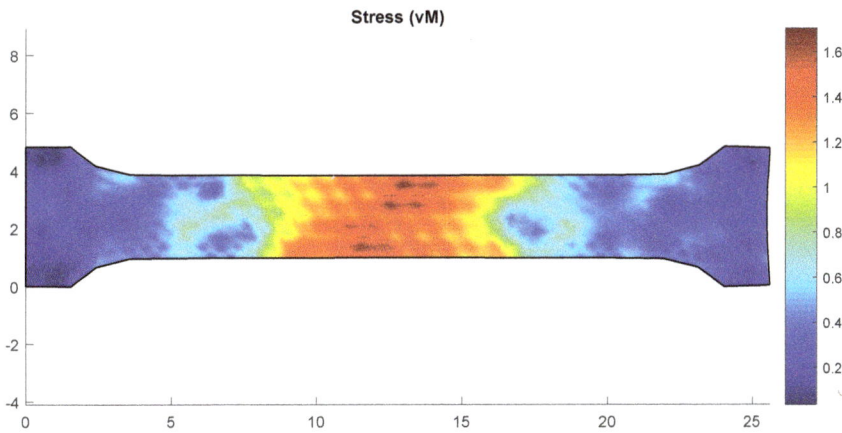

Figure 7. The von Mises stress norm at final time over the deformed configuration.

4. Conclusions

In this work, two ways of modelling damage in cortical bone were studied. The first one was a modification of a well-known damage model for concrete structures, never used for bone tissue. The second one was developed specifically for bone damage and based on a rheological model. One-dimensional simulations were performed to compare both models, reproducing a classical tensile test. Both models show similar solutions and a good agreement with experimental data. Moreover, a two-dimensional example was also considered using the Frémond–Nedjar model to show the behaviour of its solution in a more real situation. The advantage of the use of the Frémond–Nedjar model relies in its formulation, which makes it easier to couple with bone remodelling models, and it allows for a formal numerical analysis. The number of parameters required for this model is also reduced with respect to the García et al. model. These results open the possibility of using this model in bone tissue simulations.

Author Contributions: Conceptualization and Methodology J.B., J.R.F. and A.S.; Software, Formal Analysis and Data Curation J.B. and J.A.L.-C.; Validation J.B., J.R.F. and A.S.; Supervision J.R.F. and A.S.; Writing—Original Draft Preparation J.B. and J.R.F.; Writing—Review and Editing J.A.L.-C. and A.S.; Funding Acquisition J.R.F. and A.S.

Funding: This work has been partially funded by the research project PGC2018-096696-B-I00 (Ministerio de Ciencia, Innovación y Universidades, Spain). J. Baldonedo acknowledges the funding by Xunta de Galicia (Spain) under the program *Axudas á etapa predoutoral* with Ref. ED481A-2019/230. J.A. López-Campos also acknowledges the funding by Xunta de Galicia (Spain) under the program *Axudas á etapa predoutoral* with Ref. ED481A-2017/045.

Conflicts of Interest: The authors declare no conflict of interest.

References

1. Mazars, J. A description of micro- and macroscale damage of concrete structures. *Eng. Fract. Mech.* **1986**, *25*, 729–739. [CrossRef]
2. Frémond, M.; Nedjar, B. Damage, gradient of damage and principle of virtual power. *Int. J. Solids Struct.* **1996**, *33*, 1083–1103. [CrossRef]

3. Nedjar, B. Elastoplastic-damage modelling including the gradient of damage: Formulation and computational aspects. *Int. J. Solids Struct.* **2001**, *38*, 5421–5451. [CrossRef]
4. Wolff, J. *The Law of Bone Remodelling*; Springer: Berlin/Heidelberg, Germany, 1986.
5. Weinans, H.; Huiskes, R.; Grootenboer, H.J. The behavior of adaptive bone-remodeling simulation models. *J. Biomech.* **1992**, *25*, 1425–1441. [CrossRef]
6. Fondrk, M.T.; Bahniuk, E.H.; Davy, D.T. Inelastic strain accumulation in cortical bone during rapid transient tensile loading. *J. Biomech. Eng.* **1999**, *121*, 616–621. [CrossRef] [PubMed]
7. Carter, D.R.; Caler, W.E. A cumulative damage model for bone fracture. *J. Orthop. Res.* **1985**, *3*, 84–90. [CrossRef] [PubMed]
8. Pattin, C.A.; Caler, W.E.; Carter, D.R. Cyclic mechanical property degradation during fatigue loading of cortical bone. *J. Biomech.* **1996**, *29*, 69–79. [CrossRef]
9. Fondrk, M.T.; Bahniuk, E.H.; Davy, D.T. A Damage Model for Nonlinear Tensile Behavior of Cortical Bone. *J. Biomech. Eng.* **1999**, *121*, 533–541. [CrossRef] [PubMed]
10. Garcia, D.; Zysset, P.K.; Charlebois, M.; Curnier, A. A 1D elastic plastic damage constitutive law for bone tissue. *Arch. Appl. Mech.* **2009**, *80*, 543–555. [CrossRef]
11. Ramtani, S. Damaged elastic bone-column buckling theory within the context of adaptive elasticity. *Mech. Res. Commun.* **2018**, *88*, 1–6. [CrossRef]
12. Ramtani, S.; Zidi, M. Damaged-bone remodeling theory: Thermodynamical Approach. *Mech. Res. Commun.* **1999**, *26*, 701–708. [CrossRef]
13. Hosseini, H.S.; Horák, M.; Zysset, P.K.; Jirásek, M. An over-nonlocal implicit gradient-enhanced damage-plastic model for trabecular bone under large compressive strains. *Int. J. Numer. Methods Biomed. Eng.* **2015**, *31*, e02728. [CrossRef] [PubMed]
14. Martínez, G.; García-Aznar, J.M.; Doblaré, M.; Cerrolaza, M. External bone remodeling through boundary elements and damage mechanics. *Math. Comput. Simul.* **2006**, *73*, 183–199. [CrossRef]
15. Mengoni, M.; Ponthot, J.P. An enhanced version of a bone-remodelling model based on the continuum damage mechanics theory. *Comput. Methods Biomech. Biomed. Eng.* **2015**, *18*, 1367–1376. [CrossRef] [PubMed]
16. Campo, M.; Fernández, J.R.; Kuttler, K.L.; Shillor, M.; Via no, J.M. Numerical analysis and simulations of a dynamic frictionless contact problem with damage. *Comput. Methods Appl. Mech. Eng.* **2006**, *196*, 476–488. [CrossRef]
17. Ciarlet, P.G. Basic error estimates for elliptic problems. In *Handbook of Numerical Analysis*; Ciarlet, P.G., Lions, J.L., Eds.; North-Holland: Amsterdam, The Netherlands, 1993; Volume II, pp. 17–351.
18. García, D. Elastic Plastic Damage Laws for Cortical Bone. Ph.D. Thesis, Lausanne, École Polytechnique Fédérale de Lausanne, Lausanne, Switzerland, 2006.

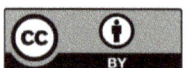

© 2019 by the authors. Licensee MDPI, Basel, Switzerland. This article is an open access article distributed under the terms and conditions of the Creative Commons Attribution (CC BY) license (http://creativecommons.org/licenses/by/4.0/).

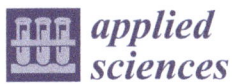

Article

Multiscale Characterisation of Cortical Bone Tissue

José A. Sanz-Herrera [1,*], Juan Mora-Macías [2], Esther Reina-Romo [1], Jaime Domínguez [1] and Manuel Doblaré [3]

1. Escuela Técnica Superior de Ingeniería, Universidad de Sevilla, 41092 Seville, Spain; erreina@us.es (E.R.-R.); jaime@us.es (J.D.)
2. Department of Mining, Mechanical, Energy and Construction Engineering, University of Huelva, Campus Universitario La Rábida, Escuela Técnica Superior de Ingeniería, Palos de la Frontera, 21007 Huelva, Spain; juan.mora@dimme.uhu.es
3. Aragon Institute of Engineering Research (I3A), University of Zaragoza, 50018 Zaragoza, Spain; mdoblare@unizar.es
* Correspondence: jsanz@us.es; Tel.: +34-954487293

Received: 28 October 2019; Accepted: 27 November 2019; Published: 1 December 2019

Featured Application: Multiscale analysis is widely applied in the field of mechanics of heterogeneous materials, as a numerical tool, to simulate both microstructure evolution and macroscopic response to loads. The potential of this technique is applied in this work to the micro- and macro-mechanical study of the cortical bone tissue, using a mixed experimental-numerical approach. Hence, the experimental characterisation of the cortical bone is used to calibrate the outcome of the multiscale analysis. This strategy provides useful information at macro- and micro scales. First, the apparent mechanical (orthotropic) behaviour of the tissue is obtained. Second, microstrain and microstress distributions are shown along the bone microstructure. The multiscale analysis presented in this paper can be a useful technique to further investigate the microstructural and local mechanical stimulus which orchestrates several bone functions, such as bone remodelling.

Abstract: Multiscale analysis has become an attractive technique to predict the behaviour of materials whose microstructure strongly changes spatially or among samples, with that microstructure controlling the local constitutive behaviour. This is the case, for example, of most biological tissues—such as bone. Multiscale approaches not only allow, not only to better characterise the local behaviour, but also to predict the field-variable distributions (e.g., strains, stresses) at both scales (macro and micro) simultaneously. However, multiscale analysis usually lacks sufficient experimental feedback to demonstrate its validity. In this paper an experimental and numerical micromechanics analysis is developed with application to cortical bone. Displacement and strain fields are obtained across the microstructure by means of digital image correlation (DIC). The other mechanical variables are computed following the micromechanics theory. Special emphasis is given to the differences found in the different field variables between the micro- and macro-structures, which points out the need for this multiscale approach in cortical bone tissue. The obtained results are used to establish the basis of a multiscale methodology with application to the analysis of bone tissue mechanics at different spatial scales.

Keywords: cortical bone; digital image correlation; multiscale analysis; micromechanics; computational mechanics

1. Introduction

The key importance of mechanical factors on the physiological functions and processes that take place in the bone tissue, in both healthy and pathological conditions, is widely accepted [1–3].

Therefore, in recent decades, important efforts have been made in the mechanical characterisation of bone tissue [4,5] (at different scales), and the mathematical modelling of its mechanical and mechanobiological behaviour [6–8].

On the one hand, the properties of the bone tissue are affected by a high number of factors, such as its morphological complexity and porosity, anisotropic orientation of trabeculae and osteons or its inherent hierarchical structure. A large number of studies characterise the structural and mechanical behaviour of the bone tissue by means of micromechanical [9,10], nano-mechanical [11] and macroscopic approaches [12], to cite a few. They all show the heterogeneity of this tissue at all scales and the difficulty of relating experimental measurements to real tissue properties. For example, Tai et al. [11] show, with atomic force microscopy experiments and computational simulations, that the nanomechanical properties and shape of cortical bone are directly related to their macroscopic mechanical behaviour, being this structure-property relation a key factor in some non-physiological behaviour of the bone tissue. Therefore, processes such as bone damage, bone remodelling and bone-related diseases (e.g., osteoporosis and fracture healing) could be better understood by relating microscale material heterogeneity to its macroscopic structural performance.

One of the techniques that allows to obtain microscopic parameters in inhomogeneous, anisotropic and non-linear materials is digital image correlation (DIC). It is particularly suitable for biological tissues and has been successfully used for measuring the strain field in bone tissue [13–15]. It consists of comparing the positions of different points of reference within a deformable loaded region that is photographed at different times. These points of reference are usually painted in the sample using a spray to create a speckles pattern. Using this method, the strain field of a region of interest within a specimen may be provided with microscopic resolution. The advantage of this method over others, such as nanoindentation [10,11], is that the whole strain field is recorded easily for different loading conditions. This technique, however, generate large amounts of data in comparison with traditional methods.

On the other hand, there is a vast literature related to modelling bone tissue in many different scenarios and at several scales. The models may be classified—according to the observation scale—as macroscopic and microscopic. At the macroscopic scale, several issues have been addressed in the last few decades, such as modelling/remodelling [16–23], poroelasticity [24,25], bone healing [26–28] or bone tissue engineering [29–32] among many others. Moreover, the driven mechanical stimulus [27,33–36] and the microstructural distribution of mechanical variables have also been studied [37–40].

The multiscale analysis is a technique initially applied in the framework of the mechanics of heterogeneous materials. Specifically, multiscale techniques have been used in the analysis of fluid circulation within a porous medium [41], plasticity [42,43], thermoelasticity or composite adhesives [44,45], to cite a few (refer to [46] for a review of multiscale analysis in different applications). On the other hand, multiscale analysis has progressively developed great potential for the combined macro-and-micro analysis of biological tissues due to their hierarchical, multiphasic and heterogeneous nature [47], such as tissue engineering processes [30,31,48]. Cancellous bone has been one the first candidates to be analysed through a multiscale approach [49–51]. However, cortical bone tissue has not been such a clear candidate, probably due to the lack of such a clear porous microstructure as compared to the cancellous bone, so it has been traditionally modelled as homogeneous, anisotropic material with directly homogenised properties [52]. However, some of the most interesting microstructures of the bone tissue are present in the cortical region including canaliculi, or Haversian and Volkmann canals [53,54].

The referred studies of the multiscale analysis of the bone tissue are developed independently of its mechanical characterization. In this paper, cortical bone is studied from a multiscale perspective to model an experimental setup specifically developed for this analysis. Therefore, the developed mathematical analysis and simulation is fed by the results recorded in the experiments providing a novel and mixed computational-experimental approach. The outcomes of the multiscale approach for the cortical tissue allow to conclude the importance of using a multiscale approach to capture the heterogeneity of the results along the microstructure, which is critical in order to understand many of the essential biological processes of bone tissue at this level.

The paper is arranged as follows: first, the experimental setup is introduced in the Section 2. Second, the mathematical multiscale approach is developed in Section 3. Both experimental and numerical results are presented in Section 4. Finally, the results are discussed and some conclusions are established at the end of the paper.

2. Materials and Methods

A cortical bone sample from the left femur of an adult male horse, aged between 15–20 years old, was used to obtain the strain maps under both longitudinal and transversal forces by means of the Digital Image Correlation (DIC) technology. Sample preparation and experimental tests were carried out as follows.

2.1. Sample Preparation

To prepare the bone sample, first, a rectangular bone piece was extracted from the mid diaphysis of the femur, lateral cranial side, by means of a band saw (Figure 1a). Second, the surface of the sample was polished with carbide papers (P600 to P4000). Colloidal silica slurry (0.04 µm) was used for the final polishing step. The sample was cleaned ultrasonically with distilled water between each polishing step. The size of the plane specimen obtained after this stage was 50 × 20 × 4 mm, with the direction of the larger side corresponding to the longitudinal direction of the bone (Figure 1b). Thirdly, the sample bone ends (10 mm approximately) were embedded in Epoxy® resin (Struers Inc, Cleveland, OH, USA) to fix them to the testing machine (Figure 1c). Finally, the spray painting was carried out with black speckles over a bright white background. It can be observed in Figure 1d that the speckles are consistent in size.

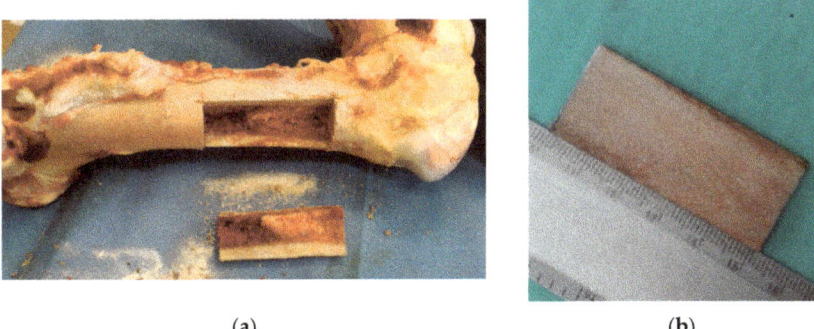

(a)　　　　　　　　　　　　　　　　(b)

Figure 1. *Cont.*

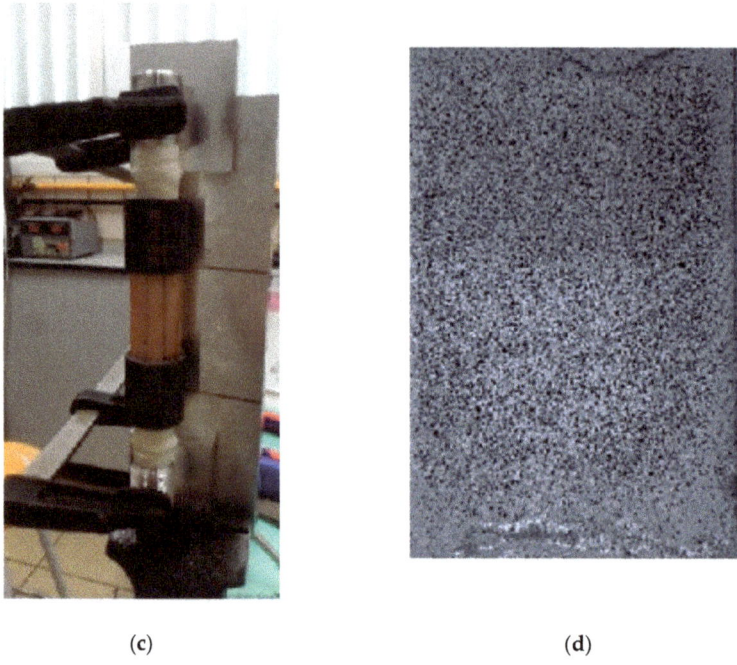

(c)   (d)

Figure 1. (a) Horse femur after extracting a piece from the mid diaphysis for machining; (b) one of the four specimens after milling; (c) embedding process; (d) spray speckle for digital image correlation strain measurements.

2.2. Experimental Tests

The experimental tests are composed of mechanical tests and strain measurements of the sample. The former consisted of applying both longitudinal compressive (F_L) and transversal compressive (F_T) forces to the prepared sample (Figure 2a). The F_L was applied in the direction of the larger side of the specimen by means of a push-pull testing machine (KEELAVITE® 50 kN) (Figure 2b). This machine consists of a hydraulic actuator directed by an automatic control (MTS 407®), which allows to apply loads up to 50 kN (Figure 2b). The longitudinal system is equipped with an Eaton Lebow 20 Klbf load cell (model: 3174-20K) for force measurement. The piston of the machine, threaded to the inferior end of the sample, compresses the sample, whose superior end is threaded to the fixed frame. In addition, a complementary device [55] allows to apply transversal compressive force (F_T) in the mid-section of the specimen as shown in Figure 2a. This device consists of a linear screw type actuator controlled manually [55], in which forces up to 1500 N are measured with a load cell connected in series (Interface 2 Klbf, model: WMC-2000).

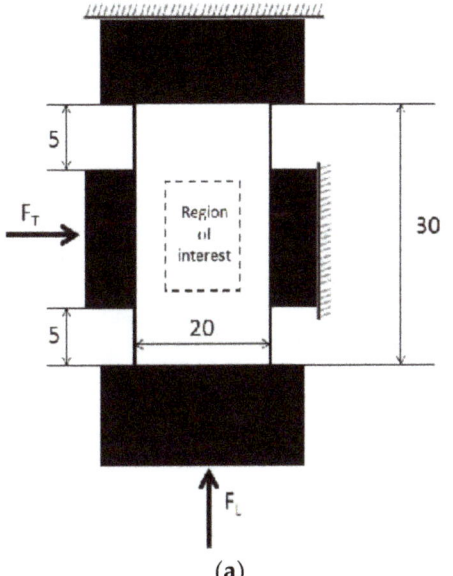
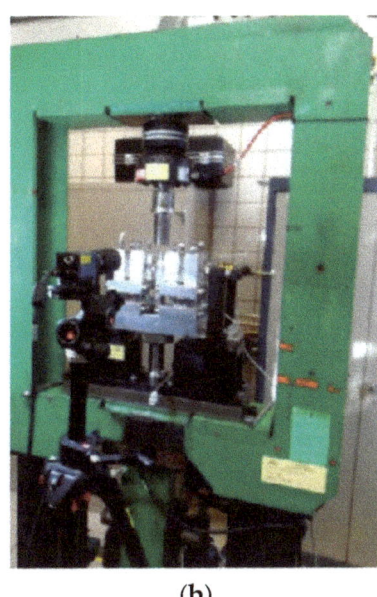

Figure 2. (a) Scheme of the loads applied to the specimen, longitudinal forces, F_L, and transversal forces, F_T; (b) picture of the system during experiments. The push-pull testing machine may be observed in the back ground. The piston and the load cell above, attached to the green frame, can be observed. The system that applies the transversal load can be seen below, while the DIC camera appears in front.

A total of eight different loading states were simulated for transversal and longitudinal force values 0, 250 and 500 N as indicated in Table 1. For each loading state, transversal and longitudinal loads were applied from 0 to the desired level of load in static conditions. The load was applied very slowly, below 10 N/s. During load application, the strain in the region of interest was measured as described below. During the 6 h required to complete the test, from the moment that the samples are taken out of the freezer, the sample was not hydrated.

Table 1. Macroscopic results of the mechanical tests.

F_L [N]	F_T [N]	$\varepsilon_L \times 10^{-3}$ [%]	$\varepsilon_T \times 10^{-3}$ [%]
0	−250	5.8	−17.6
0	−500	21.4	−35.9
−250	0	−16.5	9.5
−250	−250	−9.8	−8.8
−250	−500	0.55	−27.7
−500	0	−36.3	16.8
−500	−250	−28.2	−0.025
−500	−500	−17.9	−20.3

Note: Table notes. F_L: Overall longitudinal force. F_T: Overall transversal force. ε_L : Averaged longitudinal component of the strain tensor. ε_T : Averaged transversal component of the strain tensor.

To determine the strain of the bone sample during the biaxial test, an optical non-contact system (Limess®, Q400; Vic Snap Image Acquisition®, version 2010, build 902; and Vic2D 2009®, version 2009.1.0, build 345M) was used (Figure 3a). This system allows to obtain the history of deformations in real time on the outer surface of the sample. Strain measurements were performed in the 10 × 10 mm region of interest located in the middle of the sample (see Figure 2a). The resolution of the system allows to measure strains in points with a separation of 57 µm within the region of interest. It means that the analysed region generates a strain field of around 34,000 points. Strain maps were taken at the loading points selected with the DIC camera, which took pictures of the bone surface every 20 ms (Figure 3b). In addition, a micrograph of the region of interest in the bone sample was carried out for meshing purposes. A high resolution image with a size of 11.63 × 11.8 mm was manually generated from 54 images taken by microscopy with 5× magnification. These images were converted into a finite element model of the mineralised portion of the specimen.

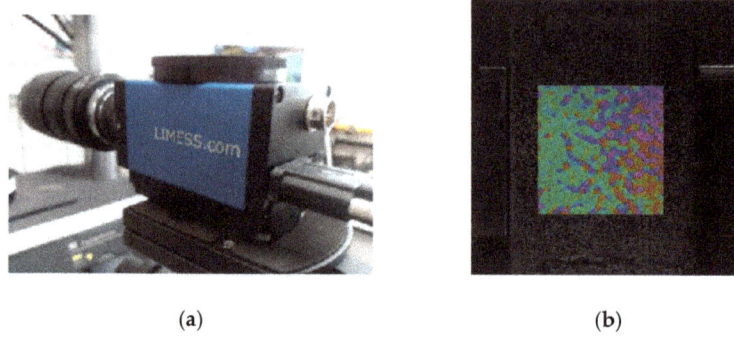

(a)   (b)

Figure 3. (a) Non-contact two-dimensional (2D) deformation system used to obtain the strain maps in the bone samples; (b) strains measured in the region of interest of the sample.

3. Mathematical Approach

The analysis of heterogeneous media involves two well-distinguished scales: the macroscopic scale (**x**), with characteristic length (L), in which the size of the heterogeneities is very small; and the microscopic scale (**y**), with characteristic length (ℓ), which is the scale of the heterogeneities. To sustain this statement, we must assume the length separation scale condition, i.e., $L \gg \ell$. In order to deal with the macroscopic scale as a continuum in a macroscopic material point, the microscopic scale is homogenised in terms of its effective behaviour over a Representative Volume Element (RVE). An RVE must statistically represent the underlying microstructure of the specimen, in such a way that every material point of the macroscopic region is featured by such RVE. Another definition of the RVE may be established as it being the smallest microstructural volume that sufficiently and accurately represents the overall macroscopic properties of interest. The minimum required RVE size also depends on the type of material behaviour, macroscopic loading path and difference of properties between heterogeneities.

In the following, the variable **x** stands in the homogeneous macroscopic body, whereas **y** describes the microscopic scale of the RVE. In the microscopic scale, the domain is composed by the (solid or bulk) bone (B) and pore (P) bodies, so that RVE $\equiv \Omega_B^\varphi \cup \Omega_P^\varphi$. The linear elastic equations are posed in the RVE domain to obtain the averaged, apparent or homogenised mechanical properties and the microscopic distribution of the stress and strain fields. Then, the primary variables are asymptotically expanded as:

$$\mathbf{u}^\varphi = \mathbf{u}^0(\mathbf{x}) + \varphi \mathbf{u}^*(\mathbf{x}, \mathbf{y}) \quad (1)$$

where $\mathbf{u}^\varphi$ is the total displacement field, $\mathbf{u}^0$ is the associated field variable averaged at the macroscopic scale and $\mathbf{u}^*$ is the perturbation (oscillating) functions due to the heterogeneity of the microscopic scale. In Equation (1), $\varphi = \ell/L$ refers to the ratio between the microscopic and macroscopic levels.

For averaging the macroscopic fields, the following operator is defined over a microscopic volume generally denoted by Θ:

$$\langle \blacksquare \rangle = \frac{1}{|\Theta|} \int_\Theta \blacksquare \, d\Theta \quad (2)$$

This expression enables us to obtain macroscopic quantities and, eventually, the macroscopic response (behaviour) induced by the underlying microstructure. This approach is called homogenisation. The inverse procedure, localisation, allows to determine the microscopic values from the macroscopic ones. Both are outlined below.

3.1. Localisation

The linear, elastic, microscopic problem in the absence of body loads reads as:

$$\begin{aligned}\nabla \cdot \sigma^\varphi &= 0 \\ \varepsilon^\varphi &= \tfrac{1}{2}\left(\nabla u^\varphi + (\nabla u^\varphi)^T\right) \\ \sigma^\varphi &= \mathbb{C}^\varphi \varepsilon^\varphi \\ \langle \varepsilon^\varphi \rangle &= \varepsilon^0 \end{aligned} \qquad (3)$$

There is an absence of boundary conditions in Equation (3). These boundary conditions must reproduce, as closely as possible, the in situ state of the RVE inside the material. Therefore, they strongly depend on the choice of the RVE itself, and particularly on its size. Amongst the classical boundary conditions considered in the literature (see Suquet [56] for further reading), Dirichlet boundary conditions are used in our problem:

$$u^\varphi = u^0 \quad \text{on } \partial \Omega_S^\varphi \qquad (4)$$

Then, the local strain $\varepsilon^\varphi(u^\varphi)$ is split into its average and fluctuating term so that:

$$\begin{aligned}\varepsilon^\varphi(u^\varphi) &= \varepsilon^0 + \varepsilon^\varphi(u^*) \\ \langle \varepsilon^\varphi(u^*) \rangle &= 0 \end{aligned} \qquad (5)$$

Let Equation (5) be substituted into the equilibrium (divergence free) equation of the stress tensor (see Equation (3)), namely:

$$\begin{aligned}\nabla \cdot (\mathbb{C}^\varphi \varepsilon^\varphi(u^*)) &= -\nabla \cdot \left(\mathbb{C}^\varphi \varepsilon^0\right) \quad \text{in } \Omega_S^\varphi(y) \\ &+ \text{boundary conditions}\end{aligned} \qquad (6)$$

where the boundary conditions are related to Equation (4). By virtue of the linearity of the problem, the solution of $\varepsilon^\varphi(u^*)$ in Equation (3) for a general macro strain ε^0 may be expressed as the superposition of elementary unit strain solutions $\varepsilon^\varphi(\chi_{kh})$ [56], such that:

$$\varepsilon^\varphi(u^*) = \varepsilon^0_{kh} \varepsilon^\varphi(\chi_{kh}) \qquad (7)$$

where χ_{kh} are the displacements associated to those elementary strain states denoted by indices kh resulting from the solution of Equation (3).

By substitution of Equation (7) into Equation (5), the micro-strains are expressed as:

$$\varepsilon^\varphi(u^\varphi) = \varepsilon^0_{kh}(I_{kh} + \varepsilon^\varphi(\chi_{kh})) \qquad (8)$$

where I_{kh} is the identity fourth order tensor with components $I_{kh} = (I_{ij})_{kh} = 1/2(\delta_{ik}\delta_{jh} + \delta_{ih}\delta_{jk})$. Equation (8) allows us to obtain the microstructural distribution of the strain field, under the aforementioned hypothesis and once the boundary conditions are established through the macroscopic ones.

3.2. Homogenisation

Once the elementary solutions $\varepsilon^\varphi(\chi_{kh})$ are obtained through (8), the macroscopic stress-strain relationship is directly obtained:

$$\sigma^0 = \langle \sigma^\varphi(u^\varphi) \rangle = \langle \mathbb{C}^\varphi \varepsilon^\varphi(u^\varphi) \rangle = \langle \mathbb{C}^\varphi (I_{kh} + \varepsilon^\varphi(\chi_{kh})) \rangle : \varepsilon^0 \qquad (9)$$

Consequently, at the macroscopic scale, the elasticity tensor is identified in Equation (9) as:

$$\mathbb{C}^0 = \langle \mathbb{C}^\varphi (I_{kh} + \varepsilon^\varphi(\chi_{kh})) \rangle \qquad (10)$$

3.3. Variational Formulation

Using the standard formulation, the variational form of Equation (6) yields to [56]:

$$\int_{\Omega_S^\varphi} \varepsilon^\varphi(w) : (\mathbb{C}^\varphi \varepsilon^\varphi(u^*)) dy = -\int_{\Omega_S^\varphi} \varepsilon^\varphi(w) : (\mathbb{C}^\varphi \varepsilon^0) dy \ \forall \ w(y) \in V_Y \qquad (11)$$

where the space V_Y is defined as:

$$V_Y : \{ w \mid w \in H^1(\Omega_S^\varphi) \} \qquad (12)$$

with $H^1(\Omega_S^\varphi)$ as the first-order Sobolev space. Using (7), Equation (11) can be further developed, namely:

$$\int_{\Omega_S^\varphi} C_{ijpq}^\varphi \frac{\partial \chi_p^{kl}}{\partial y_q} \frac{\partial \omega_i}{\partial y_j} dy = \int_{\Omega_S^\varphi} C_{ijkl}^\varphi \frac{\partial \omega_i}{\partial y_j} dy \qquad (13)$$

χ_p^{kl} represents the characteristic microstructure displacement at p directions due to an applied kl unit strain, being $k = l$ normal unit strain states and $k \neq l$ shear unit strain states. ω_i represents a virtual displacement. There are three total strain states (two normal and one shear, assuming plane stress two-dimensional (2D) modelling) corresponding to the three linear equations above (Equation (13)). Once these functions are obtained, the macroscopic stiffness tensor can be computed through Equation (10).

3.4. Multiscale Approach

The multiscale analysis of the cortical bone tissue proceeds as follows. First, at the microstructural level, the overall, apparent or homogenised properties of the macroscopic cortical bone tissue are obtained by solving the homogenisation problem, i.e., Equation (10) in the microscopic domain. The input data to solve this problem are the microstructural domain of the cortical bone tissue (Figure 4) and the mechanical properties of the mineral bone material, which are a parameters to be fitted as explained in Section 4.2.

Second, using the obtained homogenised mechanical properties, the mechanical problem is then solved at the macroscopic domain for a given loading state. Finally, strain and displacement macroscopic quantities, associated to such a loading state, are passed to the microstructure where the localisation problem is solved.

Macro and micro variables are recorded from the macroscopic and microscopic localisation problems, respectively. A sketch of the multiscale procedure can be seen in Figure 5. The details of the computational implementation can be found, as an example, in Yuan and Fish [57].

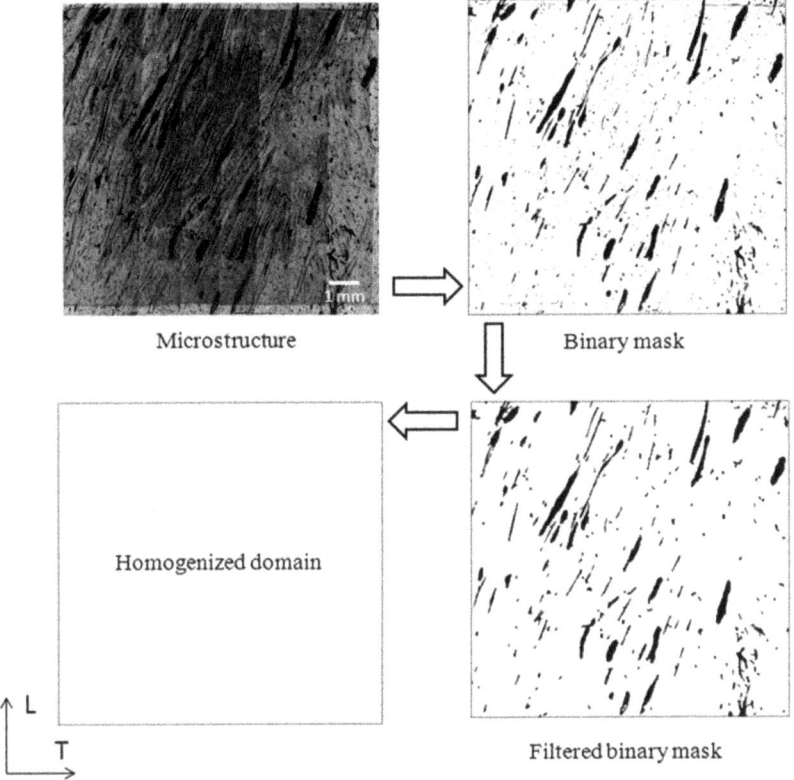

Figure 4. Workflow to generate the computational model for microstructural analysis. The porosity level of the microstructure is 6.17%.

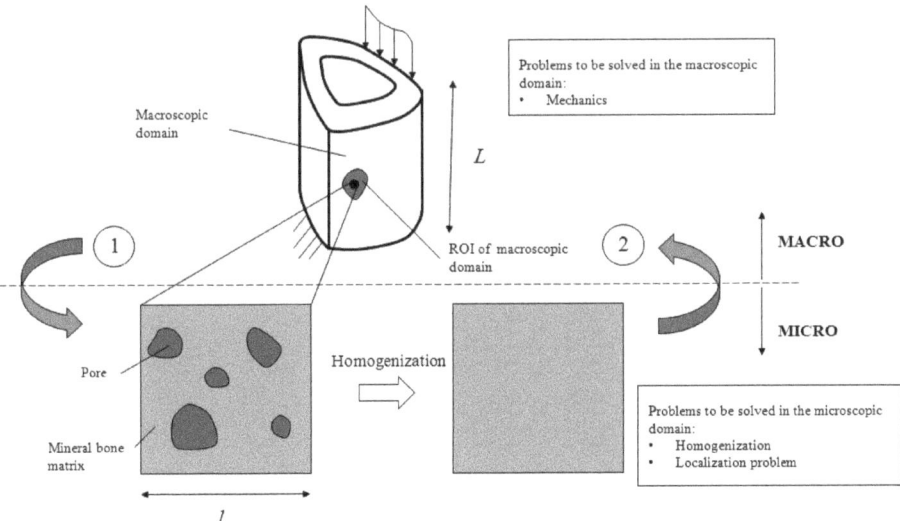

Figure 5. Sketch of the procedure followed for multiscale characterisation of cortical bone tissue.

4. Results

4.1. Computational Models

Two different levels of analysis are considered in the present multiscale approach of cortical bone tissue modelling and simulation.

First, at the macroscopic level, the experimental setup shown in Figure 2a is modelled. The model was solved using the software Abaqus Simulia® v6.17 and modelled under the plane stress hypothesis so that a 2D geometry is considered. Bilinear quadratic (plane stress) elements were selected. The model resulted in 2846 nodes and 2737 elements. Load boundary conditions are applied along the left and bottom regions of the specimen as shown in Figure 2a. Moreover, normal displacements are prescribed along the right and top regions (Figure 2a).

Second, a finite element model was developed for the microstructure presented in the region of interest (see Figure 2a). First, the microstructure image was converted into a grey level image. Then, a binary mask was created and filtered using a filter of 5 pixels (i.e., objects smaller than 5 × 5 pixels are removed). Pixels of the filtered mask were converted then to a regular quadrilateral finite element mesh with a resolution of 1358 × 1358 pixels. Matlab® R2017a was used during this process. Dirichlet boundary conditions were applied along the boundary of the domain, as a hypothesis, following the micromechanics theory [56]. The workflow of the methodology is summarised in Figure 5.

4.2. Homogenisation Macrostructural Results

4.2.1. Homogenisation

The model of the microstructure of the cortical bone tissue (see Figure 4), was used to solve the micromechanics equations presented in Section 3.2, under the finite element framework, with the objective of obtaining the homogenised mechanical properties tensor (Equation (10)) from the micromechanical analysis of the microconstituents of the microstructure.

The microstructure of the cortical bone was considered to be composed of mineral bone material and pores (voids). Mineral bone is considered at the observation scale of our model as a homogeneous material with orthotropic (2D) mechanical behaviour along the longitudinal and transversal directions, according to the literature [58,59]. After a fitting iterative procedure of the experimental results (introduced and explained below), the following values were obtained for the mechanical behaviour of bone mineral tissue: E_L = 20 GPa, E_T = 48 GPa, G_{LT} = 12.5 GPa and ν_{LT} = 0.395. These mechanical properties are associated to the following orthotropic tensor:

$$\mathbb{C}^\varphi = \begin{bmatrix} 77.0 & 30.4 & 0 \\ 30.4 & 32.0 & 0 \\ 0 & 0 & 12.5 \end{bmatrix} [\text{GPa}] \quad (14)$$

Therefore, after the homogenisation procedure, the macroscopic (or apparent) mechanical properties tensor yields to:

$$\mathbb{C}^0 = \begin{bmatrix} 23.13 & 8.63 & 1.01 \\ 8.63 & 19.54 & 0.91 \\ 1.01 & 0.91 & 6.90 \end{bmatrix} [\text{GPa}] \quad (15)$$

4.2.2. Macrostructural Results

The experimental mechanical tests (see Figure 2) provided the macroscopic results (averaged in the region of interest shown in Table 1. These results are the basis for fitting the mechanical properties of the mineral bone tissue iteratively as follows:

(i) Choose values for the mechanical properties of the mineral bone tissue (assumed as orthotropic).

(ii) Solve the homogenisation problem in the microstructural domain (Figure 4) and obtain the (homogenised) macroscopic mechanical properties.
(iii) Solve the macroscopic problem shown in Figure 2a. At the macroscopic level, bone is assumed as a homogeneous continuum medium with macroscopic (homogenised) mechanical properties derived from the micromechanics analysis of the microstructure (ii).
(iv) Obtain the average for the solution of the macroscopic problem along the ROI and compare results with Table 1.

The iterative process converged to values of the mechanical properties of the bone mineral tissue and macroscopic cortical bone tissue shown in Equations (14) and (15), respectively. The fitting of the numerical results versus the experimental ones is plotted in Figure 6.

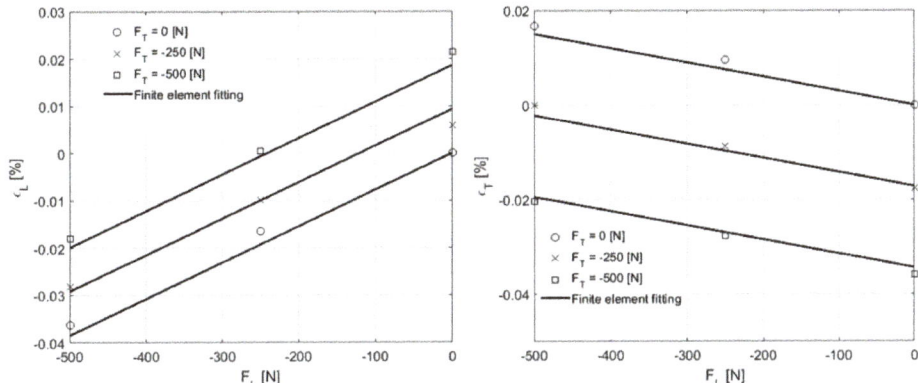

Figure 6. Fitting of the macroscopic modelling to experimental results. Left: Averaged (in the region of interest) longitudinal component of the strain tensor versus overall longitudinal force (for different values of the overall transversal force). Right: Averaged (in the region of interest) transversal component of the strain tensor versus overall longitudinal force (for different values of the overall transversal force). See macroscopic setup of the problem in Figure 2a. ROI dimensions: 10×10 mm (n = 1 specimen). Average R^2 of the fitting: 0.992.

4.3. Multiscale Results

As we have discussed throughout the paper, the proposed multiscale approach allows to obtain both the macroscopic (mechanical) solution of the problem at hand, as well as the distribution of mechanical variables along the domain of the microstructure. Therefore, micromechanical variables are recovered in the microstructure following the localisation procedure introduced in Section 3.1. On the other hand, multiscale results are obtained according to Section 3.3.

The multiscale results, i.e., results belonging to the macro geometry and microstructure, are shown in Figures 7–9 for the displacement, strain and stress fields, respectively. The microstructure of the ROI is distinguished in these figures and the results are represented both in the macroscopic (homogeneous) and microscopic (heterogeneous) domains.

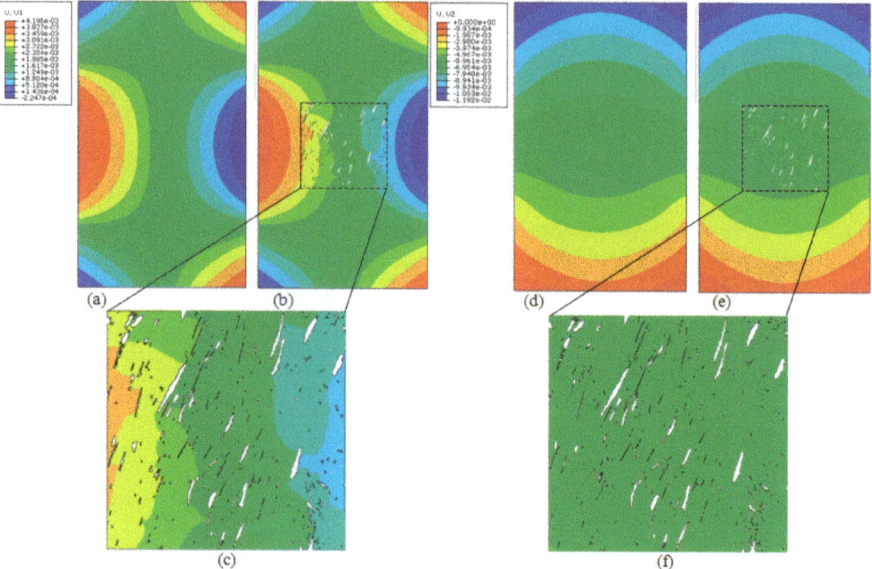

Figure 7. Displacement field [mm]. (**a**) Transversal component: macroscopic results, (**b**) transversal component: multiscale results, (**c**) transversal component: microscopic results. (**d**) Longitudinal component: macroscopic results, (**e**) longitudinal: multiscale results, (**f**) longitudinal component: microscopic results.

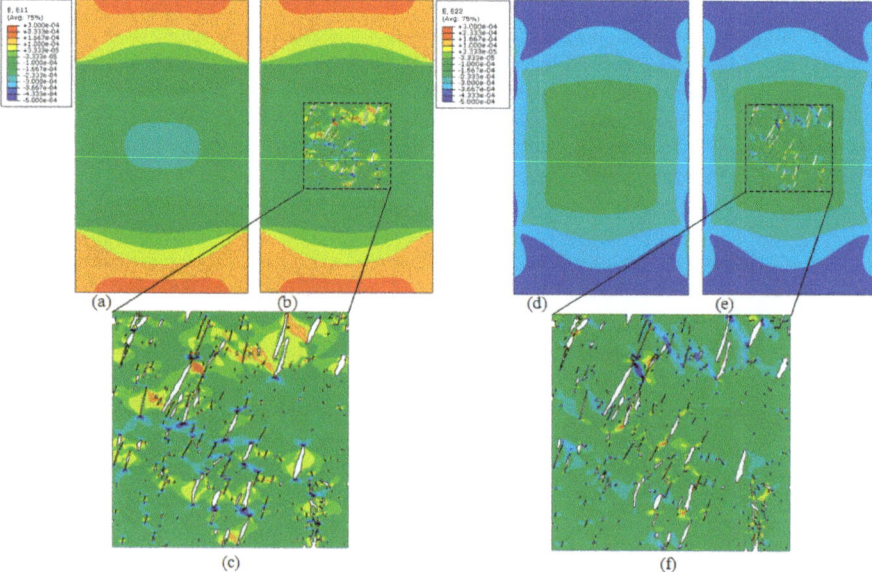

Figure 8. Strain field [-]. (**a**) Transversal component: macroscopic results, (**b**) transversal component: multiscale results, (**c**) transversal component: microscopic results. (**d**) Longitudinal component: macroscopic results, (**e**) longitudinal component: multiscale results, (**f**) longitudinal component: microscopic results.

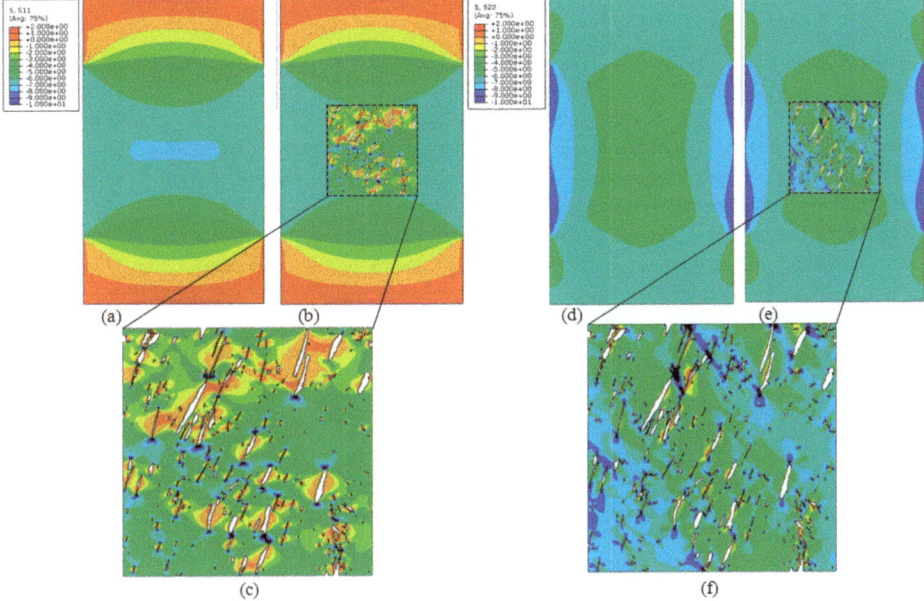

Figure 9. Stress field [MPa]. (**a**) Transversal component: macroscopic results, (**b**) transversal component: multiscale results, (**c**) transversal component: microscopic results. (**d**) Longitudinal component: macroscopic results, (**e**) longitudinal component: multiscale results, (**f**) longitudinal component: microscopic results.

5. Discussion

The multiscale characterisation and analysis of the cortical bone tissue shown in this paper included several steps of analyses at different spatial scales, namely, microscopic and macroscopic scales. The micromechanical analyses performed in the microstructure of the cortical bone tissue initially took place through a homogenisation analysis. This procedure allowed to estimate both the micromechanical properties of the mineral bone material of the matrix, as well as the homogenised apparent properties of the bone tissue. Specifically, using the information of the performed mechanical tests (Table 1), we could fit the properties of the mineral bone matrix by means of the homogenisation problem (Equation (14)), and then, the overall macroscopic or apparent behaviour (Equation (15)). Several interesting conclusions can be drawn from this analysis, as we shall reveal next.

Assuming an orthotropic mechanical behaviour of the bone mineral matrix, the microstructural arrangement of the cortical pores yields to an approximately orthotropic mechanical behaviour at the apparent level as well, along the longitudinal and transversal directions. This can be concluded from Equation (15) where it is seen that the components 1–3 and 2–3 of the matrix are one order of magnitude lower than the others. With a broad consensus, an orthotropic behaviour of the cortical bone is considered in the literature [4,58–60].

Assuming an orthotropic apparent behaviour for the bone tissue, the following values are estimated, using homogenisation, in the longitudinal and transversal directions: E_L = 16.32 GPa, E_T = 19.31 GPa, ν_{LT} = 0.373 and ν_{TL} = 0.442. These values are within the range of values measured in the literature for cortical bone tissue. For example, values in the range of 15–22 GPa are reported for the elasticity modulus of equine cortical bone [61–64]. On the other hand, for human bone tissue, values in the range of 10–25 GPa are found for the elasticity modulus, and 0.3–0.6 for the Poisson's ratio [4].

In the microstructural approach mineral bone is considered a homogeneous material without distinguishing among hydroxyapatite or collagen. A multiscale analysis may be recursively established at the microstructural level to accurately obtain the micromechanical interaction and overall behaviour of mineral bone [11,65,66].

Results referring to the multiscale approach were obtained using the fitted properties of the mineral bone matrix at the microscopic domain in the localisation problem. These results show a smooth variation along the microstructure of the displacement field (see Figure 7). Therefore, as a first approach, the displacement field may be estimated through its macroscopic modelling. However, both the strain field and—most importantly—the stress field show peak magnification of 3× versus their macroscopic and homogenised (mean) values (see Figure 9). This is an extra and important added value given by the multiscale approach. It is currently accepted that the mechanical stimulus which orchestrates many bone processes and diseases, such as osteoporosis, remodelling or consolidation, is local and microstructural [27,33–36,67–70]. In this context, a multiscale approach is critical to link mechanical loading of the bone organ with internal and microstructural evolution of the bone tissue.

Finally, as highlighted in the introduction, the low porosity level of the cortical bone makes this tissue not very attractive from a multiscale point of view, assuming a priori a similar mechanical behaviour to the mineral bone tissue matrix. However, in this work, significant differences between the macro and micro behaviours have been evidenced, highlighting the importance of considering cortical bone tissue through a multiscale approach, for a suitable characterisation of its mechanical response.

Author Contributions: Conceptualisation, J.A.S.-H., J.M.-M., E.R.-R., J.D. and M.D.; methodology, J.A.S.-H., J.M.-M., and E.R.-R.; software, J.A.S.-H.; formal analysis, J.A.S.-H., J.M.-M., E.R.-R., J.D. and M.D.; writing—original draft preparation, J.A.S.-H., J.M.-M. and E.R.-R.; writing—review and editing, J.A.S.-H., J.M.-M., E.R.-R., J.D. and M.D.; supervision, J.D. and M.D.

Funding: The authors gratefully acknowledge the Ministry of Economy and Competitiveness [Ministerio de Economía y Competitividad] of the Government of Spain (DPI2014-58233-P, DPI2017-82501-P, PGC2018-097257-B-C31) for research funding.

Conflicts of Interest: The authors declare no conflicts of interest.

References

1. Currey, J.D. The adaptation of bone to stress. *J. Theor. Biol.* **1968**, *20*, 91–106. [CrossRef]
2. Cowin, S.C.; Moss-Salentijn, L.; Moss, M.L. Candidates for the mechanosensory system in bone. *J. Biomech. Eng.* **1991**, *113*, 191–197. [CrossRef]
3. Cowin, S.C.; Sadegh, A.M.; Luo, G.M. An evolutionary Wolff's law for trabecular architecture. *J. Biomech. Eng.* **1992**, *114*, 129–136. [CrossRef]
4. Skalak, R.; Chien, S. *Handbook of Bioengineering*; McGraw-Hill: New York, NY, USA, 1987.
5. Currey, J.D. *Bones: Structure and Mechanics*; Princeton University Press Editions: Princeton, NJ, USA, 2006.
6. Cowin, S.C.; Hegedus, D.H. Bone remodeling i: A theory of adaptive elasticity. *J. Elast.* **1976**, *6*, 313–326. [CrossRef]
7. Huiskes, R.; Ruimerman, R.; van Lenthe, G.H.; Janssen, J.D. Effects of mechanical forces on maintenance and adaptation of form in trabecular bone. *Nature* **2000**, *405*, 704–706. [CrossRef]
8. Christen, P.; Ito, K.; Ellouz, R.; Boutroy, S.; Sornay-Rendu, E.; Chapurlat, R.D.; van Rietbergen, B. Bone remodelling in humans is load-driven but not lazy. *Nat. Commun.* **2014**, *5*, 4855. [CrossRef] [PubMed]
9. Bouxsein, M.L.; Boyd, S.K.; Christiansen, B.A.; Guldberg, R.E.; Jepsen, K.J.; Müller, R. Guidelines for assessment of bone microstructure in rodents using micro-computed tomography. *J. Bone Miner. Res.* **2010**, *25*, 1468–1486. [CrossRef] [PubMed]
10. Mora-Macías, J.; Pajares, A.; Miranda, P.; Domínguez, J.; Reina-Romo, E. Mechanical characterization via nanoindentation of the woven bone developed during bone transport. *J. Mech. Behav. Biomed. Mater.* **2017**, *74*, 236–244. [CrossRef] [PubMed]
11. Tai, K.; Dao, M.; Suresh, S.; Palazoglu, A.; Ortiz, C. Nanoscale heterogeneity promotes energy dissipation in bone. *Nat. Mater.* **2007**, *6*, 454–462. [CrossRef]
12. Schaffler, M.B.; Burr, D.B. Stiffness of compact bone: Effects of porosity and density. *J. Biomech.* **1998**, *21*, 13–16. [CrossRef]

13. Thompson, M.S.; Schell, H.; Lienau, J.; Duda, G.N. Digital image correlation: A technique for determining local mechanical conditions within early bone callus. *Med. Eng. Phys.* **2007**, *29*, 820–823. [CrossRef] [PubMed]
14. Carriero, A.; Abela, L.; Pitsillides, A.A.; Shefelbine, S.J. Ex vivo determination of bone tissue strains for an in vivo mouse tibial loading mode. *J. Biomech.* **2014**, *47*, 2490–2497. [CrossRef] [PubMed]
15. Gustafsson, A.; Mathavan, N.; Turunen, M.J.; Engqvist, J.; Khayyeri, H.; Hall, S.A.; Isaksson, H. Linking multiscale deformation to microstructure in cortical bone using in situ loading, digital image correlation and synchrotron X-ray scattering. *Acta Biomater.* **2018**, *69*, 323–331. [CrossRef] [PubMed]
16. Carter, D.R.; Orr, T.E.; Fyhrie, D.P. Relationships between loading history and femoral cancellous bone architecture. *J. Biomech.* **1989**, *22*, 231–244. [CrossRef]
17. Hernandez, C.J.; Beaupre, G.S.; Carter, D.R. A model of mechanobiologic and metabolic influences on bone adaptation. *J. Rehabil. Res. Dev.* **2000**, *37*, 235–244. [PubMed]
18. Hazelwood, S.J.; Martin, R.B.; Rashid, M.M.; Rodrigo, J.J. A mechanistic model for internal bone remodeling exhibits different dynamic responses in disuse and overload. *J. Biomech.* **2001**, *34*, 299–308. [CrossRef]
19. Garcia-Aznar, J.M.; Rueberg, T.; Doblare, M. A bone remodelling model coupling micro-damage growth and repair by 3D BMU-activity. *Biomech. Model. Mechanobiol.* **2005**, *4*, 147–167. [CrossRef] [PubMed]
20. Beaupre, G.S.; Orr, T.E.; Carter, D.R. An approach for time-dependent bone modelling and remodelling: Theoretical development. *J. Orthop. Res.* **1990**, *8*, 651–661. [CrossRef] [PubMed]
21. Beaupre, G.S.; Orr, T.E.; Carter, D.R. An approach for time-dependent bone modeling and remodeling-application: A preliminary remodeling simulation. *J. Orthop. Res.* **1990**, *8*, 662–670. [CrossRef] [PubMed]
22. Jacobs, C.R. Numerical Simulation of Bone Adaptation to Mechanical Loading. Ph.D. Thesis, Stanford University, Stanford, CA, USA, 1994.
23. Wittkowske, C.; Reilly, G.C.; Lacroix, D.; Perrault, C.M. In Vitro Bone Cell Models: Impact of Fluid Shear Stress on Bone Formation. *Front. Bioeng. Biotechnol.* **2016**, *15*, 4–87. [CrossRef] [PubMed]
24. Cowin, S.C. Bone poroelasticity. *J. Biomech.* **1999**, *32*, 217–238. [CrossRef]
25. Cowin, S.C.; Gailani, G.; Benalla, M. Hierarchical poroelasticity: Movement of interstitial fluid between porosity levels in bones. *Philos. Trans. A Math. Phys. Eng. Sci.* **2009**, *367*, 3401–3444. [CrossRef] [PubMed]
26. Bailon-Plaza, A.; van der Meulen, C.H. A mathematical framework to study the effects of growth factor influences on fracture healing. *J. Theor. Biol.* **2001**, *212*, 191–200. [CrossRef] [PubMed]
27. Lacroix, D.; Prendergast, P.J. A mechano-regulation model for tissue differentiation during fracture healing: Analysis of gap size and loading. *J. Biomech.* **2002**, *35*, 1163–1171. [CrossRef]
28. Wang, M.; Yang, N.; Wang, X. A review of computational models of bone fracture healing. *Med. Biol. Eng. Comput.* **2017**, *55*, 1895–1914. [CrossRef] [PubMed]
29. Byrne, D.P.; Lacroix, D.; Planell, J.A.; Kelly, D.J.; Prendergast, P.J. Simulation of tissue differentiation in a scaffold as a function of porosity, Young's modulus and dissolution rate: Application of mechanobiological models in tissue engineering. *Biomaterials* **2007**, *28*, 5544–5554. [CrossRef] [PubMed]
30. Sanz-Herrera, J.A.; Garcia-Aznar, J.M.; Doblare, M. A mathematical model for bone tissue regeneration inside a specific type of scaffold. *Biomech. Model. Mechanobiol.* **2008**, *7*, 355–366. [CrossRef]
31. Sanz-Herrera, J.A.; Garcia-Aznar, J.M. A mathematical approach to bone tissue engineering. *Philos. Trans. A Math. Phys. Eng. Sci.* **2009**, *367*, 2055–2078. [CrossRef]
32. Guyot, Y.; Papantoniou, I.; Chai, Y.C.; Van Bael, S.; Schrooten, J.; Geris, L. A computational model for cell/ECM growth on 3D surfaces using the level set method: A bone tissue engineering case study. *Biomech. Model. Mechanobiol.* **2014**, *13*, 1361–1371. [CrossRef]
33. Claes, L.E.; Heigele, C.A. Magnitudes of local stress and strain along bony surfaces predict the course and type of fracture healing. *J. Biomech.* **1999**, *32*, 255–266. [CrossRef]
34. Isaksson, H.; Comas, O.; van Donkelaar, C.C.; Mediavilla, J.; Wilson, W.; Huiskes, R.; Ito, K. Bone regeneration during distraction osteogenesis: Mechano-regulation by shear strain and fluid velocity. *J. Biomech.* **2007**, *40*, 2002–2011. [CrossRef] [PubMed]
35. Reina-Romo, E.; Gomez-Benito, M.J.; Garcia-Aznar, J.M.; Dominguez, J.; Doblare, M. Modeling distraction osteogenesis: Analysis of the distraction rate. *Biomech. Model. Mechanobiol.* **2009**, *8*, 323–335. [CrossRef] [PubMed]

36. Reina-Romo, E.; Gomez-Benito, M.J.; Dominguez, J.; Niemeyer, F.; Wehner, T.; Simon, U.; Claes, L.E. Effect of the fixator stiffness on the young regenerate bone after bone transport: Computational approach. *J. Biomech.* **2011**, *44*, 917–923. [CrossRef] [PubMed]
37. Adachi, T.; Tsubota, K.I.; Tomita, Y.; Hollister, S.J. Trabecular surface remodelling simulation for cancellous bone using microstructural voxel finite element models. *J. Biomech. Eng. T ASME* **2001**, *123*, 403–409. [CrossRef] [PubMed]
38. Adachi, T.; Osako, Y.; Tanaka, M.; Hojo, M.; Hollister, S.J. Framework for optimal design of porous scaffold microstructure by computational simulation of bone regeneration. *Biomaterials* **2006**, *27*, 3964–3972. [CrossRef]
39. Kelly, D.J.; Prendergast, P.J. Prediction of the optimal mechanical properties for a scaffold used in osteochondral defect repair. *Tissue Eng.* **2006**, *12*, 2509–2519. [CrossRef]
40. Schulte, F.A.; Ruffoni, D.; Lambers, F.M.; Christen, D.; Webster, D.J.; Kuhn, G.; Muller, R. Local mechanical stimuli regulate bone formation and resorption in mice at the tissue level. *PLoS ONE* **2013**, *8*, e62172. [CrossRef]
41. Terada, K.; Kikuchi, N. A class of general algorithms for multi-scale analyses of heterogeneous media. *Comput. Methods Appl. Mech. Eng.* **2001**, *190*, 5427–5464. [CrossRef]
42. Kouznetsova, V.; Geers, M.G.D.; Brekelmans, W.A.M. Multi-scale constitutive modelling of heterogeneous materials with a gradient-enhanced computational homogenization scheme. *Int. J. Numer. Meth. Eng.* **2002**, *54*, 1235–1260. [CrossRef]
43. Miehe, C.; Bayreuther, C.G. On multiscale FE analyses of heterogeneous structures: From homogenization to multigrid solvers. *Int. J. Numer. Methods Eng.* **2007**, *71*, 1135–1180. [CrossRef]
44. Kulkarni, M.G.; Matous, K.; Geubelle, P.H. Coupled multi-scale cohesive modeling of failure in heterogeneous adhesives. *Int. J. Numer. Methods Eng.* **2010**, *84*, 916–946. [CrossRef]
45. Reina-Romo, E.; Sanz-Herrera, J.A. Multiscale simulation of particle-reinforced elastic-plastic adhesives at small strains. *Comput. Methods Appl. Mech. Eng.* **2011**, *200*, 2211–2222. [CrossRef]
46. Montero-Chacon, F.; Sanz-Herrera, J.A.; Doblare, M. Computational multiscale solvers for continuum approaches. *Materials* **2019**, *12*, 691. [CrossRef] [PubMed]
47. Webster, D.; Muller, R. In silico models of bone remodeling from macro to nano–from organ to cell. *Wiley Interdiscip. Rev. Syst. Biol. Med.* **2010**, *3*, 241–251. [CrossRef]
48. Nguyen, T.K.; Carpentier, O.; Monchau, F.; Chai, F.; Hornez, J.C.; Hivart, P. Numerical optimization of cell colonization modelling inside scaffold for perfusion bioreactor: A multiscale model. *Med. Eng. Phys.* **2018**, *57*, 40–50. [CrossRef]
49. Sanz-Herrera, J.A.; Garcia-Aznar, J.M.; Doblare, M. Micro–macro numerical modelling of bone regeneration in tissue engineering. *Comput. Meth. Appl. Mech. Eng.* **2008**, *197*, 3092–3107. [CrossRef]
50. Sanz-Herrera, J.A.; Garcia-Aznar, J.M.; Doblare, M. On scaffold designing for bone regeneration: A computational multiscale approach. *Acta Biomater.* **2009**, *5*, 219–229. [CrossRef]
51. Colloca, M.; Blanchard, R.; Hellmich, C.; Ito, K.; van Rietbergen, B. A multiscale analytical approach for bone remodeling simulations: Linking scales from collagen to trabeculae. *Bone* **2014**, *64*, 303–313. [CrossRef]
52. Garcia, D.; Zysset, P.K.; Charlebois, M.; Curnier, A. A three-dimensional elastic plastic damage constitutive law for bone tissue. *Biomech. Model. Mechanobiol.* **2009**, *8*, 149–165. [CrossRef]
53. Yoon, Y.J.; Cowin, S.C. The estimated elastic constants for a single bone osteonal lamella. *Biomech. Model. Mechanobiol.* **2008**, *7*, 1–11. [CrossRef]
54. Gailani, G.; Benalla, M.; Mahamud, R.; Cowin, S.C.; Cardoso, L. Experimental determination of the permeability in the lacunar-canalicular porosity of bone. *J. Biomech. Eng.* **2009**, *131*, 101007. [CrossRef] [PubMed]
55. Vazquez, J.; Navarro, C.; Dominguez, J. Analysis of fretting fatigue initial crack path in Al7075-T651 using cylindrical contact. *Tribol. Int.* **2017**, *108*, 87–94. [CrossRef]
56. Suquet, P.M. Elements of homogenization for inelastic solid mechanics, trends and applications of pure mathematics to mechanics. In *Homogenization Techniques for Composite Media, Lecture Notes in Physics*; Sanchez-Palencia, E., Zaoui, A., Eds.; Springer: Berlin, Germany, 1985; Volume 272, pp. 193–278.
57. Yuan, Z.; Fish, J. Toward realization of computational homogenization in practice. *Int. J. Numer. Meth. Eng.* **2008**, *73*, 361–380. [CrossRef]

58. Taylor, W.R.; Roland, E.; Ploeg, H.; Hertig, D.; Klabunde, R.; Warner, M.D.; Hobatho, M.C.; Rakotomanana, L.; Clift, S.E. Determination of orthotropic bone elastic constants using FEA and modal analysis. *J. Biomech.* **2002**, *35*, 767–773. [CrossRef]
59. Bernard, S.; Grimal, Q.; Laugier, P. Accurate measurement of cortical bone elasticity tensor with resonant ultrasound spectroscopy. *J. Mech. Behav. Biomed. Mater.* **2013**, *18*, 12–19. [CrossRef] [PubMed]
60. Reilly, D.; Burstein, A. The elastic and ultimate properties of compact bone tissue. *J. Biomech.* **1975**, *8*, 393–405. [CrossRef]
61. Schryver, H.F. Bending properties of cortical bone of the horse. *Am. J. Vet. Res.* **1978**, *39*, 25–28.
62. Riggs, C.M.; Vaughan, L.C.; Evans, G.P.; Lanyon, L.E.; Boyde, A. Mechanical implications of collagen fibre orientation in cortical bone of the equine radius. *Anat. Embryol.* **1993**, *187*, 239–248. [CrossRef]
63. Reilly, G.C.; Currey, J.D. The development of microcracking and failure in bone depends on the loading mode to which it is adapted. *J. Exp. Biol.* **1999**, *202*, 543–552.
64. Batson, E.L.; Reilly, G.C.; Currey, J.D.; Balderson, D.S. Post-exercise and positional variation in mechanical properties of the radius in young horses. *Equine Vet.* **2000**, *32*, 95–100. [CrossRef]
65. Hellmich, C.; Barthelemy, J.; Dormieux, L. Mineral-collagen interactions in elasticity of bone ultrastructure—A continuum micromechanics approach. *Eur. J. Mech. A Solids* **2004**, *23*, 783–810. [CrossRef]
66. Fritsch, A.; Hellmich, C. 'Universal' microstructural patterns in cortical and trabecular, extracellular and extravascular bone materials: Micromechanics-based prediction of anisotropic elasticity. *J. Theor. Biol.* **2007**, *244*, 597–620. [CrossRef] [PubMed]
67. Carter, D.R.; Blenman, P.; Beaupre, G.S. Correlations between mechanical stress history and tissue differentiation in initial fracture healing. *J. Orthop. Res.* **1988**, *6*, 736–748. [CrossRef] [PubMed]
68. Cowin, S.C. Mechanosensation and fluid transport in living bone. *J. Musculoskelet. Neuronal Interact.* **2002**, *2*, 256–260.
69. Van Rietbergen, B.; Huiskes, R.; Eckstein, F.; Ruegsegger, P. Trabecular bone tissue strains in the healthy and osteoporotic human femur. *J. Bone Miner. Res.* **2003**, *18*, 1781–1788. [CrossRef]
70. Shefelbine, S.J.; Carter, D.R. Mechanobiological predictions of growth front morphology in developmental hip dysplasia. *J. Orthop. Res.* **2004**, *22*, 346–352. [CrossRef]

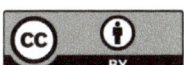 © 2019 by the authors. Licensee MDPI, Basel, Switzerland. This article is an open access article distributed under the terms and conditions of the Creative Commons Attribution (CC BY) license (http://creativecommons.org/licenses/by/4.0/).

Article

Biomechanical Evaluation of the Effect of Mesenchymal Stem Cells on Cartilage Regeneration in Knee Joint Osteoarthritis

Yong-Gon Koh [1], Jin-Ah Lee [2], Hwa-Yong Lee [2], Hyo-Jeong Kim [3] and Kyoung-Tak Kang [2,*]

[1] Joint Reconstruction Center, Department of Orthopaedic Surgery, Yonsei Sarang Hospital, 10 Hyoryeong-ro, Seocho-gu, Seoul 06698, Korea; osygkoh@gmail.com
[2] Department of Mechanical Engineering, Yonsei University, 50 Yonsei-ro, Seodaemun-gu, Seoul 03722, Korea; gna0812@gmail.com (J.-A.L.); au0707@gmail.com (H.-Y.L.)
[3] Department of Sport and Healthy Aging, Korea National Sport University, 1239 Yangjae-dearo, Songpa-gu, Seoul 05541, Korea; knsu.hjkim@gmail.com
* Correspondence: tagi1024@gmail.com; Tel.: +82-2-2123-4827; Fax: +82-2-362-2736

Received: 28 March 2019; Accepted: 25 April 2019; Published: 7 May 2019

Abstract: Numerous clinical studies have reported cell-based treatments for cartilage regeneration in knee joint osteoarthritis using mesenchymal stem cells (MSCs). However, the post-surgery rehabilitation and weight-bearing times remain unclear. Phenomenological computational models of cartilage regeneration have been only partially successful in predicting experimental results and this may be due to simplistic modeling assumptions and loading conditions of cellular activity. In the present study, we developed a knee joint model of cell and tissue differentiation based on a more mechanistic approach, which was applied to cartilage regeneration in osteoarthritis. First, a phenomenological biphasic poroelastic finite element model was developed and validated according to a previous study. Second, this method was applied to a real knee joint model with a cartilage defect created to simulate the tissue regeneration process. The knee joint model was able to accurately predict several aspects of cartilage regeneration, such as the cell and tissue distributions in the cartilage defect. Additionally, our results indicated that gait cycle loading with flexion was helpful for cartilage regeneration compared to the use of simple weight-bearing loading.

Keywords: stem cell; cartilage; finite element

1. Introduction

Osteoarthritis (OA) of the knee is the most common result of arthritis that leads to pain, stiffness and decreased mobility, with this disease being one of the major causes of disability among non-institutionalized adults [1,2]. OA is a process of cartilage degeneration that involves the immune system, in which local inflammatory responses are observed with the production of proinflammatory cytokines [3,4]. The articular cartilage possesses limited reparative abilities and the associated osteochondral defects present in young patients generally do not heal but usually progress to degeneration of the surrounding cartilage [5]. There are a limited number of treatment options available to improve or reverse the process [3,4]. Additionally, with the exception of joint replacement, the most common treatments for OA are not widely applied and can be associated with substantial adverse events, high costs or both [6].

Mesenchymal stem cells (MSCs) have been proposed to possess potential in the cell-based treatment of cartilage lesions [7]. These cells show great promise as a therapeutic agent in regenerative medicine due to their multilineage potential, immunosuppressive activities, limited immunogenicity and relative ease of growth in culture [7]. Additionally, MSCs represent an autologous cell source that reduces the chance for rejection and disease transmission they are also less tumorigenic than their embryonic counterparts [8]. However, there are no studies that have quantitatively evaluated the degree of rehabilitation of an OA knee joint after injection or transplantation of MSCs.

Mechano-regulation algorithms have been suggested to evaluate the possible relationship between mechanical stimulation and the differentiation of cells and tissues [9–15]. These phenomenological computational models, however, have several problems, particularly regarding the general simplification, such as loading condition and simplified geometry [9–12]. Recently we studied to predict the mechanical properties of an optimum scaffold required for cartilage regeneration using three-dimensional knee joint developed from medical imaging and mechano-regulation theory [16].

Therefor, the aim of the present study was to investigate cartilage regeneration in OA or cartilage defects based on the knee joint mechano-regulation of MSC differentiation theory using a realistic model based on three-dimensional (3D) medical imaging. This model considers the effect of mechanical stimuli on cell mitosis and death and it also incorporates the influence of the tissues on cell dispersal rate We hypothesized that the prediction of mechano-regulated tissue differentiation would differ with respect to the loading conditions.

2. Materials and Methods

To investigate individual cellular model parameters of cartilage regeneration, a mechano-biological tissue-differentiation model that included theoretical descriptions of cellular processes was used according to a previous validation method [17]. This model has been employed to simulate the major aspects of normal conditions and cartilage regeneration [17,18]. Mechano-regulation processes are driven by the mechanical environment in the vicinity of the cell. A computational approach, such as finite element (FE) modeling, enables the evaluation of the mechanical stimuli within the extracellular matrix of a regenerating tissue. In this study, a cartilage defect within the knee joint was investigated using a poroelastic FE model. Briefly, the entire callus was assumed to consist of granulation tissue at the beginning of the stimulation regimen. Generally, once the subchondral bone is penetrated, MSCs invade the defect in the bone marrow. Given this, the stem cells were assumed to originate from the periosteum, outer cortical surface and medullary canal in a previous study [18]. This method was applied to generate the first phenomenological model. In the second model, adipose synovium-derived MSCs were used for cartilage defect implantation because we have had successful clinical experience with this approach [19–21].

To simulate the diffusion of stem cells throughout the callus, a diffusion coefficient was selected to predict 99% stem cell coverage at six weeks after implantation [12]. After this, the differentiation of the granulation tissue in a given element towards the fibrous tissue, cartilage or bone was determined by the stimulus factor (S) according to Equation (1):

$$S = \frac{\gamma}{a} + \frac{v}{b} \quad (1)$$

where γ is the octahedral shear strain, v is the fluid velocity and a (3.75%) and b (3 µm/s) are the scaling factors for each stimulus. Based on the mechano-regulation theory, $S > 3$ is predicted as fibrous connective tissue, $1 < S < 3$ indicates cartilage, $0.53 < S < 1$ indicates immature woven bone, $0.01 < S < 0.53$ indicates mature woven bone and $0 < S < 0.01$ indicates bone resorption [4,12,13,18,19,22].

Poroelastic material properties were updated according to a rule of mixtures based on the concentration of cells in a given element (n_c), the volume fractions (φ_j) and material properties of the granulation tissue and j types of differentiated tissues in that element. For example, Young's modulus (E) for a given element was calculated according to Equation (2):

$$E = \frac{(n_c^{max} - n_c)}{n_c^{max}} E_{granulation} + \frac{n_c}{n_c^{max}} \sum_{j=1}^{n_t} E_j \varphi_j \quad (2)$$

where n_c^{max} is the maximum number of cells that can occupy any single element and Ej is Young's Modulus of the jth differentiated tissue. The volume fraction φ_j of a given type of differentiated tissue was evaluated as the fraction of the last ten iterations for which this particular differentiated tissue type was predicted in the element. This enabled the material properties to change gradually and prevented instability in the algorithm [23]. Material property was calculated for each element by this formula using a custom FORTRAN script.

The two poroelastic FE models were developed to simulate in vivo mechnical conditions within knee joint OA mechano-regulation under different loading conditions. The first phenomenological axi-symmetric FE model of the knee was created, which included a meniscus, femoral condyle and articular cartilage layer to validate this approach (Figure 1). The pore fluid pressure was adjusted to zero at free. The meniscus and the cartilage surface could not penetrate each other in the axial direction. However, the surfaces were allowed to slide relative to each other. The cartilage defect size and depth were set at 5 mm each. Complete integration was assumed between the repair tissue and normal tissue. An axial ramp load of 800 N was applied for 0.5 s. All tissues were modeled as being biphasic based on the poroelastic theory. The material properties used for each tissue type are shown in Table 1. The meniscus was modeled as transversely isotropic and poroelastic with a higher stiffness in the circumferential direction [12].

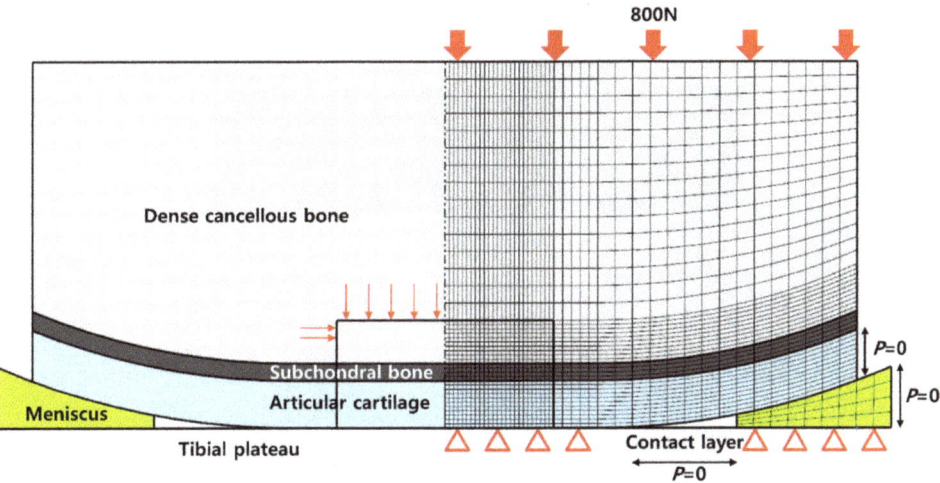

Figure 1. Schematic of the phenomenological axi-symmetric FE model of the knee including a femoral condyle, articular cartilage layer and meniscus for validation.

Table 1. Material properties used in this simulation.

	Granulation Tissue	Fibrous Tissue	Cartilage	Immature Bone	Mature Bone	Cortical Bone
Young's modulus (MPa)	0.2	2	10	1000	6000	17,000
Poisson's ratio (ν)	0.167	0.167	0.167	0.3	0.3	0.3
Permeability ($m^4/N_s \times 10^{-14}$)	1	1	0.5	0.1	0.37	0.001
Porosity	0.8	0.8	0.8	0.8	0.8	0.04
Diffusion coefficient (mm^2/iteration)	0.8	0.1	0.05	0.01	0.01	-

The second poroelastic FE model of the knee joint (Figure 2c) was developed from real medical imaging based on a previously reported model [24–26] that was further developed. Briefly, a 3D FE model of a normal knee joint was developed using data from computed tomography (CT) (Figure 2a) and magnetic resonance imaging (MRI) scans (Figure 2b) of a healthy 37-year-old male subject. The CT and MRI models were developed with a slice thickness of 0.1 mm and 0.4 mm, respectively. Unlike the phenomenological model, this model was developed specifically for the tibial cartilage to describe an actual clinical situation. Contact was modeled between the femoral cartilage and the meniscus, the meniscus and the tibial cartilage and the femoral cartilage and the tibial cartilage for both the medial and lateral sides, which resulted in a total of six contact pairs. In short, the components were not penetrating. The second model developed at 64 mm^2 with a depth of 3 mm. Two loading conditions were applied. The first condition was an axial ramp load of 1750 N, which was the same as that applied in the phenomenological model, and the second was a stance-phase gait cycle derived from the ISO14,243-1 standard [27]. All FE analyses were completed using ABAQUS 6.5 (Abaqus, Inc., East Providence, RI, USA) and the mechano-regulation theory was a user-defined subroutine constructed by the FORTRAN code.

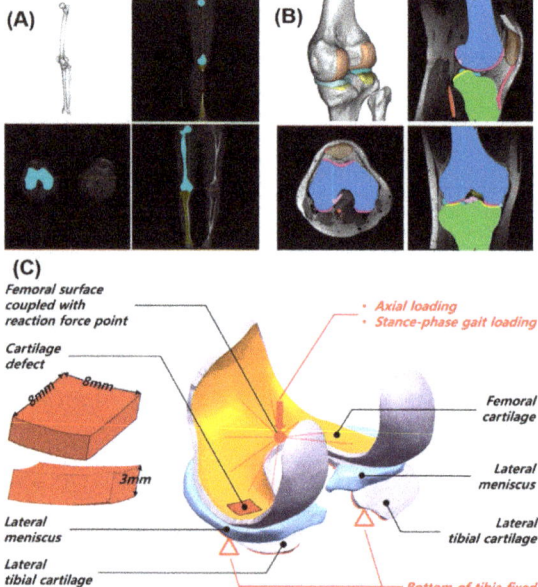

Figure 2. A realistic 3D knee joint model developed using data from (**a**) CT and (**b**) MRI scans. (**c**) Schematic representations of the cartilage defect model and the boundary conditions for cartilage regeneration prediction.

3. Results

Figure 3 presents the phenomenological computational model of predicted patterns of tissue differentiation in cartilage defects. This results in higher cell death predictions in the superficial layer of the repair tissue as MSCs differentiate into fibroblasts and undergo death in the high-strain environment. This trend was also observed in a previous study [9].

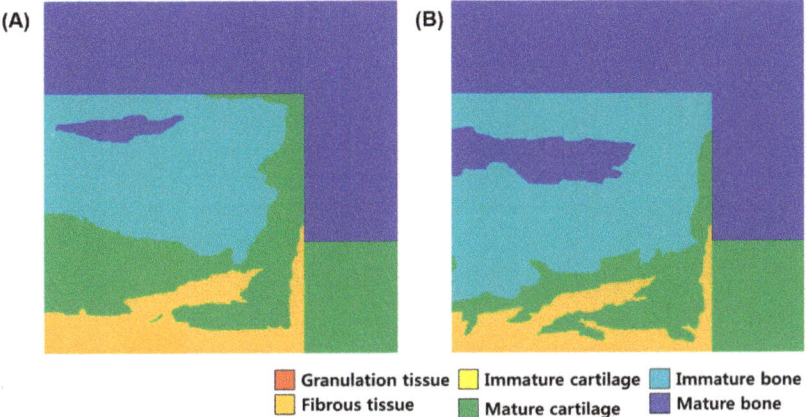

Figure 3. Predicted patterns of tissue differentiation with 5 mm cartilage defect in a simulation of (**a**) 25 iterations and (**b**) 50 iterations.

The cell concentration and each tissue type formation observed in this study and Kelly and Prendergast's study were compared in Figure 4 [9]. A minor difference was observed, but the overall trend is consistent. In particular, there were similar predictions for the simulated fibrous tissue formation (18% in the present study and 16% in the previous study) and bone formation (61% in the present study and 64% in the previous study) [9].

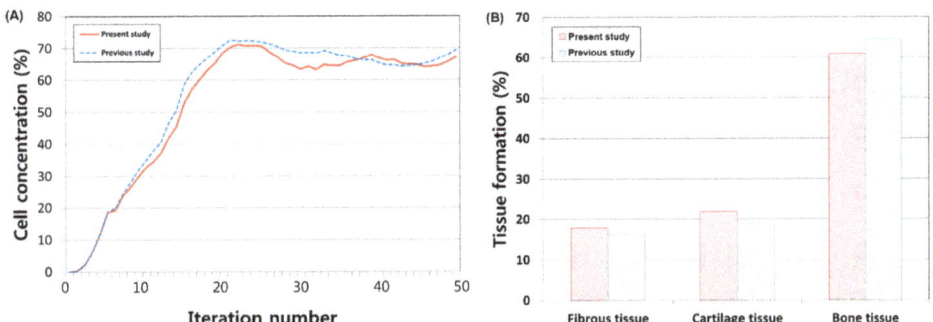

Figure 4. Comparison of prediction of (**a**) cell concentration at the articular surface and (**b**) percentage of tissue types between this study and a previous study [9] for validation.

Figure 5 shows the pattern of regeneration of the cartilage defect in the knee joint model for axial and stance-phase gait cycle loadings. The predicted patterns of tissue differentiation after MSC implantation in the stance-phase gait cycle condition model were found to be remarkably different from those predicted by the axial force model. The stance-phase gait model was predicted to support early chondrogenesis, with the chondral region of the defect consisting primarily of immature cartilage tissue. Increased cartilage formation was predicted as the simulation of the defect repair progressed and a remarkably greater proportion of the defect consisted of cartilage tissue. A strong uniform band of fibrous tissue was maintained at the articular cartilage. Additionally, the remainder of the chondral portion of the defect consisted of cartilage tissue. However, in the axial force model, the simulations showed that the defect was partially shielded by the adjacent intact cartilage and the stimulus within the defect was low. As the regenerated tissue begins to stiffen, it begins to support loads and chondrogenesis is favored within the center of the defect. After a given period of time, increased bone formation is predicted to occur by endochondral ossification and particular regions of cartilage begin to differentiate into fibrous tissue, ultimately resulting in a reduction in the amount of cartilage within the defect. Figure 6 showed cell concentration in axial force model and stance phase gait model. Axial force model cell death was found in articular surface, but stance phase gait model cell death was prevented because rotation or translation because controlled axial force was exerted only at the defect region. Figure 7 shows tissue type formation after 40 iterations in axial force model in stance phase gait model. In 40 iterations, greater amounts of cartilage tissue formation were predicted, with 56% in the stance-phase gait model and 29% in the axial force model.

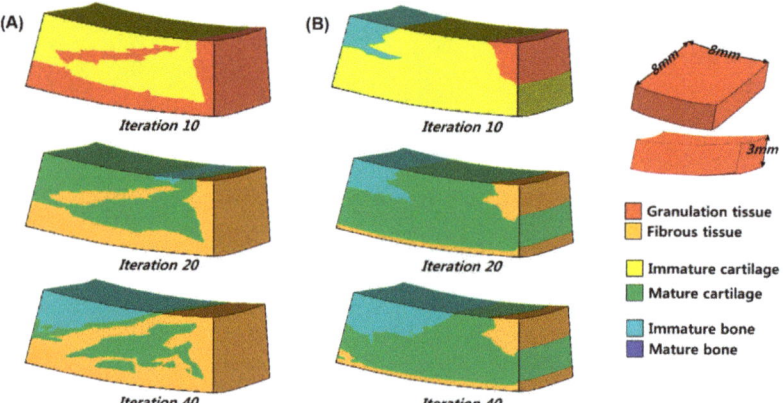

Figure 5. Pattern of regeneration of the cartilage defect in the knee joint model in 10, 20 and 40 iterations for (**a**) axial and (**b**) stance-phase gait cycle loading.

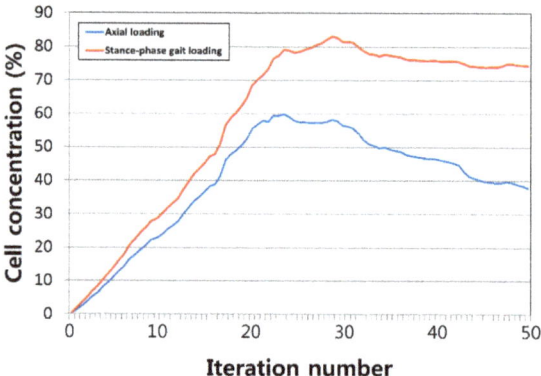

Figure 6. Comparison of the prediction of cell concentration between the axial loading and the stance-phase gait loading model.

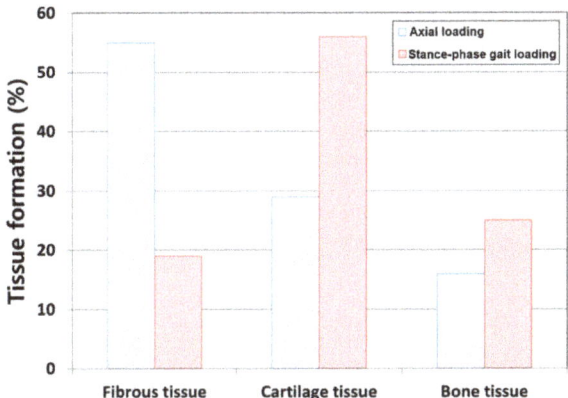

Figure 7. Percentage of each tissue type formation in the axial loading and the stance-phase gait loading model after 40 iterations.

4. Discussion

The most important finding of this study was that different results were found with respect to the loading conditions in a real knee joint model for mechano-biological tissue differentiation.

Cartilage defects possess a very limited intrinsic healing capacity. Curl et al. described 53,569 hyaline cartilage lesions in 19,827 patients that received total knee arthroplasty [28]. Similarly, a more recent prospective survey of 993 consecutive knee arthroscopies showed evidence of articular cartilage abnormality in 66% of the patients [29]. Several techniques for articular cartilage defect treatment have been described recently with various results and indications [24,30]. Microfracture represents a widely used technique for the repair of symptomatic articular cartilage defects of the knee [31,32]. The penetration of the subchondral bone plate in these defects causes clot formation in the defect. This clot contains pluripotent, marrow-derived MSCs, which can induce fibrocartilage repair as they possess varying amounts of type II collagen [30]. However, the microfracture technique is limited for treating large-sized defects. Small defects can spontaneously undergo repair with the hyaline cartilage, while larger defects undergo repair only with fibrous tissue or fibrocartilage, which are biochemically and biomechanically different from normal hyaline cartilage [3]. A recent review paper indicated that osteochondral autograft transfer may achieve higher activity levels and a lower risk of failure compared to the microfracture technique for cartilage lesions greater than 3 cm^2, although there was no significant difference for lesions smaller than 3 cm^2 at midterm [33]. Therefore, degeneration may occur, which can subsequently progress to osteoarthritic changes [34].

Recently, MSCs have been recommended for use in the cell-based treatment of cartilage lesions. Chondrogenesis of MSCs was primarily reported by Ashton et al. [35] and a defined medium for the in-vitro chondrogenesis of MSCs was primarily reported by Johnstone et al. [36], who used micromass culture with transforming growth factor-beta and dexamethasone. With regard to the in-vivo studies, the transplantation of MSCs into full-thickness articular cartilage defects has been attempted under various conditions. Some studies recently reported that adipose-derived MSCs therapy for young and even elderly patients with knee OA was effective with respect to cartilage healing, reducing pain and improving function [19–21]. Additionally, Kim et al. demonstrated that the implantation of MSCs for knee OA resulted in improved clinical and second-look arthroscopic outcomes compared to those reported after an injection of MSCs [37]. Another recent study recommended that non-weight-bearing conditions with only toe-touching for 8 weeks may have similar effects to those achieved within the period used in other treatments for cartilage regeneration when MSCs were injected to OA patients [38]. However, the authors also stated that although this prolonged period of non-weight-bearing may enable some native repair, it decreased and delayed the recovery of knee function after injections as evidenced by an initial decline of the Knee Society Clinical Rating System function score [38]. Therefore, an optimal rehabilitation protocol for the injection and implantation of MSCs should be further investigated and determined.

To date, the Prendergast mechano-regulation theory has been applied to a number of different scenarios of bone healing and cartilage regeneration and it has displayed tremendous promise as a theory that could accurately describe the course of mesenchymal tissue differentiation in response to a wide spectrum of mechanical conditions [12,17,18]. However, all of these studies performed simulations from a microfracture perspective [12,17,18,39]. Moreover, the stem cells were assumed to originate from the periosteum, the outer cortical surface and medullary canal according to mechano-regulation tissue differentiation [12,17,18,39].

The objective of the present study was to perform a robust test of this theory by applying it to a MSC implantation model in knee OA where different mechanical loadings were used to alter the cartilage regeneration response. One of the main strengths of this study is that the modeling technique used to test the mechano-regulation theory is dissimilar to those typically used to investigate the mechano-regulation of cartilage regeneration. Many previous computational studies examining the mechano-biology of cartilage regeneration only investigated the physiological axial load. Additionally, they described boundary and contact conditions that do not accurately reflect clinical situations using simple phenomenological computational models. Our knee joint model that was developed from real medical imaging could successfully predict the patterns of cellular differentiation in osteochondral defect regeneration. A previous study demonstrated regeneration through both endochondral and direct intramembranous ossification in the base of the defect, with cartilage formation occurring at the center of the defect and fibrous tissue formation superficially [40]. This pattern of repair was also found in the present model. We also found that gait cycle loading was better than vertical loading for cartilage regeneration. However, in the simple vertical loading model, increased bone formation was predicted to occur via endochondral ossification and particular regions of the cartilage began to differentiate into fibrous tissue, ultimately leading to a reduction in the amount of cartilage within the defect. Due to an increase in the magnitude of fluid flow within the defect, the stimulus for fibrous tissue formation is increased [41]. This increase in strain also promotes cell death at the articular surface [41]. Thus, preventing this fibrous tissue formation superficially and any subsequent cell death by an appropriate rehabilitation protocol would be beneficial in avoiding long-term failure of tissue repair.

There are also several limitations to this study. First, we assumed that cell movement can be described using a diffusion equation of a non-linear relationship that exists between mitosis/cell death and the magnitude of strain experienced by cells; and that tissue differentiation is regulated by a combination of the magnitude of octahedral shear strain and fluid flow within the tissue, which may not be completely accurate. Second, we did not account for the rate at which cells differentiate and produce a matrix and we did not attempt to model the effects of growth factors, such as transforming growth factor-beta. Third, we did not model the scaffold. The MSCs are not actually injected directly but should rather be implanted in combination with a scaffold.

Fourth, our model could not be validated using experimental data. It is very challenging to find experimental data with identical conditions. There are also advantages of using computational simulations to predict the results in this way. In addition, we validated it with previous computational results.

Finally, the developed models did not consider cells that only migrate into the defect from the exposed cancellous bone and it was instead assumed that MSCs could only enter the defect through implantation.

Developments of computational technology have now enabled researchers to perform simulations from a patient- or subject-specific perspective in the orthopedic field. Our results were obtained using a 3D model developed from real medical imaging and our results demonstrate that stance-phase loading was better than axial loading for cartilage regeneration. This is because simple vertical loading may cause excessive strain, while a stance-phase gait cycle prevents this strain at the cartilage defect due to the relationship with other loadings. The advantage of using such an approach is that it is one of the key features of computational methods in tissue engineering that enables the expedition of the testing of new constructs and the development of strategies for identifying the optimal therapy for each patient [42]. From this perspective, our results could provide patient-specific rehabilitation guidelines for the implantation of MSCs.

In conclusion, we developed a computational approach to simulate tissue differentiation that was tested by attempting to simulate cartilage regeneration and the results yielded tissue formation patterns similar to those observed clinically. Although we found that a stance-phase gait was better than axial loading in the context of cartilage regeneration, a more complex study protocol is required for future investigations and such a protocol should include consideration of the effects of passive flexion after axial force or crutches in weight-bearing.

Author Contributions: Y.G.K. designed the study, evaluated the FEA results and wrote the paper; J.A.L. developed the 3D model; K.T.K. supervised the study and analyzed the data; H.Y.L. confirmed data; H.Y.K. review the paper.

Funding: This research received no external funding.

Acknowledgments: No external funding was received for the study.

Conflicts of Interest: The authors declare no conflicts of interest.

References

1. Lawrence, R.C.; Felson, D.T.; Helmick, C.G.; Arnold, L.M.; Choi, H.; Deyo, R.A.; Gabriel, S.; Hirsch, R.; Hochberg, M.C.; Hunder, G.G.; et al. Estimates of the prevalence of arthritis and other rheumatic conditions in the united states. Part ii. *Arthritis Rheum.* **2008**, *58*, 26–35. [CrossRef]
2. Dillon, C.F.; Rasch, E.K.; Gu, Q.; Hirsch, R. Prevalence of knee osteoarthritis in the united states: Arthritis data from the third national health and nutrition examination survey 1991–94. *J. Rheumatol.* **2006**, *33*, 2271–2279.
3. Koh, Y.G.; Choi, Y.J. Infrapatellar fat pad-derived mesenchymal stem cell therapy for knee osteoarthritis. *Knee* **2012**, *19*, 902–907. [CrossRef] [PubMed]
4. Mankin, H.J. The response of articular cartilage to mechanical injury. *J. Bone Jt. Surg.* **1982**, *64*, 460–466. [CrossRef]
5. Kim, H.K.; Moran, M.E.; Salter, R.B. The potential for regeneration of articular cartilage in defects created by chondral shaving and subchondral abrasion. An experimental investigation in rabbits. *J. Bone Jt. Surg. Am. Vol.* **1991**, *73*, 1301–1315. [CrossRef]
6. Lohmander, L.S.; Roos, E.M. Clinical update: Treating osteoarthritis. *Lancet (Lond. Engl.)* **2007**, *370*, 2082–2084. [CrossRef]
7. Beitzel, K.; McCarthy, M.B.; Cote, M.P.; Chowaniec, D.; Falcone, L.M.; Falcone, J.A.; Dugdale, E.M.; Deberardino, T.M.; Arciero, R.A.; Mazzocca, A.D. Rapid isolation of human stem cells (connective progenitor cells) from the distal femur during arthroscopic knee surgery. *Arthrosc. J. Arthrosc. Relat. Surg. Off. Publ. Arthrosc. Assoc. N. Am. Int. Arthrosc. Assoc.* **2012**, *28*, 74–84. [CrossRef]
8. Raghunath, J.; Salacinski, H.J.; Sales, K.M.; Butler, P.E.; Seifalian, A.M. Advancing cartilage tissue engineering: The application of stem cell technology. *Curr. Opin. Biotechnol.* **2005**, *16*, 503–509. [CrossRef] [PubMed]
9. Kelly, D.J.; Prendergast, P.J. Mechano-regulation of stem cell differentiation and tissue regeneration in osteochondral defects. *J. Biomech.* **2005**, *38*, 1413–1422. [CrossRef] [PubMed]
10. Ament, C.; Hofer, E.P. A fuzzy logic model of fracture healing. *J. Biomech.* **2000**, *33*, 961–968. [CrossRef]
11. Prendergast, P.J.; Huiskes, R.; Søballe, K. Biophysical stimuli on cells during tissue differentiation at implant interfaces. *J. Biomech.* **1997**, *30*, 539–548. [CrossRef]
12. Isaksson, H.; van Donkelaar, C.C.; Huiskes, R.; Ito, K. A mechano-regulatory bone-healing model incorporating cell-phenotype specific activity. *J. Theor. Biol.* **2008**, *252*, 230–246. [CrossRef] [PubMed]
13. Nagel, T.; Kelly, D.J. Mechano-regulation of mesenchymal stem cell differentiation and collagen organisation during skeletal tissue repair. *Biomech. Model. Mechanobiol.* **2010**, *9*, 359–372. [CrossRef] [PubMed]
14. O'Reilly, A.; Kelly, D.J. Role of oxygen as a regulator of stem cell fate during the spontaneous repair of osteochondral defects. *J. Orthop. Res. Off. Publ. Orthop. Res. Soc.* **2016**, *34*, 1026–1036. [CrossRef] [PubMed]

15. O'Reilly, A.; Kelly, D.J. A computational model of osteochondral defect repair following implantation of stem cell-laden multiphase scaffolds. *Tissue Eng. Part A* **2017**, *23*, 30–42. [CrossRef]
16. Koh, Y.G.; Lee, J.A.; Kim, Y.S.; Lee, H.Y.; Kim, H.J.; Kang, K.T. Optimal mechanical properties of a scaffold for cartilage regeneration using finite element analysis. *J. Tissue Eng.* **2019**, *10*, 2041731419832133. [CrossRef] [PubMed]
17. Lacroix, D.; Prendergast, P.J.; Li, G.; Marsh, D. Biomechanical model to simulate tissue differentiation and bone regeneration: Application to fracture healing. *Med. Biol. Eng. Comput.* **2002**, *40*, 14–21. [CrossRef]
18. Hayward, L.N.; Morgan, E.F. Assessment of a mechano-regulation theory of skeletal tissue differentiation in an in vivo model of mechanically induced cartilage formation. *Biomech. Model. Mechanobiol.* **2009**, *8*, 447–455. [CrossRef] [PubMed]
19. Kim, Y.S.; Choi, Y.J.; Suh, D.S.; Heo, D.B.; Kim, Y.I.; Ryu, J.S.; Koh, Y.G. Mesenchymal stem cell implantation in osteoarthritic knees: Is fibrin glue effective as a scaffold? *Am. J. Sports Med.* **2015**, *43*, 176–185. [CrossRef] [PubMed]
20. Koh, Y.G.; Choi, Y.J.; Kwon, O.R.; Kim, Y.S. Second-look arthroscopic evaluation of cartilage lesions after mesenchymal stem cell implantation in osteoarthritic knees. *Am. J. Sports Med.* **2014**, *42*, 1628–1637. [CrossRef] [PubMed]
21. Kim, Y.S.; Choi, Y.J.; Koh, Y.G. Mesenchymal stem cell implantation in knee osteoarthritis: An assessment of the factors influencing clinical outcomes. *Am. J. Sports Med.* **2015**, *43*, 2293–2301. [CrossRef] [PubMed]
22. Isaksson, H.; Van Donkelaar, C.C.; Huiskes, R.; Yao, J.; Ita, K. Determining the most important cellular characteristics for fracture healing using design of experiments methods. *J. Theor. Biol.* **2008**, *255*, 26–39. [CrossRef]
23. Lacroix, D.; Prendergast, P.J. A homogenization procedure to prevent numerical instabilities in poroelastic tissue differentiation models. In Proceedings of the Eighth Annual Symposium: Computational Methods in Orthopaedic Biomechanics, Lake Buena Vista, FL, USA, 11 March 2000.
24. Kang, K.T.; Kim, S.H.; Son, J.; Lee, Y.H.; Chun, H.J. Computational model-based probabilistic analysis of in vivo material properties for ligament stiffness using the laxity test and computed tomography. *J. Mater. Sci. Mater. Med.* **2016**, *27*, 183. [CrossRef]
25. Koh, Y.G.; Son, J.; Kwon, S.K.; Kim, H.J.; Kwon, O.R.; Kang, K.T. Preservation of kinematics with posterior cruciate-, bicruciate- and patient-specific bicruciate-retaining prostheses in total knee arthroplasty by using computational simulation with normal knee model. *Bone Jt. Res.* **2017**, *6*, 557–565. [CrossRef] [PubMed]
26. Kang, K.T.; Koh, Y.G.; Son, J.; Kim, S.J.; Choi, S.; Jung, M.; Kim, S.H. Finite element analysis of the biomechanical effects of 3 posterolateral corner reconstruction techniques for the knee joint. *J. Arthrosc.* **2017**, *33*, 1537–1550. [CrossRef]
27. 14243-1, I. Implants for surgery—wear of total knee-joint prostheses—part 1: Loading and displacement parameters for wear-testing machines with load control and corresponding environmental conditions for test. 2009.
28. Curl, W.W.; Krome, J.; Gordon, E.S.; Rushing, J.; Smith, B.P.; Poehling, G.G. Cartilage injuries: A review of 31,516 knee arthroscopies. *Arthrosc. J. Arthrosc. Relat. Surg. Off. Publ. Arthrosc. Assoc. N. Am. Int. Arthrosc. Assoc.* **1997**, *13*, 456–460. [CrossRef]
29. Aroen, A.; Loken, S.; Heir, S.; Alvik, E.; Ekeland, A.; Granlund, O.G.; Engebretsen, L. Articular cartilage lesions in 993 consecutive knee arthroscopies. *Am. J. Sports Med.* **2004**, *32*, 211–215. [CrossRef]
30. Mithoefer, K.; Williams, R.J., 3rd; Warren, R.F.; Potter, H.G.; Spock, C.R.; Jones, E.C.; Wickiewicz, T.L.; Marx, R.G. The microfracture technique for the treatment of articular cartilage lesions in the knee. A prospective cohort study. *J. Bone Jt. Surg. Am. Vol.* **2005**, *87*, 1911–1920. [CrossRef]
31. Steadman, J.R.; Briggs, K.K.; Rodrigo, J.J.; Kocher, M.S.; Gill, T.J.; Rodkey, W.G. Outcomes of microfracture for traumatic chondral defects of the knee: Average 11-year follow-up. *Arthrosc. J. Arthrosc. Relat. Surg. Off. Publ. Arthrosc. Assoc. N. Am. Int. Arthrosc. Assoc.* **2003**, *19*, 477–484. [CrossRef] [PubMed]
32. Steadman, J.R.; Rodkey, W.G.; Rodrigo, J.J. Microfracture: Surgical technique and rehabilitation to treat chondral defects. *Clin. Orthop. Relat. Res.* **2001**, *S391*, S362–S369. [CrossRef]
33. Pareek, A.; Reardon, P.J.; Macalena, J.A.; Levy, B.A.; Stuart, M.J.; Williams, R.J., 3rd; Krych, A.J. Osteochondral autograft transfer versus microfracture in the knee: A meta-analysis of prospective comparative studies at midterm. *Arthrosc. J. Arthrosc. Relat. Surg. Off. Publ. Arthrosc. Assoc. N. Am. Int. Arthrosc. Assoc.* **2016**, *32*, 2118–2130. [CrossRef]

34. Shelbourne, K.D.; Jari, S.; Gray, T. Outcome of untreated traumatic articular cartilage defects of the knee: A natural history study. *J. Bone Jt. Surg. Am. Vol.* **2003**, *85A* (Suppl. 2), 8–16. [CrossRef]
35. Ashton, B.A.; Allen, T.D.; Howlett, C.R.; Eaglesom, C.C.; Hattori, A.; Owen, M. Formation of bone and cartilage by marrow stromal cells in diffusion chambers in vivo. *Clin. Orthop. Relat. Res.* **1980**, *151*, 294–307. [CrossRef]
36. Johnstone, B.; Hering, T.M.; Caplan, A.I.; Goldberg, V.M.; Yoo, J.U. In vivo chondrogenesis of bone marrow-derived mesenchymal progenitor cells. *Exp. Cell Res.* **1998**, *238*, 265–272. [CrossRef] [PubMed]
37. Kim, Y.S.; Kwon, O.R.; Choi, Y.J.; Suh, D.S.; Heo, D.B.; Koh, Y.G. Comparative matched-pair analysis of the injection versus implantation of mesenchymal stem cells for knee osteoarthritis. *Am. J. Sports Med.* **2015**, *43*, 2738–2746. [CrossRef] [PubMed]
38. Jo, C.H.; Lee, Y.G.; Shin, W.H.; Kim, H.; Chai, J.W.; Jeong, E.C.; Kim, J.E.; Shim, H.; Shin, J.S.; Shin, I.S.; et al. Intra-articular injection of mesenchymal stem cells for the treatment of osteoarthritis of the knee: A proof-of-concept clinical trial. *Stem Cells (Dayt. Ohio)* **2014**, *32*, 1254–1266. [CrossRef] [PubMed]
39. Lacroix, D.; Prendergast, P.J. A mechano-regulation model for tissue differentiation during fracture healing: Analysis of gap size and loading. *J. Biomech.* **2002**, *35*, 1163–1171. [CrossRef]
40. Shapiro, F.; Koide, S.; Glimcher, M.J. Cell origin and differentiation in the repair of full-thickness defects of articular cartilage. *J. Bone Jt. Surg. Am. Vol.* **1993**, *75*, 532–553. [CrossRef]
41. Kelly, D.J.; Prendergast, P.J. Prediction of the optimal mechanical properties for a scaffold used in osteochondral defect repair. *Tissue Eng.* **2006**, *12*, 2509–2519. [CrossRef] [PubMed]
42. Semple, J.L.; Woolridge, N.; Lumsden, C.J. In vitro, in vivo, in silico: Computational systems in tissue engineering and regenerative medicine. *Tissue Eng.* **2005**, *11*, 341–356. [CrossRef] [PubMed]

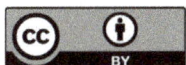

© 2019 by the authors. Licensee MDPI, Basel, Switzerland. This article is an open access article distributed under the terms and conditions of the Creative Commons Attribution (CC BY) license (http://creativecommons.org/licenses/by/4.0/).

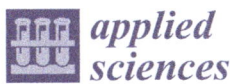

Article

Biomechanical Evaluation of a New Fixation Type in 3D-Printed Periacetabular Implants using a Finite Element Simulation

Dae Woo Park [1], Aekyeong Lim [1], Jong Woong Park [2], Kwon Mook Lim [3] and Hyun Guy Kang [1,2,*]

1. Innovative Medical Engineering & Technology, National Cancer Center, Goyang 10408, Korea; bigrain@ncc.re.kr (D.W.P.); aklim@ncc.re.kr (A.L.)
2. Orthopaedic Oncology Clinic, Specific Organs Cancer Branch, National Cancer Center, Goyang 10408, Korea; jwpark82@ncc.re.kr
3. Research & Development Center, Medyssey Co., Ltd, Jecheon-Si 27116, Korea; lkm@medyssey.com
* Correspondence: ostumor@ncc.re.kr; Tel.: +82-31-920-1665

Received: 14 January 2019; Accepted: 18 February 2019; Published: 26 February 2019

Abstract: Pelvic implants require complex geometrical shapes to reconstruct unusual areas of bone defects, as well as a high mechanical strength in order to endure high compressive loads. The electron beam melting (EBM) method is capable of directly fabricating complex metallic structures and shapes based on digital models. Fixation design is important during the 3D printing of pelvic implants, given that the fixation secures the pelvic implants to the remaining bones, while also bearing large amounts of the loads placed on the bone. In this study, a horseshoe-shaped plate fixation with a bridge component between two straight plates is designed to enhance the mechanical stability of pelvic implants. The aim of this study is to investigate the biomechanics of the horseshoe-shaped plate fixation in a 3D-printed pelvic implant using a finite element (FE) simulation. First, computed tomography (CT) scans were acquired from a patient with periacetabular bone tumors. Second, 3D FE implant models were created using the patient's Digital Imaging and Communications in Medicine (DICOM) data. Third, a FE simulation was conducted and the stress distribution between a conventional straight-type plate model, and the horseshoe-shaped plate model was compared. In both of the models, high-stress regions were observed at the iliac fixation area. In contrast, minimal stress regions were located at the pubic ramus and ischium fixation area. The key finding of this study was that the maximal stress of the horseshoe-shaped plate model (38.6 MPa) was 21% lower than that of the straight-type plate model (48.9 MPa) in the iliac fixation area. The clinical potential for the application of the horseshoe-shaped plate fixation model to the pelvic implant has been demonstrated, although this is a pilot study.

Keywords: Pelvis; Bone tumor; 3D-printed implant; Fixation design; von Mises stress

1. Introduction

Pelvic implants require complex geometrical shapes to reconstruct unusual areas of bone defects, as well as mechanical strength to endure high compressive loads [1]. For limb salvage procedures, custom pelvic prostheses have been utilized for reconstruction after the resection of bone tumors [1,2]. Custom pelvic prostheses have been fabricated by machining a solid titanium block, and this requires intensive labor and a long fabrication time [2]. Electron-beam melting (EBM), a type of 3D printing technology, can directly fabricate complex metallic structures with excellent material properties (almost no porosity) [3] and shapes, on the basis of digital models [4]. Thus, the EBM has been utilized to fabricate orthopedic components such as knee, hip, and jaw replacements, and maxillofacial plates [5–8].

For custom pelvic implants, fixation design is important, considering that the fixation secures the pelvic implants to the remaining bones, and should bear substantial loads as well [9]. A double column plating or a single column plating combined with lag screws has been commonly utilized to fix pelvic bones. The double column plating is effective to fix the complex fractures of pelvic bones [10]. However, the double column plating requires more screws for penetration during surgery, and this often results in a serious traumatic complication [11,12] that can lead to the development of osteoarthritis [11]. The single column plating combined with lag screws was regarded as the preferred technique, as it produces minimal exposure and devascularization of the pelvis [13], with comparable stability to the double column plating [13,14]. Therefore, in pelvic implants, two or three straight column platings combined with lag screws have been conventionally utilized for fixation [15,16]. These fixation types reportedly incur high traumatic fracture risks under compressive loading conditions [16,17]. Enhancements of the mechanical stability using spinal rod connectors, which have a bridge component between two straight connectors, have been reported in spine surgery publications [18,19]. Thus far, this bridge component design has not been utilized for pelvic implant fixation. We designed a horseshoe-shaped plate fixation with a bridge component between two straight plates, in an effort to enhance the mechanical stability of pelvic implants. Several studies have evaluated the strength of a conventional straight-type plate fixation for the posterior wall or transverse acetabular fractures [20–23]. In pelvic implants, there have been no studies comparing the biomechanical stabilities of the new horseshoe-shaped plate fixation with the conventional straight-type plate fixation consisting of column plates and lag screws.

The aim of this study is to investigate the biomechanics of the horseshoe-shaped plate fixation in a 3D-printed pelvic implant, using a finite element (FE) simulation. First, computed tomography (CT) scans were acquired from a patient suffering from periacetabular bone tumors. Second, 3D FE implant models, in this case a conventional straight-type plate model and the horseshoe-shaped plate model, were created using the patient's Digital Imaging and Communications in Medicine (DICOM) data. Third, a FE simulation was performed, and the stress distribution between the straight-type plate and the horseshoe-shaped plate models was compared.

2. Materials and Methods

2.1. Patient Information

The patient was a 53-year-old woman with a height of 157 cm, weighing 50 kg. She had a recurrent high-grade spindle cell sarcoma in the left pelvic bone and proximal femur. After a type II resection, reconstruction surgery was planned using a 3D-printed titanium periacetabular implant.

2.2. 3D-Reconstruction of the Pelvic Implant Model

Figure 1 shows the anterior view of the radiographic (Figure 1a) and 3D CT (Figure 1b) images obtained from the patient. The sarcoma resection areas were represented in red dashed circles. The patient's pelvis model was constructed using Digital Imaging and Communications in Medicine (DICOM) data based on computerized tomography (CT) scans. The DICOM data comprise a series of slices through the patient's left pelvis, each approximately 1.0 mm thick. A 3D model of the intact pelvis was constructed using a mirror image of the right pelvis, from a series of slices.

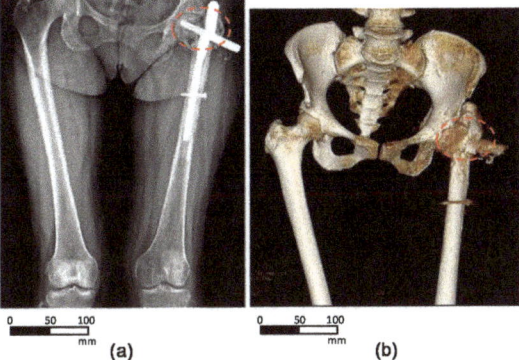

Figure 1. Pre-operative medical images of the pelvis area obtained from the patient: (**a**) plain radiograph and (**b**) 3D computed tomography (CT) images.

Figure 2 presents the 3D implant model developed from the pelvic bone model using the offset function in the software MIMICS (Version 20.0, Materialise Company, Leuven, Belgium). The pelvic bone and implant are shown in grey and light yellow, respectively. For the implant fixation, the straight-type plates (Figure 2a) and the horseshoe-shaped plates (Figure 2b) were designed. The sizes of the holes in the fixation were designed to fit cannulated screw holes (D = 3.0 mm). The final implant design was completed by smoothing the rough surfaces of the implant model using the software 3-Matic (Version 13.0, Materialise Company, Leuven, Belgium). The design was stored as a Standard Triangle Language (STL) file.

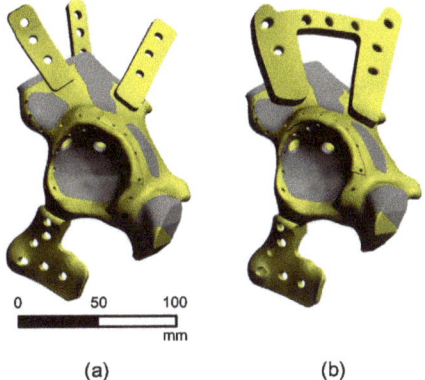

Figure 2. 3D model of the periacetabular implant and femur shaft area. The implant fixation models with (**a**) the straight-type plates and (**b**) the horseshoe-shaped plates.

2.3. Finite Element Simulation of a Pelvic Implant Model

The FE simulation was performed using the software ANSYS (Workbench 18.0, ANSYS Inc., Canonsburg, PA, USA). Figure 3 shows the pelvic implant FE models created using the straight-type plate fixation (Figure 3a) and the horseshoe-shaped plate fixation (Figure 3b). The volume mesh was created on the implant models using the software ANSYS (Workbench 18.0, ANSYS Inc., Canonsburg, PA, USA). The straight-type plate model and horseshoe-shaped plate model consist of 215,838 and 222,488 tetrahedral elements, respectively. Here, the cortical bone, cancellous bone, straight-type plate model, and horseshoe-shaped plate model are represented in yellow, blue, purple, and orange, respectively. Table 1 summarizes the material properties of the cortical bone, cancellous bone, and titanium, chosen from previous mechanical measurements [24]. Both the cortical bone and cancellous bone were assumed to be isotropic and homogeneous. The boundary conditions were defined such that the hemi-pelvis was fixed in all directions by the pubis symphysis and femoral head, represented as the green surface laid over the FE models. The contact type between the pelvis and implant was set to "bonded", and the contact surface between the femoral head and the acetabulum was set to "frictionless." A distributed compressive force of 4.9 kN was applied to the iliac crest, represented by the red surface laid over the FE models, along the vertical axis of the pelvis, based on the maximal load exerted by the patient's weight [25].

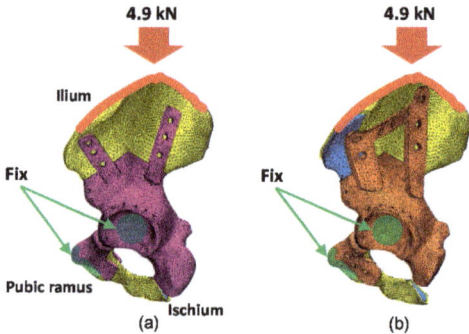

Figure 3. Boundary conditions of finite element (FE) models with (**a**) the straight-type plate fixation and (**b**) the horseshoe-shaped plate fixation.

Table 1. Material properties used for the finite element simulation.

Material	Density (g/cm^3)	Young's Modulus (MPa)	Poisson's Ratio (v)	Tensile Strength (MPa)	Compressive Strength (MPa)
Cortical bone	1.64	16,700	0.26	106	157
Cancellous bone	0.16	155	0.30	6	6
Ti-6Al-4V	4.62	96,000	0.36	1070	1070

3. Results

Figure 4 presents the von Mises stress distribution of the FE models with the straight-type plate fixation and the horseshoe-shaped plate fixation. In the straight-type plate model and the horseshoe-shaped plate model, a high-stress region was observed at the iliac fixation area. In contrast, low-stress regions were located at the pubic ramus and ischium fixation areas. For the straight-type plate model, the proportions of the stress concentration in the ilium, pubic ramus, and ischium were 17.8%, 2.3%, and 0.5%, respectively. For the horseshoe-shaped plate model, the corresponding stress concentration proportions were 19.8%, 2.3%, and 0.6%. In the iliac fixation area, the maximal stress of the horseshoe-shaped plate model (38.6 MPa) was 21% lower than that of the straight-type plate model (48.9 MPa).

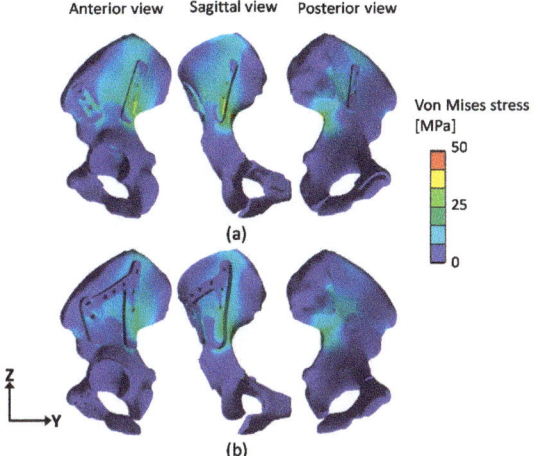

Figure 4. The von Mises stress distribution of the finite element (FE) models with (**a**) the straight-type plate fixation and (**b**) the horseshoe-shaped plate fixation.

The horseshoe-shaped plate model was fabricated for the patient's reconstruction surgery, using EBM with the following process parameters: beam power of 3000 W, beam scan speed of 8000 m/s, beam spot size of 0.2 mm, build rate of 55 mm^3/h, and a build thickness of 50 µm, on all sides of the scanning strategy. Figure 5 shows the horseshoe-shaped plate model fabricated with medical-grade titanium (Ti-6Al-4V-ELI per ASTM 136) using a powder-based EBM 3D printer (model: ARCAM A1, Arcam AB, Mölndal, Sweden) [26].

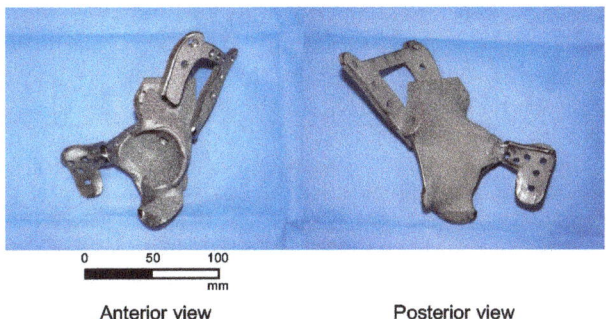

Figure 5. 3D-printed titanium periacetabular implant with the horseshoe-shaped plates.

Figure 6 presents the medical images of the pelvis area obtained from the patient after the implantation surgery. The post-operative radiograph (Figure 6a) and 3D CT (Figure 6b) images demonstrated that the pelvis showed a satisfactory implant alignment and no evidence of implant loosening. In the postoperative evaluation, the patient was allowed to walk with underarm crutches two weeks after the surgery, and her feedback was positive.

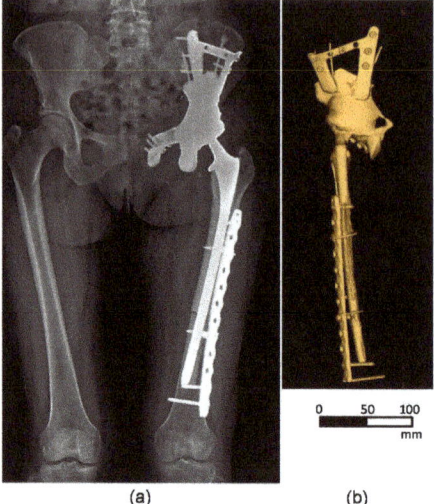

Figure 6. Post-operative medical images of the pelvis area obtained from a patient: (**a**) plain radiograph and (**b**) 3D CT images.

4. Discussion

The FE simulation results indicated that a high-stress concentration existed in the iliac fixation area. In contrast, a low-stress region was found at the pubis and ischium fixation area (Figure 4). This high-stress concentration at the iliac fixation area has been previously reported [27,28]. Based on this stress distribution, we could conclude that the iliac fixation area bore most of the compressive load, and thus that the region of the ilium required more stable fixation with the implant than the pubis and ischium regions after type II tumor resection.

The important finding of this study was that the bridge component in the horseshoe plate model reduced the stress concentration by as much as 21% at the iliac fixation area (Figure 4). This indicates that the bridge component dissipated a large portion of the compressive load to the surrounding bones, and thus reduced the risk of fracture at the iliac fixation area. While this is the FE simulation result from only one patient's pelvic implant, this study suggests that the bridge component of the periacetabular implant fixation would enhance the mechanical stability after type II resection. In future work, the mechanical stability of the horseshoe-shaped plate model should be evaluated in order to determine the suitability of this model for periacetabular implants in more patients.

This study demonstrated that the horseshoe-shaped plate model exhibited a more stable fixation than the conventional straight-type plate model in the pelvic implant fixation. For the fixation of a pelvic bone fracture, previous investigators have developed various fixation systems by incorporating screws or another plate into the fixation system with a column plate [13,14,29,30]. In addition to the pelvic implant fixation, our horseshoe-shaped plate model could be beneficial to enhance the stabilities of the fixation system in the pelvic bone fracture. In future studies, we will investigate stable fixation systems for the pelvic bone fracture by comparing the biomechanical stabilities between the horseshoe-shaped plate model and other conventional fixation systems.

In this study, the porous structure was applied on the surface of the titanium implants in order to reduce the stress shielding effect. The titanium implant is much stiffer than the surrounding bones, and the stress transfer between an implant device and a bone is not homogeneous [31]. The surrounding bone is then stress shielded and experiences abnormally low levels of stress, which can lead to the resorption of the bone, and again, loosening of the implant [32]. The porous titanium material has the advantages of enhancing the bone–implant interface strength by promoting bone and soft tissue ingrowth, and of reducing the bone–implant strength mismatch [33]. In future studies, the porous design, such as pores, holes, or lattice structure, should be investigated in order to enhance the mechanical properties as well as osteointegration.

Our FE simulation approach has several limitations. First, the FE simulation model was created with a uniform thickness of the cortical bone. In an actual pelvic bone, the thickness of the cortical bone varies across the pelvic bone in order to adjust to load transfers [28]. This variable thickness of the cortical bone would affect the stress distribution in the pelvic bone and the implant. Therefore, the mechanical stability of the horseshoe-shaped plate model should be evaluated further with various cortical bone thicknesses via FE simulations. Second, in the FE model, the contact type between the pelvis and implant was set to "bonded", and the effects of the screws on the stress distribution in the pelvis bone were not considered. In future research, the stress concentration at the screw holes should be investigated with the horseshoe-shaped plate model. Third, the FE simulation was performed while only considering compressive loading conditions. We assumed that the compressive load of the patient's weight was the most influential loading condition in the pelvis area. However, pelvic bones normally experience complex mechanical loading conditions [34]. More in-depth investigations should be performed while considering complex loading conditions in order to validate the stress distribution results in this study. Fourth, we undertook an FE simulation using a simplified FE model without including ligaments. This FE model produced sufficient results for a stress distribution comparison between the straight-type plate model and the horseshoe-shaped plate model. However, the stress distribution obtained from this FE model may not fully represent the actual loading conditions. Fifth, only the von Mises stress results were analyzed to compare the stress distribution between the conventional model and the horseshoe-shaped plate model within the scope of this study. In future studies, more parameters, such as principle stresses and strains, should be investigated in order to validate the mechanical stability of the horseshoe-shaped plate model.

5. Conclusions

The horseshoe-shaped plate fixation demonstrated an enhanced mechanical stability in a 3D-printed titanium periacetabular implant. The horseshoe-shaped plate fixation model may have clinical potential and thus warrants more extensive clinical investigations.

Author Contributions: Conceptualization, D.W.P. and H.G.K.; methodology, D.W.P.; software, A.L.; validation, A.L. and D.W.P.; formal analysis, A.L. and D.W.P.; investigation, D.W.P.; resources, J.W.P. and K.M.L.; data curation, A.L. and D.W.P.; writing (original draft preparation), D.W.P.; writing (review and editing), J.W.P. and H.G.K.; visualization, D.W.P.; supervision, H.G.K.; project administration, H.G.K.

Funding: This study was supported by a grant from the Korea Health Technology R&D Project through the Korea Health Industry Development Institute (KHIDI), and was funded by the Ministry of Health and Welfare, Republic of Korea (grant number HI17C1823).

Acknowledgments: The technical support of the finite element software was provided by the Medical Device Development Center of the Daegu-Gyeongbuk Medical Innovation Foundation.

Conflicts of Interest: The authors declare no conflict of interest.

References

1. Wong, K.C.; Kumta, S.M.; Geel, N.V.; Demol, J. One-step reconstruction with a 3D-printed, biomechanically evaluated custom implant after complex pelvic tumor resection. *Comput. Aided. Surg.* **2015**, *20*, 14–23. [CrossRef] [PubMed]
2. Fan, H.; Fu, J.; Li, X.; Pei, Y.; Li, X.; Pei, G.; Guo, Z. Implantation of customized 3-D printed titanium prosthesis in limb salvage surgery: A case series and review of the literature. *World J. Surg. Oncol.* **2015**, *13*, 308. [CrossRef] [PubMed]
3. Sing, S.L.; An, J.; Yeong, W.Y. Laser and electron-beam powder-bed additive manufacturing of metallic implants: A review on processes, materials and designs. *J. Orthop. Res.* **2015**, *34*, 369–385. [CrossRef] [PubMed]

4. Rengier, F.; Mehndiratta, A.; von Tengg-Kobligk, H.; Zechmann, C.M.; Unterhinninghofen, R.; Kauczor, H.U.; Giesel, F.L. 3D printing based on imaging data: Review of medical applications. *Int. J. Comput. Assist. Radiol. Surg.* **2010**, *5*, 335–341. [CrossRef] [PubMed]
5. Cronskär, M.; Bäckström, M.; Rännar, L.-E. Production of customized hip stem prostheses—A comparison between conventional machining and electron beam melting (EBM). *Rapid Prototyp. J.* **2013**, *19*, 365–372.
6. Mazzoli, A.; Germani, M.; Raffaeli, R. Direct fabrication through electron beam melting technology of custom cranial implants designed in a PHANToM-based haptic environment. *Mater. Des.* **2009**, *30*, 3186–3192. [CrossRef]
7. Jardini, A.L.; Larosa, M.A.; de Carvalho Zavaglia, C.A.; Bernardes, L.F.; Lamber, C.S. Customised titanium implant fabricated in additive manufacturing for craniomaxillofacial surgery. *Virtual Phys. Prototyp.* **2014**, *9*, 115–125. [CrossRef]
8. Jardini, A.L.; Larosaemail, M.A.; Filho, R.M.; de Carvalho Zavaglia, C.A.; Bernardes, L.F.; Lambert, C.S.; Calderoni, D.R.; Kharmandayan, P. Cranial reconstruction: 3D biomodel and custom-built implant created using additive manufacturing. *J. Craniomaxillofac. Surg.* **2014**, *42*, 1877–1884. [CrossRef] [PubMed]
9. Lei, J.; Dong, P.; Li, Z.; Zhu, F.; Wang, Z.; Cai, X. Biomechanical analysis of the fixation systems for anterior column and posterior hemi-transverse acetabular fractures. *Acta Orthopaedica et Traumatologica Turcica* **2017**, *51*, 248–253. [CrossRef] [PubMed]
10. Wolf, H.; Wieland, T.; Pajenda, G.; Vecsei, V.; Mousavi, M. Minimally invasive ilioinguinal approach to the acetabulum. *Injury* **2007**, *38*, 1170–1176. [CrossRef] [PubMed]
11. Russell, G.V.; Nork, S.E.; Chip, R.M.L. Perioperative complications associated with operative treatment of acetabular fractures. *J. Trauma Acute Care Surg.* **2001**, *51*, 1098–1103. [CrossRef]
12. Ebraheim, N.A.; Savolaine, E.R.; Hoeflinger, M.J.; Jackson, W.T. Radiological diagnosis of screw penetration of the hip joint in acetabular fracture reconstruction. *J. Orthop. Trauma* **1989**, *3*, 196–201. [CrossRef] [PubMed]
13. Sawaguchi, T.; Brown, T.D.; Rubash, H.E.; Mears, D.C. Stability of acetabular fractures after internal fixation: A cadaveric study. *Acta Orthop.* **1984**, *55*, 601–605. [CrossRef]
14. Schopfer, A.; DiAngelo, D.; Hearn, T.; Powell, J.; Tile, M. Biomechanical comparison of methods of fixation of isolated osteotomies of the posterior acetabular column. *Int. Orthop.* **1994**, *18*, 96–101. [CrossRef] [PubMed]
15. Singh, V.A.; Elbahri, H.; Shanmugam, R. Biomechanical analysis of a novel acetabulum reconstruction technique with acetabulum reconstruction cage and threaded rods after type II pelvic resections. *Sarcoma* **2016**, *2016*, 1–7. [CrossRef] [PubMed]
16. Plessers, K.; Mau, H. Stress analysis of a Burch-Schneider cage in an acetabular bone defect: A case study. *Reconstr. Rev.* **2016**, *6*, 37–42. [CrossRef]
17. Atik, F.; Ataç, M.S.; Özkan, A.; Kilinç, Y.; Arslan, M. Biomechanical analysis of titanium fixation plates and screws in mandibular angle fractures. *Niger. J. Clin. Pract.* **2016**, *19*, 386–390. [PubMed]
18. Zhang, B.C.; Liu, H.B.; Kai, X.H.; Wang, Z.H.; Xu, F.; Kang, H.; Ding, R.; Luo, X.Q. Biomechanical comparison of a novel transoral atlantoaxial anchored cage with established fixation technique—A finite element analysis. *BMC Musculoskelet. Disord.* **2015**, *16*, 216. [CrossRef] [PubMed]
19. Goel, V.K.; Mehta, A.; Jangra, J.; Faizan, A.; Kiapour, A.; Hoy, R.W.; Fauth, A.R. Anatomic facet replacement system (AFRS) restoration of lumbar segment mechanics to intact: A finite element study and in vitro cadaver investigation. *SAS J.* **2007**, *1*, 46–54. [CrossRef]
20. Chang, J.K.; Gill, S.S.; Zura, R.D.; Krause, W.R.; Wang, G.J. Comparative strength of three methods of fixation of transverse acetabular fractures. *Clin. Orthop. Relat. Res.* **2001**, *392*, 433–441. [CrossRef]
21. Shazar, N.; Brumback, R.J.; Novak, V.P.; Belkoff, S.M. Biomechanical evaluation of transverse acetabular fracture fixation. *Clin. Orthop. Relat. Res.* **1998**, *352*, 215–222. [CrossRef]
22. Xin-wei, L.; Shuo-gui, X.; Chun-cai, Z.; Qing-ge, F.; Pan-feng, W. Biomechanical study of posterior wall acetabular fracture fixation using acetabular tridimensional memory alloy-fixation system. *Clin. Biomech.* **2010**, *25*, 312–317. [CrossRef] [PubMed]
23. Olson, S.A.; Bay, B.K.; Chapman, M.W.; Sharkey, N.A. Biomechanical consequences of fracture and repair of the posterior wall of the acetabulum. *J. Bone Joint Surg. Am.* **1995**, *77*, 1184–1192. [CrossRef] [PubMed]
24. Aziz, M.S.R.; Dessouki, O.; Samiezadeh, S.; Bougherara, H.; Schemitsch, E.H.; Zero, R. Biomechanical analysis using FEA and experiments of a standard plate method versus three cable methods for fixing acetabular fractures with simultaneous THA. *Med. Eng. Phys.* **2017**, *46*, 71–78. [CrossRef] [PubMed]

25. Bergmann, G.; Graichen, F.; Rohlmann, A. Hip joint loading during walking and running, measured in two patients. *J. Biomech.* **1993**, *26*, 969–990. [CrossRef]
26. Harrysson, O.L.A.; Cansizoglu, O.; Marcellin-Little, D.J.; Cormier, D.R.; West II, H.A. Direct metal fabrication of titanium implants with tailored materials and mechanical properties using electron beam melting technology. *Mater. Sci. Eng. C* **2008**, *28*, 366–373. [CrossRef]
27. Shen, F.H.; Mason, J.R.; Shimer, A.L.; Arlet, V.M. Pelvic fixation for adult scoliosis. *Eur. Spine J.* **2013**, *22* (Suppl. 2), 265–275. [CrossRef] [PubMed]
28. Thompson, M.S.; Northmore-Ball, M.D.; Tanner, K.E. Effects of acetabular resurfacing component material and fixation on the strain distribution in the pelvis. *Proc. Inst. Mech. Eng.* **2002**, *216*, 237–245. [CrossRef] [PubMed]
29. Wu, Y.; Cai, X.; Liu, X.; Zhang, H. Biomechanical analysis of the acetabular buttressplate: Are complex acetabular fractures in the quadrilateral area stable after treatment with anterior construct plate-1/3 tube buttress plate fixation? *Clinics* **2013**, *68*, 1028e1033. [CrossRef]
30. Andersen, R.C.; O'Toole, R.V.; Nascone, J.W.; Sciadini, M.F.; Frisch, H.M.; Turen, C.W. Modified stoppa approach for acetabular fractures with anterior and posterior column displacement: Quantification of radiographic reduction and analysis of interobserver variability. *J. Orthop. Trauma* **2010**, *24*, 271e278. [CrossRef] [PubMed]
31. Niinomi, M.; Nakai, M. Titanium-Based Biomaterials for Preventing Stress Shielding between Implant Devices and Bone. *Int. J. Biomater.* **2011**, *2011*, 836587. [CrossRef] [PubMed]
32. Black, J. *Biological Performance of Materials, Fundamentals of Biocompatibility*, 3rd ed.; Marcel Dekker: New York, NY, USA, 1999.
33. Thelen, S.; Barthelat, F.; Brinson, L.C. Mechanics considerations for microporous titanium as an orthopedic implant material. *J. Biomed. Mater. Res. A* **2004**, *69A*, 601–610. [CrossRef] [PubMed]
34. Dalstra, M.; Huiskes, R.; van Erning, L. Development and validation of a three-dimensional finite element model of the pelvic bone. *J. Biomech. Eng.* **1995**, *117*, 272–278. [CrossRef] [PubMed]

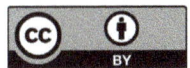

© 2019 by the authors. Licensee MDPI, Basel, Switzerland. This article is an open access article distributed under the terms and conditions of the Creative Commons Attribution (CC BY) license (http://creativecommons.org/licenses/by/4.0/).

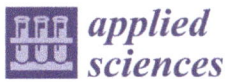

Article

FEM-Based Compression Fracture Risk Assessment in Osteoporotic Lumbar Vertebra L1

Algirdas Maknickas [1,*], Vidmantas Alekna [2], Oleg Ardatov [1], Olga Chabarova [3], Darius Zabulionis [4], Marija Tamulaitienė [2] and Rimantas Kačianauskas [1,4]

1. Institute of Mechanics, Vilnius Gediminas Technical University, 03224 Vilnius, Lithuania
2. Faculty of Medicine, Vilnius University, 03101 Vilnius, Lithuania
3. Department of Applied Mechanics, Vilnius Gediminas Technical University, 10223 Vilnius, Lithuania
4. Department of Information Systems, Vilnius Gediminas Technical University, 10223 Vilnius, Lithuania
* Correspondence: algirdas.maknickas@vgtu.lt

Received: 27 June 2019; Accepted: 24 July 2019; Published: 26 July 2019

Abstract: This paper presents a finite element method (FEM)-based fracture risk assessment in patient-specific osteoporotic lumbar vertebra L1. The influence of osteoporosis is defined by variation of parameters such as thickness of the cortical shell, the bone volume–total volume ratio (BV/TV), and the trabecular bone score (TBS). The mechanical behaviour of bone is defined using the Ramberg–Osgood material model. This study involves the static and nonlinear dynamic calculations of von Mises stresses and follows statistical processing of the obtained results in order to develop the patient-specific vertebra reliability. In addition, different scenarios of parameters show that the reliability of the proposed model of human vertebra highly decreases with low levels of BV/TV and is critical due to the thinner cortical bone, suggesting high trauma risk by reason of osteoporosis.

Keywords: bone tissue; elastoplasticity; finite element method; fracture risk; osteoporosis; trabeculae; trabecular bone score; vertebra

1. Introduction

Spinal bones can be affected by several diseases, but spinal brittleness is mainly caused by osteoporosis. Due to the importance of studying this disease and its consequences, various social and medical aspects of osteoporosis have been investigated all over the world [1–4]. A comprehensive discussion of the role of computational biomechanical modeling is presented in a review article by Doblare et al. [5]. The paper emphasized numerical modeling as the main directions for future research. The adequacy of the modeling of finite elements strongly depends on the selection of the mechanical properties, the geometrical form of the numerical model, and mesh making possibilities.

With regard to considerable difficulties in the assignment of the anatomical geometry to the model, most researches are focused on simplifications. Some developments are restrained to small fragments of the vertebra [6,7], but most studies concerning the vertebral body in isolation [8–11] also use a simplified form, excluding the posterior elements [12,13].

A two-scale modeling approach was proposed in a series of papers where the macroscopic defining behavior is defined by the influence of the microstructure. For example, the work of McDonald et al. used a microscopic lattice network [12]. A similar approach was applied by Reference [14]. In contrast, a more comprehensive method of modeling was used in Reference [15] where the porous trabecular cell in the cancellous bone is considered as three-dimensional solid.

To determine the level of stress and bone strength, classical criteria for fluidity at the continuum level are often applied. Thus, the von Mises yield criterion is the most frequently used [11]

criterion used for the trabecular bone of a vertebra, but a tissue-dependent orthotropic yield criterion Tsai–Wu [16] was proposed also.

In most cases, studies were perfomed by using static loads, while the number of investigations with dynamic loads are rather limited [13,17]. Also, the computational biomechanics can provide the ability to assess fracture risk and can serve as a useful diagnostic tool for analysing the state of osteoporotic bones. One of the most effective modern indicators used to verify vertebral fragility is the the trabecular bone score (TBS). This method involves the measurment of gray level texture, which shows the average state of trabecular bone microarchitecture [18], closely related to the ratio volume–total bone volume (BV/TV) [19]. Although TBS is a rough estimate of the strength properties of bone tissue, it can also be provided to study bone fragility and predict bone fractures.

There are several developed methods which employ bone mineral density (BMD) to predict the long-term fracture risk. BMD is usually assessed by dual-energy X-ray absorptiometry (DXA), and some studies have shown that a decrease of BMD is bonded with a higher risk for future fracture [20–22]. In addition, modern techniques of medical diagnostics also dispose computer-based algorithms, such as FRAX [23], which calculate fracture probability from clinical risk factors, such as age and body mass index(BMI), and dichotomized risk factors comprising prior fragility fracture, parental history of hip fracture, currently smoking tobacco, long-term oral glucocorticoid use, rheumatoid arthritis, other causes of secondary osteoporosis, and alcohol consumption [24]. In contrast, these methods do not verify the complicated relationship between the important parameters such as BV/TV, the thickness of the cortical shell, and the external load. The finite element method (FEM)-based continuum models can supply the additional patient-specific data to define the risk of fracture by additionally applying the reliability theory.

One of the aims of present work is numerical investigation of the osteoportic affect on strength properties of the proposed vertebrae model including the time-dependent load. The evaluation results might be useful for the medical diagnostics of the osteoporosis and for verifying the strength properties of the bone tissue of the patient. The main aim of this study is proposing the structural mechanics-based method of calculating fracture risk based on statistically processed results obtained by the numerical investigation of strength properties of the lumbar vertebral L1 body with various grades of osteoporotic degradation.

2. Methods and Materials

2.1. Problem Formulation

In order to model bone tissue as elastoplastic three-dimensional solid, the Ramberg–Osgood stress–strain equation was applied [25]:

$$\varepsilon = \frac{\sigma}{E_0 \dot{\varepsilon}^d} + \alpha \left(\frac{\sigma}{K}\right)^n \dot{\varepsilon}^b \tag{1}$$

where E_0 is the modulus of elasticity, K is the strain hardening coefficient, n is the strain-hardening exponent, and α is the yield offset, where $\dot{\varepsilon} = 1$ equality was used. According to research [25], the loading rate of cortical bone influences the behaviour of the stress–strain relation. Therefore, our model of risk evaluation should be treated as the upper risk limit for load rates, which do not exceed rates of $\dot{\varepsilon} \leq 1$.

In this work, the von Mises–Hencky criterion is chosen to predict the fracture of the model. It is defined in Equation (2): There, σ_1, σ_2 and σ_3 are the maximum, intermediate and minimum principal stresses. σ_Y presents yield stress (40 MPa) [26].

$$\sqrt{\frac{(\sigma_1 - \sigma_2)^2 + (\sigma_2 - \sigma_3)^2 + (\sigma_3 - \sigma_1)^2}{2}} = \sigma_Y \tag{2}$$

In the case of nonlinear analysis, the equilibrium equations are presented at time step $t + \Delta t$:

$$\mathbf{M}^{t+\Delta t}\mathbf{U}''^{(i)} + \mathbf{C}^{t+\Delta t}\mathbf{U}'^{(i)} + {}^{t+\Delta t}\mathbf{K}^{(i)t+\Delta t}\Delta\mathbf{U}^{(i)} = {}^{t+\Delta t}\mathbf{R} - {}^{t+\Delta t}\mathbf{F}^{(i-1)} \qquad (3)$$

where $\mathbf{M}$ is the mass matrix, $\mathbf{C}$ is the damping matrix, ${}^{t+\Delta t}\mathbf{K}^{(i)}$ is the stiffness matrix, ${}^{t+\Delta t}\mathbf{R}$ is the vector of nodal loads, ${}^{t+|deltat}\mathbf{F}^{(i-1)}$ is the vector of nodal forces in case of iteration iteration $(i-1)$, ${}^{t+\Delta t}\Delta\mathbf{U}^{(i)}$ is the vector nodal displacements while the iteration is (i), ${}^{t+\Delta t}\mathbf{U}'^{(i)}$ is the vector of total velocities while the iteration is (i), and $\mathbf{M}^{t+\Delta t}\mathbf{U}''^{(i)}$ is the vector of total accelerations while the iterations is (i). Using an implicit time integration Newmark–Beta scheme and employing Newton's iterative method, the presented equations are cast in the following form:

$$^{t+\Delta t}\mathbf{K}^{(i)t+\Delta t}\Delta\mathbf{U}^{(i)} = {}^{t+\Delta t}\mathbf{R} \qquad (4)$$

where ${}^{t+\Delta t}\mathbf{R}^{(i)}$ is the effective load vector and ${}^{t+\Delta t}\mathbf{K}^{(i)}$ is the effective stiffness matrix. The three-dimensional static and dynamic analyses were performed using Abaqus (c) [27] software.

2.2. Structure and Geometrical Properties of the Model

The inhomogeneous model is made of two basic parts members: the lumbar body with posterior elements and intervertebral disks. The lumbar geometrical form is extracted by processing DICOM format data and then converted into a numerical model using Slice3D software. It is presented in Figure 1a.

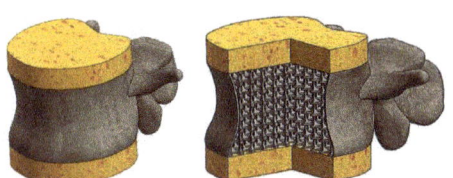

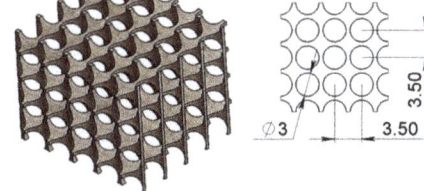

(a) The view of lumbar vertebra model with intervertebral disks.

(b) The fragment of the trabecular network and its geometrical parameters.

Figure 1. Geometrical models of vertebra.

The trabecular network is formed by cylindrical cuts which are extruded from vertical and horizontal planes. This method allowed the creation of the characteristic structure made of rod-like and plate-like trabeculas, and a fragment of the trabecular lattice is shown in Figure 1b.

2.3. Mechanical Properties

The nonlinear stress–strain diagram of bone is presented in Figure 2. On the other hand, the intervertebral disks were considered as isotropic and perfectly elastic. The material constants of the listed components were taken from data reported by Reference [10] and presented in table Table 1.

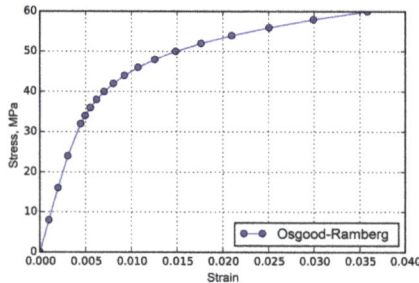

Figure 2. Osgood–Ramberg stress–strain relation for cortical bone.

Table 1. Elasticity constants of model components.

Property	Lumbar Body	Intervertebra Disc
Young modulus, MPa	8000	10
Ulimate strength, MPa	60	-
Yield strength, MPa	40	-
Poisson's ratio	0.30	0.40

2.4. The Parameters of Osteoporosis Impact

The effect of osteoporotic degradation is implemented by thickening the cortical bone and by varying the TBS, which depending on BV/TV. This research proposes the investigation of three parametric models with various cortical thicknesses of 0.2, 0.4, and 0.5 mm first offered in References [12,14]. Also, the relation of the BV/TV as well as the TBS value is typical for a high level of osteoporosis. The data taken from References [18,19] is presented in Table 2.

Table 2. The parameters of a healthy and osteoporotic model.

Model	Thickness, mm	BV/TV	TBS
Healthy	0.5	0.35	1.45
Ostseopenea	0.4	0.20	1.33
Osteoporosis	0.2	0.10	1.20

To make a profound investigation, the parameters in Table 2 were combined in different cases of calculations that were performed for both static and dynamic analyses (Table 3).

Table 3. The parameters of different lumbar body models.

Cortical Shell Thickness, mm	BV/TV	TBS
0.20	0.10	1.28
0.40	0.10	1.28
0.50	0.10	1.28
0.20	0.20	1.33
0.40	0.20	1.33
0.50	0.20	1.33
0.20	0.35	1.45
0.40	0.35	1.45
0.50	0.35	1.45

2.5. Boundary Conditions and Mesh

The model was tested by the external loads in the range of 0.15–0.75 MPa which arise in the results of daily motions [14]. The conditions of loading are reflected in Figure 3. Also, in the case of the nonlinear problem, the load direction is bonded with the displacement values and, during the test, follows the deformed shape of the model.

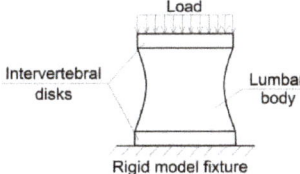

Figure 3. Load conditions of the compression test.

The time curve of the load is presented in Figure 4 and simulates the bearing of dynamic load. The time curve character comes from experimental data reported by Reference [28].

The model is meshed with tetrahedral finite elements and characterized by 306,435, 277,896, and 256,438 mesh elements for BV/TV ratios of 0.35, 0.20, and 0.1 or TBS values of 1.45, 1.33, and 1.2, respectively.

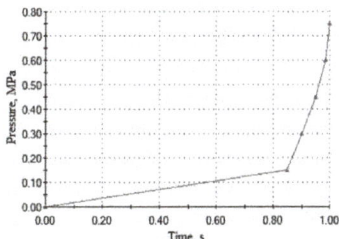

Figure 4. Time curve of dynamic load.

The contact between vertebra and intervertebral disks is treated as no penetration-bonded contact.

2.6. Risk Evaluation

The following three random variables were used to evaluate risk: external load P, the cortical shell thickness of lumbar vertebra Δ, and bone volume to total volume ratio β_{BVTV} which was obtained from TBS interdependence. In contrast, TBS was obtained from the 2-D vertebra CT scan. These variables were used for solving the FEM for the proposed mechanical model strength of the lumbar vertebra. Finally, the obtained set of points values for different combinations of independent variables were used for least square fitting by cubic polynomial as follows

$$\sigma_s(\beta, \delta, p) = \sum_{i,j,k=0}^{i+j+k \leq 3} a_{ijk} \beta^i \delta^j p^k \quad (5)$$

where p is the external load, δ is the cortical shell thickness, and β is the BV/TV ratio.

Furthermore, the approximation was obtained by using logarithmic values of FEM stresses $\log(\sigma_{vonMises})$ by searching minima of the following expression:

$$\min \left| \sum_{i,j,k} \log(\sigma_{vonMises}(i,j,k)) - \sigma_s(\beta_i, \delta_j, p_k) \right| \quad (6)$$

where indexes i, j, k denote values of discrete independent variables used in FEM computations.

Fracture risk F_R of lumbar vertebra can be expressed in term of reliability:

$$R = P(Z \leq 0) = 1 - F_R(Z \leq 0), \tag{7}$$

where $Z = X_\sigma - Y_{\sigma_Y}$, X_σ is max stress, and Y_{σ_Y} is yield strength. The general expression for the fracture risk of a stress–strength system has the following cumulative density function (CDF) [29]:

$$F_R = 1 - P(Z \leq 0) = 1 - \int_0^\infty \int_0^\infty f_{X_\sigma}(\sigma + z) f_{Y_{\sigma_Y}}(\sigma) d\sigma dz \tag{8}$$

where f_{X_σ} and $f_{Y_{\sigma_Y}}$ are probability density functions (PDFs) of the random values X_σ and Y_{σ_Y} of the maximum stress caused by the external load p and the strength, respectively.

3. Numerical Results and Discussion

Important parameters that impact the state of lumbar body, such as the thickness of the cortical shell and the BV/TV relation, were combined between themselves and investigated due to various values of external load. Also, the numerical results of both static and dynamic analysis and the discussion of the results are presented in the following section.

3.1. Static Analysis

Contours of the deformed shape of the model were generated, and stress distribution on the model is shown in Figure 5. The figure shows that the highest von Mises stresses occurred in the middle of the cortical shell on the front side of the model and that the deformations are scaled by a factor of 20 for visualization purposes. Figure 5b shows a relation between the von Mises stress versus the BV/TV ratio and the external load. The results show that maximal calculated stress reaches 38% of yield stress due to a 0.75 MPa load on the model with the lowest BV/TV ratio (0.1). Figure 5c,d shows the von Mises stress for models with thicknesses of cortical shell of 0.4 and 0.2 mm, respectively. In the case of a cortical shell with a thickness of 0.4 mm, maximal stress is about 17 MPa due to the minimal BV/TV ratio and the maximum external load (0.75 MPa), reaching 43% of the yield stress.

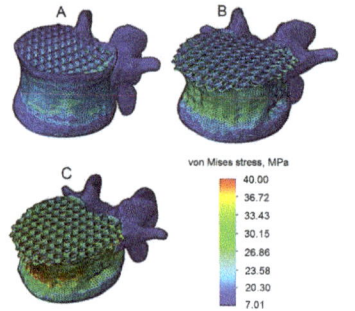

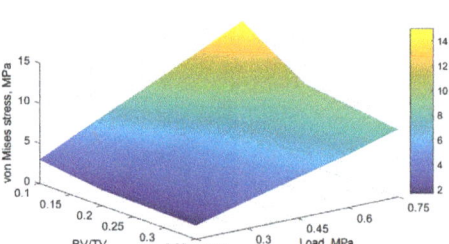

(a) Von Mises stress on the vertebra model: (A) when BV/TV is 35% and cortical shell thickness is 0.5 mm; (B) when BV/TV is 20% and the cortical shell thickness is 0.4 mm; and (C) as BV/TV is 10% and the cortical shell thickness is 0.2 mm. The cortical shell thickness is 0.5 mm

(b) A relation between the von Mises stress versus the BV/TV ratio and the external load. The thickness of cortical shell is 0.4 mm

Figure 5. *Cont.*

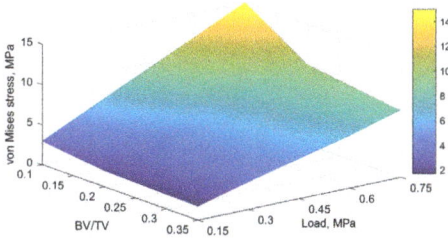 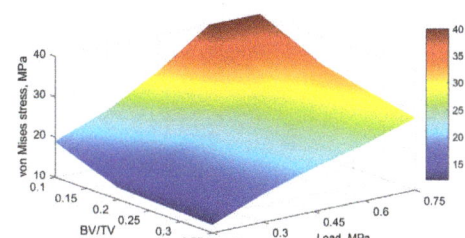

(c) Maximum von Mises stress versus the BV/TV ratio and the external load. The thickness of cortical shell is 0.5 mm

(d) Maximum von Mises stress versus the BV/TV ratio and the external load. The thickness of cortical shell is 0.2 mm

Figure 5. Results of the static analysis.

Figure 5d shows that the strength load is 0.60 MPa (the yield stress is exceeded), while the BV/TV ratio is 0.1. The obtained results agree well with the research of Kim et al., [14], with a difference about 5–10% for the model with a low apparent density and a cortical shell thickness of 0.2 mm, while McDonald [12] reports this value up to 0.99 MPa.

3.2. Dynamic Analysis

The stress distribution in the lumbar vertebra during dynamical analysis was computed, and the analysis shows that the stress concentrators have greater differences than seen in the static analysis. The highest value of stress appeared in the middle of the cortical shell and agrees well with clinical observations [1–4,30]. Also, the distribution of the von Mises stress on the cortical shell of the model is shown in Figure 6a. Figure 6b–d presents a relation of the von Mises stress on the model versus the BV/TV ratio and the external load. Figure 6d shows that yield stress is exceeded due to the 0.45 MPa load while the BV/TV ratio is less than 0.1. The relations between the von Mises stress on the cortical shell of the model with thicknesses of 0.4 and 0.2 mm versus the BV/TV ratios and the external load are presented in Figure 6c,d, respectively.

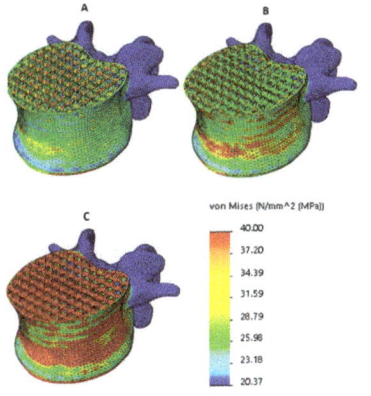 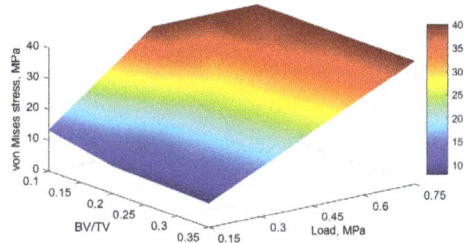

(a) Von Mises stress on the vertebra model: (A) when BV/TV is 35% and cortical shell thickness is 0.5 mm; (B) when BV/TV is 20% and the cortical shell thickness is 0.4 mm; and (C) as BV/TV is 10% and the cortical shell thickness is 0.2 mm

(b) Maximum von Mises stress versus the BV/TV ratio and the external load. The cortical shell thickness is 0.5 mm

Figure 6. Cont.

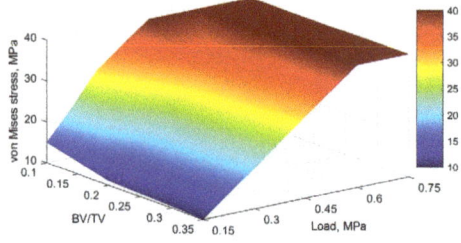 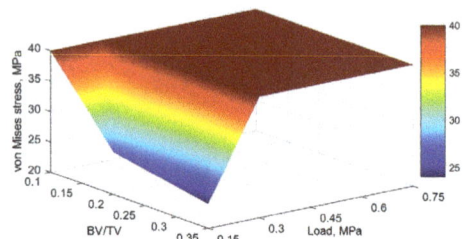

(c) Maximum von Mises stress versus the BV/TV ratio and the external load. The cortical shell thickness is 0.4 mm

(d) Maximum von Mises stress versus the BV/TV ratio and the external load. The cortical shell thickness is 0.2 mm

Figure 6. Results of the dynamic analysis.

As shown in Figure 6c, the excess yield stress is expected due to the 0.45 MPa load, while the BV/TV ratio is minimal. In the case of a high BV/TV ratio, the excess yield stress was identified due to the load of 0.6 MPa in terms of the average thickness of the cortical shell (0.4 mm). Figure 6d shows that yield stress is exceeded almost in every sample of bone tissue if the load is higher than 0.3 MPa. In addition, if the load grows increases 0.3 MPa, the yield stress is reached even in the case of a sufficient BV/TV ratio (0.35). This effect can be explained by the low thickness of the cortical shell (0.2 mm).

3.3. Estimation of the Fracture Risk

The risk of fracture of the lumbar vertebra can be estimated by the Monte Carlo method as a probability $Pr_f = Pr(Z \leq 0)$, where $Z = Y_{p,R} - X_{p,E}$ and $X_{p,E}$ and $Y_{p,R}$ are external pressure p imposed on the vertebra and the load-bearing capacity of the vertebra random variables respectively. It is assumed that the load-bearing capacity of the vertebra p_R equals the minimum pressure p at which the maximum von Mises stresses equal the yield stress σ_Y, that is, for the given δ and β, the load-bearing capacity r.v. $p_R = min\{p : g_{FEM}(\delta, \beta, p) \geq \sigma_Y\}$. It is assumed that $X_{p,E}$ and $Y_{p,R}$ are independent random variables. To evaluate the fracture risk Pr_f, the random numbers of the acting pressure random variable $X_{p,E}$ can be generated directly, while the generation of the random numbers of the load-bearing capacity $Y_{p,R}$ is more complicated since it is known that the cortical shell thickness and BV/TV are dependent random variables. In addition, the load-bearing capacity function of the lumbar vertebra $p_R = h(\delta, \beta, \sigma_Y, ...)$ dependent of all variables must be known. Then, the r.v. of the load-bearing capacity $Y_{p,R}$ can be obtained as a transformation $Y_{p,R} = h(X_\delta, X_\beta, X_{\sigma,Y}, ...)$, where $X_\delta, X_\beta, X_{\sigma,Y}, ...$ are random variables affecting the load-bearing capacity of the lumbar vertebra: for example, the cortical shell thickness, BV/TV ratio, the yield stress, geometry, and so on. It is evident that it is not possible to generate the sample of the realizations of the load-bearing capacity r.v. $Y_{p,R}$ directly by calculating each random number by FEM. Therefore, in the present article, another approach is adopted: to approximate the maximum von Mises stresses of the vertebra by the polynomial $\hat{g}$ and then, by solving this polynomial as an equation $\sigma_Y = \hat{g}(\delta, \beta, p)$, to obtain the pressure p that corresponds to the given variables δ, β, and the maximum von Mises stress σ_Y.

3.3.1. Approximation of the Maximum von Mises Stress

The approximation of the calculated maximum von Mises stresses of the lumbar vertebra was conducted by using the program "R studio" [31] and the package "nlme" [32] over the set $\mathbb{D} \times \mathbb{B} \times \mathbb{P}$, where $\mathbb{D}$, $\mathbb{B}$, and $\mathbb{P}$ are sets of values of the cortical shell thickness δ, BV/TV ratio β, and the external load p, respectively: $\delta \in \mathbb{D} = \{0.5, 0.4, 0.2\}$ mm, $\beta \in \mathbb{B} = \{0.1, 0.2, 0.35\}$, and $p \in \mathbb{P} = \{0.15, 0.30, 0.45, 0.60, 0.75\}$ MPa. The set of 45 points of the maximum von Mises stresses

$\mathbb{D} \times \mathbb{B} \times \mathbb{P}$ of the static analysis obtained by the finite element method that were used to obtain the approximating polynomial is given in Table 4.

Table 4. The maximum von Mises stresses of the static analysis calculated by finite element method (FEM) at different δ, β, and p

Analysis	Thickness, mm, δ	BV/TV, β	External Load, MPa, p				
			0.15	0.30	0.45	0.60	0.75
Static	0.5	0.10	2.9	6.1	9.3	12.3	15.2
		0.20	2.0	4.1	6.1	8.2	8.5
		0.35	1.6	3.4	5.0	6.7	8.5
	0.4	0.10	3.4	6.7	10.2	14.1	17.0
		0.20	2.1	4.2	6.3	8.4	10.5
		0.35	1.8	3.5	5.4	7.3	9.1
	0.2	0.10	18.9	24.1	31.3	40.8	49.4
		0.20	13.3	18.4	23.2	28.1	33.5
		0.35	12.1	17.4	21.0	24.5	28.0

The approximating polynomial of the maximum von Mises stresses of the static analysis is as follows:

$$\sigma \approx \hat{g}(p, \beta, \delta) = a_0 + a_1 p + a_2 \beta + a_3 \delta + a_{11} p^2 + a_{33} \delta^2 + a_{12} p \beta + a_{13} p \delta + a_{123} p \beta \delta + \\ a_{112} p^2 \beta + a_{113} p^2 \delta + a_{221} \beta^2 p + a_{223} \beta^2 \delta + a_{331} \delta^2 p + a_{332} \delta^2 \beta + a_{12233} p \beta^2 \delta^2 + \\ a_{11233} p^2 \beta \delta^2, \delta \in [0.2, 0.5] \text{ mm}, \beta \in [0.1, 0.35], p \in [0.15, 0.75] \text{ MPa} \quad (9)$$

where the coefficients are as follows: $a_0 = 40.095$, $a_1 = 109.545$, $a_2 = -33.064$, $a_3 = -153.799$, $a_{11} = 56.976$, $a_{33} = 152.808$, $a_{12} = -410.969$, $a_{13} = -348.377$, $a_{123} = 704.586$, $a_{112} = -153.953$, $a_{113} = -117.969$, $a_{221} = 737.456$, $a_{223} = 97.428$, $a_{331} = 361.940$, $a_{332} = 56.473$, $a_{12233} = -2913.652$, and $a_{11233} = 702.954$.

It should be noted that only the coefficients a_i for which the statistical hypothesis $H_0 : a_i = 0$ is rejected and the alternative $H_1 : a_i \neq 0$ is accepted are present in the given approximating polynomial Equation (9). The hypotheses were tested using the Student t-test. The maximum and minimum residuals are as follows: $max\{g_{FEM}(p_i, \beta_i, \delta_i) - \hat{g}(p_i, \beta_i, \delta_i)\} = 0.883$ MPa and $min\{g_{FEM}(p_i, \beta_i, \delta_i) - \hat{g}(p_i, \beta_i, \delta_i)\} = -0.838$ MPa, where $(p_i, \beta_i, \delta_i) \in \mathbb{D} \times \mathbb{B} \times \mathbb{P}$ and $g_{FEM}(p_i, \beta_i, \delta_i)$ stand for the stress values calculated by the FEM. The relative residuals $(\hat{g}(p_i, \beta_i, \delta_i) - g_{FEM}(p_i, \beta_i, \delta_i))/g_{FEM}(p_i, \beta_i, \delta_i)$ versus the stresses calculated by FEM are depicted in Figure 7.

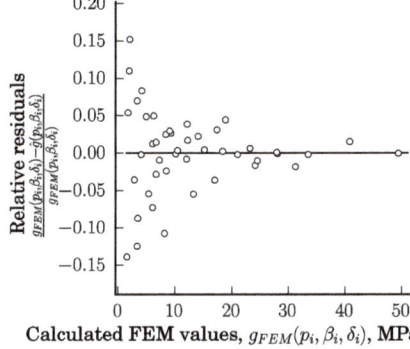

Figure 7. Relative residuals versus calculated values of the maximum von Mises stress.

The obtained polynomial $\hat{g}$, given in Equation (9), can be treated as a quadratic equation $\sigma_Y = \hat{g}(p, \beta, \delta)$ with respect to the pressure p when the other two variables δ and β are treated as known quantities or, in other words, as the parameters. Then, the solution of the obtained polynomial $\hat{g}$, given in Equation (9), gives two roots: One of them is the load-bearing capacity p_R corresponding to the given δ, β, and the yield stress σ_Y:

$$p_R \approx \hat{h}(\beta, \delta) = \frac{-b_1(\beta, \delta) + \sqrt{b_1(\beta, \delta)^2 - 4b_2(\beta, \delta)(b_0(\beta, \delta) - \sigma_Y)}}{2b_2\beta, \delta} \qquad (10)$$

where $b_0(\beta, \delta) = a_{332}\beta\delta^2 + a_{33}\delta^2 + a_{223}\beta^2 x_3 + a_3\delta + a_2\beta + a_0$, $b_1(\beta, \delta) = a_{12233}\beta^2\delta^2 + a_{331}\delta^2 + a_{123}\beta\delta + a_{13}\delta + a_{221}\beta^2 + a_{12}\beta + a1$ and $b_2(\beta, \delta) = a_{11233}\beta\delta^2 + a_{113}\delta + a_{112}\beta + a_{11}$.

Then, the load-bearing capacity r.v. $Y_{p,R}$ can be modelled as the transformation $Y_{p,R} = \hat{h}(X_\beta, X_\delta)$ of r.vs. X_β and X_δ by assuming that the yield stress σ_Y is the deterministic predefined quantity.

3.3.2. Stochastic Models and for the Risk Modelling

It is well-known that osteoporosis of the trabecular bone also entails decreasing of the thickness of the cortical shell of the lumbar vertebra δ. Therefore, BV/TV and the cortical shell thickness are dependent random variables. In addition, decreasing BV/TV also entails decrease of the cortical shell thickness δ [33,34]. Therefore, the correlation coefficient of these r.vs. is positive. For example in Reference [33], it is obtained that the statistically significant coefficient of correlation between the cortical shell thickness and BV/TV is 0.5, when the significance level is 0.05. According to Reference [34], the coefficient of correlation between BV/TV and the cortical shell thickness is 0.29; however, it is statistically insignificant. To generate the load-bearing capacity $X_{p,R}$ random numbers, it is assumed that the BV/TV ratio and the cortical shell thickness form a bivariate correlated truncated Gaussian random variable $(X_\beta, X_\delta)^T \in [M(G_\beta) - 3\sqrt{D(G_\beta)}, M(G_\beta) + 3\sqrt{D(G_\beta)}] \times [M(G_\delta) - 3\sqrt{D(G_\delta)}, M(G_\beta) + 3\sqrt{D(G_\beta)}]$; where $\times$ is the Cartesian product of two sets; $M(G_\beta)$, $D(G_\beta)$, $M(G_\delta)$, and $D(G_\delta)$ are the means and variances of the correlated untruncated normal random variables G_β and G_δ, respectively, that also form a bivariate Gaussian random variable $(G_\beta, G_\delta)^T \sim N(\vec{\mu}, \Sigma)$ of which the mean vector is $\vec{\mu} = (M(G_\beta), M(G_\delta))^T$ and the covariance matrix is

$$\Sigma = \begin{bmatrix} D(G_\beta) & Cor(G_\beta, G_\delta)\sqrt{D(G_\beta)D(G_\delta)} \\ Cor(G_\delta, G_\beta)\sqrt{D(G_\delta)D(G_\beta)} & D(G_\delta) \end{bmatrix} \qquad (11)$$

where $Cor(G_\beta, G_\delta)$ and $Cor(G_\delta, G_\beta)$ are the correlation coefficients between r.vs. G_β and G_δ, $Cor(G_\beta, G_\delta) = Cor(G_\delta, G_\beta)$.

R.v. $Y_{p,R}$ can be estimated by the empirical cumulative distribution function (ECDF) and by the empirical quantile function (EQF). Usually, ECDF is defined as follows: $Pr(Y_{p,R} \leq y) \approx \hat{F}_{Y,p,R}(y) = \frac{1}{n}\sum_{i=1}^{n} I(y_i \leq y)$, where I is the indicator function, n is the sample size, y_i is the realization i of r.v. $Y_{p,R}$; while EQF of r.v. $Y_{p,R}$ is usually defined as $Q(p) = inf\{y : F_{Y,p,R}(y) \geq p\}$, where p is the required probability.

For the evaluation of the fracture risk as the probability $Pr_f = Pr(Y_{p,R} - X_{p,E} \leq 0)$, the external pressure independent r.v. $X_{p,E}$ can distributed according to various laws. In the present article, it is assumed that the external load r.v. $X_{p,E}$ is also truncated normal r.v. attaining values from the interval $X_{p,E} \in [M(G_{p,E}) - 3\sqrt{D(G_{p,E})}, M(G_{p,E}) + 3\sqrt{D(G_{p,E})}]$, where $M(G_{p,E})$ and $D(G_{p,E})$ are the mean and the variances of the untruncated external pressure normal r.v. $G_{p,E}$.

The fracture risk of the lumbar vertebra can be expressed as $Pr_f = Pr(Y_{p,R} - X_{p,E} \leq 0) = Pr(Z \leq 0) \approx \hat{F}_Z(0)$, where $\hat{F}_Z$ is the ECDF of r.v. $Z = Y_{p,R} - X_{p,E}$: $\hat{F}_Z(z) = \frac{1}{n}\sum_{i=1}^{n} I(y_{p,R,i} - x_{p,E,i} \leq z)$, where n is the sample size and $y_{p,R,i}$ and $x_{p,E,i}$ are realization i

of r.vs. $Y_{p,R}$ and $X_{p,E}$, respectively. It should be noted that the fracture risk can be also evaluated according to the following known integral [29]:

$$Pr_f = P(Z \leq 0) = \int_{-\infty}^{0} \int_{-\infty}^{+\infty} f_{Y,p,R}(p+z) f_{X,p,E}(p) dp dz \qquad (12)$$

where $f_{Y,p,R}$ and $f_{X,p,E}$ are probability density functions (PDFs) of the load-bearing capacity r.v. $Y_{p,R}$ and the external presure r.v. $X_{p,E}$, respectively.

For the following analysis of the reliability of the vertebra, the concrete parameters of the r.v. G_β, G_δ, and $G_{p,E}$ must be adopted. In the case of the Gaussian r.vs., only the means, variances, and covariances are required. The coefficient of variation $Cvar(G_\beta)$ of BV/TV can vary in a wide range, for example, from about 18% [18,33] up to 37% [34] or even up to 42% for the normal bones [26]. There is less literature on the coefficient of the variation of the cortical shell thickness δ. We found that the coefficient of variation is also big, for example, 24.5% [33] or even 62.4%, according to Reference [34]. For the patient-specific cases, the variability of these parameters should be less. However, since the BV/TV ratio is determined indirectly, the variability of r.v. X_β cannot be very low.

As it was already mentioned, the r.vs. X_β and X_δ are dependent [33,34]. In the case of the Gaussian bivariate r.v. (G_β, G_δ), the correlation coefficient $Cor(G_\delta, G_\beta)$ is used in the covariance matrix given in Equation (11) and it is determined that $Cor(G_\delta, G_\beta)$ may equal 0.5 [33] or 0.29 [34]. The external load $X_{p,E}$ acting on the vertebra is a random variable depending mainly on the mechanical loads. For example, according to Reference [28], the ground reaction of a human may vary from 750 N in the rest state and increases up to 2000 N in the squat jump. The ground reaction of the rest state shows that the mass of the investigated human body in Reference [28] is about 75 kg. Then, in the squat jump, the weight of the body increases $2000/750 = 2.66(7)$ times. It should be mentioned that not all the weight of a body is imposed on the lumbar vertebra. On the basis of the data given in Reference [35], it is possible to conclude that a lumbar vertebra sustains about 60% of the total load. By taking into account the area of the loaded surface of the vertebra under investigation, $A = 1210$ mm^2, we can conclude that, for the person of article [28], the external load varies within an interval $[p_{min}, p_{max}] = [0.372, 0.992]$ MPa.

3.3.3. Fracture Risk Modelling Data, Results, and Discussion

On the basis of the above given review, for the probabilistic estimations of the load-bearing capacity of the lumbar vertebra $Pr(Y_{p,R} \leq y_p) = \hat{F}_{Y,p,R}(y_p)$ and the failure risk $Pr_f = Pr(Z \leq 0) = F_Z(0)$, the following two cases were considered. For the first case (Case I), the following values are adopted: the mean of BV/TV $M(G_\beta) = 0.1$ and the mean of the cortical shell thickness $M(G_\delta) = 0.2$ mm; the coefficients of variation $Cvar(G_\beta) = \sqrt{D(G_\beta)}/M(G_\beta) = 0.2$ and $Cvar(G_\delta) = 0.2$; the correlation coefficient $Cor(G_\beta, G_\delta) = 0.35$; the mean of the external load $G_{p,E}$ attains three values $M(G_{p,E}) \in \{p_{min}, 1.5p_{min}, 2.5p_{min}\}$, where $p_{min} = 0.372$ Mpa; and the coefficient of variation for all external pressures is constant: $Cvar(G_{p,E}) = 0.20$. For the second case (Case II), the following values are adopted: means $M(G_\beta) = 0.25$ and $M(G_\delta) = 0.2$ mm; the coefficients of variation $Cvar(G_\beta) = 0.2$ and $Cvar(G_\delta) = 0.2$; the correlation coefficient $Cor(G_\beta, G_\delta) = 0.35$; mean of the external load $G_{p,E}$ attains three values $M(G_{p,E}) \in \{p_{min}, 1.5p_{min}, 2.5p_{min}\}$, where $p_{min} = 0.372$ Mpa; and the coefficient of variation for all external pressures is constant: $Cvar(G_{p,E}) = 0.2$. Thus, for both Cases I and II, the external load $G_{p,E}$ attains the same three different means and the coefficient of variation is constant, and for both cases, the coefficient of the correlation between the cortical shell thickness and BV/TV is the same, 0.35. It should be noted that for Cases I and II the mean of the external pressure $M(G_{p,E}) = 0.372$ MPa approximately corresponds to the external load of the lumbar vertebra of a person of mass 75 kg in rest, while $M(G_{p,E}) = 2.5p_{min} = 0.93$ MPa is close to the maximum load during the squat jump of the person. Totally, 10^6 random values of the r.vs. G_β and G_δ were generated. However, due to the truncation the samples of the realizations of the r.vs. X_β, X_δ, $X_{p,E}$, and $Y_{p,R}$ were smaller than 10^6 but bigger than 9×10^5. All analyses were performed by the program "R studio" [31]. The bivariate Gaussian random numbers were generated using the package "MASS" [36].

The realizations of the histograms of the r.vs. X_β, X_δ and $Y_{p,R}$ are shown in Figure 8. The realizations of the histograms of the truncated BV/TV ratio r.v. X_β are depicted in Figure 8a,d and the realizations of the truncated cortical shell thickness r.v. X_δ are depicted in Figure 8b,e while realizations of the histograms of the load-bearing capacity r.v. $Y_{p,R}$ as well as the 0.05 and 0.95 empirical quantiles of r.v. $Y_{p,R}$ are depicted in Figure 8c,f. It should be noticed that the histograms depicted in Figure 8a,b,d,e show entire ranges of the random numbers of the r.vs. X_β and X_δ, while Figure 8c,d show truncated ones from the right of the intervals of r.vs. $Y_{p,R}$.

As we can see from Figure 8c,f, the probability density function of the load-bearing capacity r.v. $Y_{p,R}$ can have a positive skew. However, there are such cases of $M(X_\beta)$, $M(X_\delta)$, $D(X_\beta)$, and $D(X_\delta)$ in which the histograms of r.v. $Y_{p,R}$ have a negative skew. It was also observed that at the small values of variances $D(X_\beta)$ and $D(X_\delta)$, the histograms of the r.v. $Y_{p,R}$ are symmetrical and the histograms are very similar to the normal distribution probability density function with mean $M(Y_{p,R})$ and variance $D(Y_{p,R})$. However, the given Figure 8c,f shows a counterexample, and in general, we cannot state that r.v. $Y_{p,R}$ is normal provided that r.vs. X_β and X_δ are symmetrically truncated dependent normal random variables with nonnegative correlation coefficient. As we can see from Figure 8c,f, the 0.05 quantiles of the load-bearing capacity of the vertebra r.v. $Y_{p,R}$ increase from $p_{0.050} = 0.355$ MPa for Case I up to $p_{0.05} = 0.638$ MPa for Case II. Analogously, the 0.95 quantiles increase from $p_{0.95} = 0.913$ MPa up to $p_{0.95} = 2.364$ MPa. The quantiles of the load-bearing capacity r.v. $Y_{p,R}$ can serve as extra information on the fracture risk of the lumbar vertebra. It should be noted that the correlation between r.vs. X_β and X_δ in general is important for r.v. $Y_{p,E}$. For example, for the considered Case I, the increase of the correlation coefficient $Cor(G_\beta, G_{delta})$ from 0.35 up to 0.5 decreases the small quantiles of the load-bearing capacity r.v. $Y_{p,R}$ from $p_{0.05} = 0.355$ up to $p_{0.05} = 0.347$ and increases the big quantiles from $p_{0.05} = 0.913$ up to $p_{0.95} = 0.929$. For Case II, the increase the correlation coefficient from $Cvar(G_\beta, G_\delta) = 0.35$ up to $Cvar(G_\beta, G_\delta) = 0.5$ also entails a decrease of small value quantiles of r.v. $Y_{p,R}$ from $p_{0.05} = 0.638$ up to $p_{0.05} = 0.620$, but the increase in the correlation coefficient also increases the big quantile values from $p_{0.95} = 2.364$ up to $p_{0.95} = 2.423$.

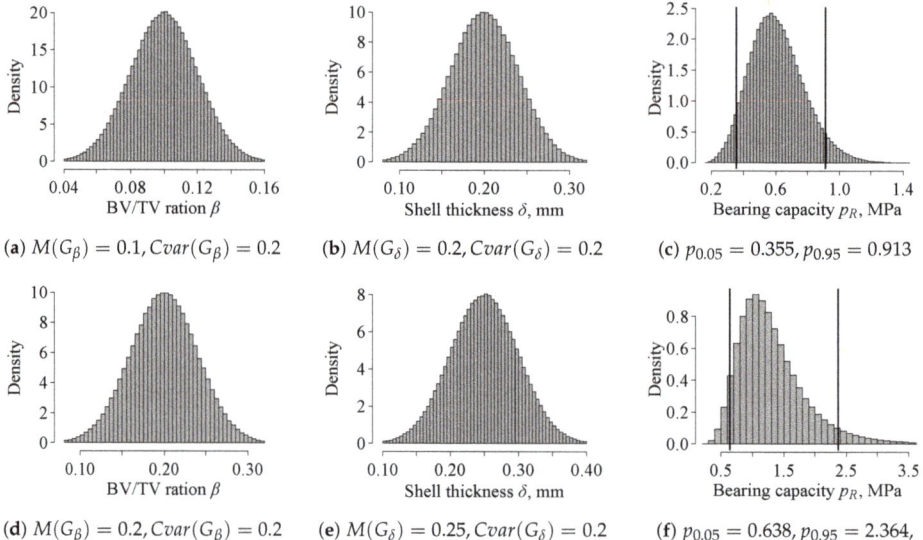

(a) $M(G_\beta) = 0.1$, $Cvar(G_\beta) = 0.2$
(b) $M(G_\delta) = 0.2$, $Cvar(G_\delta) = 0.2$
(c) $p_{0.05} = 0.355$, $p_{0.95} = 0.913$
(d) $M(G_\beta) = 0.2$, $Cvar(G_\beta) = 0.2$
(e) $M(G_\delta) = 0.25$, $Cvar(G_\delta) = 0.2$
(f) $p_{0.05} = 0.638$, $p_{0.95} = 2.364$,

Figure 8. Realizations of the probability density functions of the random variables X_β (a,d); r.v. X_δ (b,e); and r.v. $Y_{p,R}$ (c,f).

The fracture risks of static vertebra loads of Case I and Case II as well histograms of r.vs. $Y_{p,R}$, $X_{p,E}$, and $Z = Y_{p,R} - X_{p,E}$ can be seen in Figure 9. It was obtained that with increasing the cortical shell thickness from $\delta = 0.2$ (Case I) to $\delta = 0.25$ (Case II) and the BV/TV ratio from $\beta = 0.1$ (Case I) to $\beta = 0.2$ (Case II), the failure risk Pr_f decreases from 0.0904 to $2.752 \cdot 10^{-3}$ for $M(G_{p,E}) = p_{min} = 0.372$ MPa; from 0.417 to 0.0337 for $M(G_{p,E}) = 1.5 p_{min} = 0.558$ MPa; and from 0.897 to 0.260 for $M(G_{p,E}) = 2.5 p_{min} = 0.93$ MPa. The obtained results suggest that, for the considered supposed person, the squat jump inevitably would lead to the fracture of a lumbar vertebra, while a relatively small increasing BV/TV and the cortical shell thickness δ significantly decrease the fracture risk Pr_f.

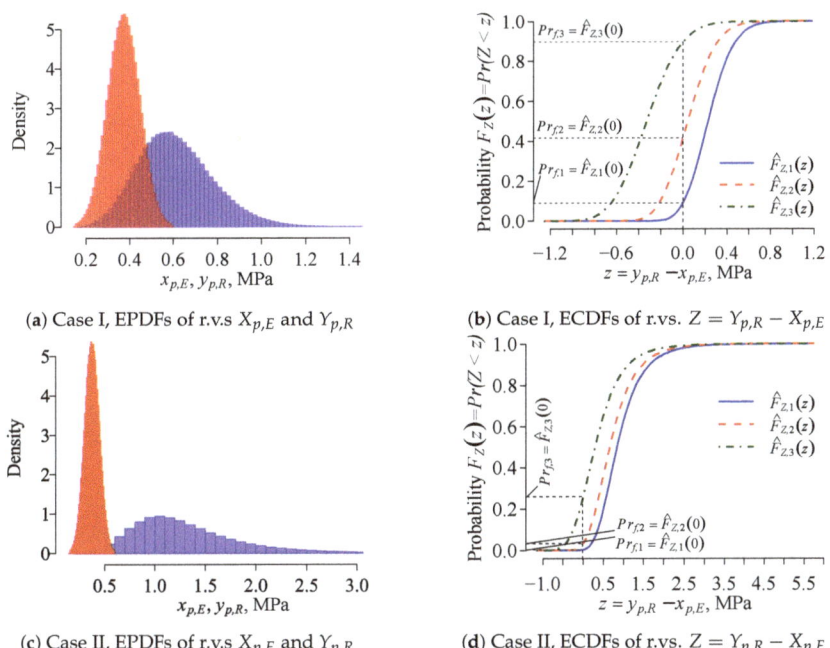

Figure 9. Realizations of the probability density functions of the random variables $X_{p,E}$ and $Y_{p,R}$ (**a**) for Case I and (**c**) for Case II; and empirical cumulative distribution functions $\hat{F}_{Z,i}(z)$ of r.v. $Z = Y_{p,E} - X_{p,E}$ and failure risks $Pr_{f,i}$, $i \in \{1, 2, 3\}$ for Case I (**b**) and for Case II (**d**): $\hat{F}_{Z,1}(z)$ and $pr_{f,1}$ when $M(G_{p,E}) = p_{min}$; $\hat{F}_{Z,2}(z)$ and $pr_{f,2}$ when $M(G_{p,E}) = 1.5 p_{min}$; $\hat{F}_{Z,3}(z)$ and $pr_{f,3}$ when $M(G_{p,E}) = 2.5 p_{min}$, where correlation coefficient $Cvar(G_{p,E}) = 0.2$ for all $Pr_{f,i}$, $\hat{F}_{Z,i}(z)$, $i \in \{1, 2, 3\}$.

The correlation between r.vs. X_β and X_δ is also important for the fracture risk Pr_f. For example, for the considered Case I, the increase of the correlation coefficient $Cor(G_\beta, G_\delta)$ from 0.35 up to 0.5 increases the fracture risk from $Pr_f = 0.0904$ up to $Pr_f = 0.0963$ and from $Pr_f = 0.417$ up to $Pr_f = 0.418$ at small values of the loading, i.e., as $M(G_{p,E}) \in \{p_{min}, 1.5 p_{min}\} = \{0.372, 0.558\}$ MPa. However, at big load values, the increasing correlation coefficient decreases the fracture risk from $Pr_f = 0.897$ up to $Pr_f = 0.892$ as $M(G_{p,E}) = 2.5 p_{min} = 0.93$ MPa. For Case II, the increase in the correlation coefficient from $Cvar(G_\beta, G_\delta) = 0.35$) up to $Cvar(G_\beta, G_\delta) = 0.5$ increases the fracture risk from $Pr_f = 0.002752$ up to $Pr_f = 0.00387$ as $M(G_{p,E}) = p_{min} = 0.372$ MPa; from $Pr_f = 0.0337$ up to $Pr_f = 0.0392$ as $M(G_{p,E}) = 1.5 p_{min} = 0.558$ MPa; and from $Pr_f = 0.260$ up to $Pr_f = 0.270$ as $M(G_{p,E}) = 2.5 p_{min} = 0.93$ MPa.

It should be noted that the probabilistic evaluation of the fracture risk demands information on the probability distribution functions of the many variables that affect the failure of a lumbar vertebra such as BV/TV ratio, the cortical shell thickness, yield strength of bone, geometric parameters, and so on. These variables should be treated as the random variables, and in addition, as it was already mentioned, these random variable are dependent. Therefore, at least the correlation coefficients or covariances between these random variables should be known. However, we could not find any information about the probability distribution laws of the mentioned variables that affect lumbar vertebra fracture. Therefore, the Gaussian laws were applied to the modelling.

The proposed model can be used to determine the fracture risk of individual patients by applying the peculiar anatomical properties of lumbar vertebrae, such as TBS or BV/TV. So, the proposed evaluation scheme of assessing fracture risk includes the model of a vertebra with cancellous bone and the cortical shell, in-silico numerical results obtained by using FEM software, and the basic expressions of evaluating the fracture risk of a mechanical system. In case of the existence of other universally recognized methods, our proposed method can be used as a supplementary method with other known fracture risk evaluation methods.

3.4. Influence of Vertebra Cortical Shell Buckling

Mechanical properties. Different properties are assigned for particular phases. The dense cortical shell phase is characterised by volume density $\rho_{cor} = 1850 \, \text{kg/m}^3$ [37,38], while the density of fully degenerated cancellous bone is $\rho_{can} = 100 \, \text{kg/m}^3$. The cortical phase is modelled as an isotropic elastic-plastic continuum. The elastic properties are defined by elasticity modulus $E_{cor} = 8.0 \, \text{GPa}$, and the Poisson's ratio is $\nu_{cor} = 0.3$ [14,39]. The plastic properties are defined on the basis of perfect plasticity and obey the von Mises yield criteria. The yield stress is $\sigma_Y = 64 \, \text{MPa}$ [14]. This value is further used as the ultimate strength constant. The trabecular phase is modelled as an elastic orthotropic continuum. The elastic modulus of the trabecular bone in the vertical (longitudinal) direction is calculated according to the formula given in Reference [40] as follows:

$$E_{can,zz} = 4.73 \rho_{can}^{1.56} \tag{13}$$

Thereby, the transverse elastic modulus is assumed to be the fraction of the longitudinal modulus, thus

$$E_{can,xx} = E_{can,yy} = 0.1 E_{can,zz} \tag{14}$$

The Poisson's ratio is $\nu_{can,xy} = 0.3$, and $\nu_{can,xz} = \nu_{can,yz} = 0.2$.

Finite element method. The thin-walled domain of the cortical shell was discretised by shell finite elements. The shell element applied is a four-node element with six degrees of freedom at each node. Such an element is associated with plasticity and larger strain and describes structure buckling. It is suitable for analysing thin to moderately thick shell structures. The finite element mesh of cortical shells contains 3094 nodes and 2976 shell elements.

A cancellous bone, endplates, and posterior bone models were meshed with volumetric finite elements. This type of solid element is a higher-order 3-D 20-node solid element that allows quadratic displacement behaviour. The element supports plasticity, large deflection, and large strain capabilities. Finally, the solid phase was described by a 3-D mesh containing 348,138 nodes and 147,814 solid elements. The meshed model is presented in Figure 10a.

Shell and volumetric domains may be connected in a different manner, and two computational finite element models were finally generated. The first model reflects a healthy cortex state. A connection between the cortical wall and trabecular phase is implemented as a contact of two solids (Figure 10b). In the perfect case, the connection is modelled as a bonded contact, where no sliding or separation between faces or edges is allowed. For the shell-solid constraint option, an internal set of force-distributed constraints between nodes on the shell edges and nodes on the solid surface is created. In the model, each shell node acts as the master node and associated solid nodes act as slave nodes.

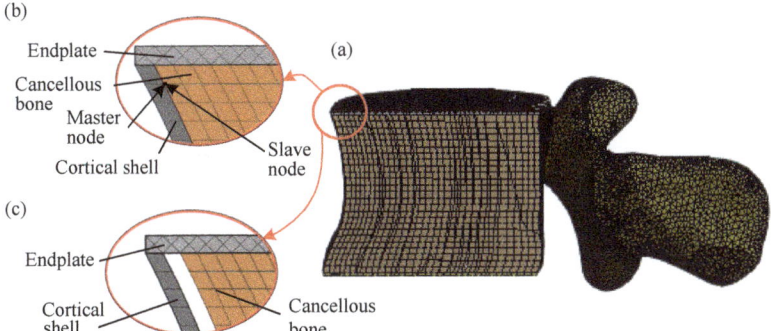

Figure 10. Cross-sectional view of the 3-D finite element model of the vertebra in the sagittal plane (**a**); bonded and unbonded, with a gap and cortical shells (**b**,**c**) respectively.

In the case of osteoporotic degradation, the bond is weakened. The second model reflects the limit case with a fully degenerated interface. The degradation effect could be evaluated by removing the connecting bond, and the gap was imposed between the shell and the solid (Figure 10c). Therewithin, integrity of the body was held by connecting the edge of the shell by endplates.

Numerical results. The physical nature of different models is qualitatively illustrated by deformed shapes, and a colour plot of the displacement magnitude of the cortical shell is shown in Figure 11. The displacement values, defined in millimetres, are illustrated in a unified colour scale. The first line of subfigures (Figure 11a–c) illustrates bonded shell-solid contact, while the next line of subfigures (Figure 11d–f) illustrates unbonded contact. The first column (Figure 11a,d) reflects results obtained with the large thickness equal to 0.5 mm, while the third column (Figure 11c,f) reflects results for most degradation of cortical shell. Characterising deformation shapes in a colour scale clearly illustrates the degradation degree. Unbonded contact leads to the occurrence of two higher-order deformation modes. Extremely high displacement, which exceeds nominal values by more than 1.5 times, is observed in the vicinity of point B. This result indicates buckling of the shell in the vicinity of this point.

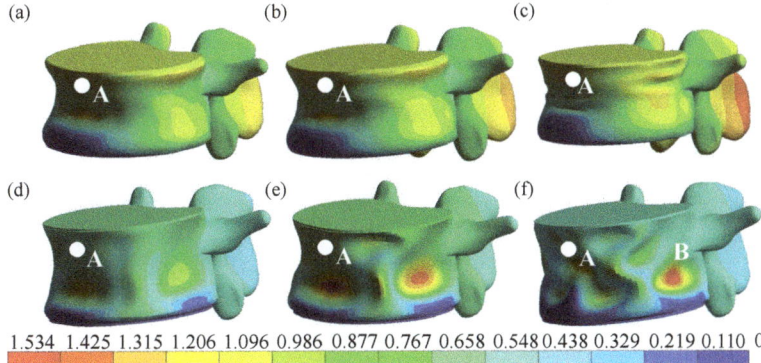

Figure 11. Deformed shape effect at the first bifurcation point A. Figure a–c for the bonded trabecular bone (Figure 10b): (**a**) when $\delta = 0.5$, $t = 0.86 t_{max}$, (**b**) when $\delta = 0.4$ mm and $t = 0.85 t_{max}$, (**c**) when $\delta = 0.2$ mm and $t = 0.58 t_{max}$. Figure d–f for the unbounded trabecular bone (Figure 10c): (**d**) when $\delta = 0.5$ mm and $t = 0.32 t_{max}$, (**e**) when $\delta = 0.4$ mm and $t = 0.32 t_{max}$, (**f**) when $\delta = 0.2$ mm and $t = 0.38 t_{max}$.

The most important results of the mechanical analyses are illustrated by considering the relative variation of vertebrae height h, %. According to medical practice [41], this parameter is used as a deformity grade. It is used as a fracture risk indicator. The normal state of vertebrae is characterised by deformability grade 0 which corresponds to variation $0 \leq h \leq 20\%$. It is worth noting that the obtained values of $h = 1.26 - 3\%$ are below the threshold value. The h threshold is 20%. Furthermore, the first bifurcation points of investigated vertebrae cortical shell is approximately twice higher than the maximum external loads applied in the proposed model (Figure 12). Therefore, it is obvious that buckling can be avoided in the current fracture risk model.

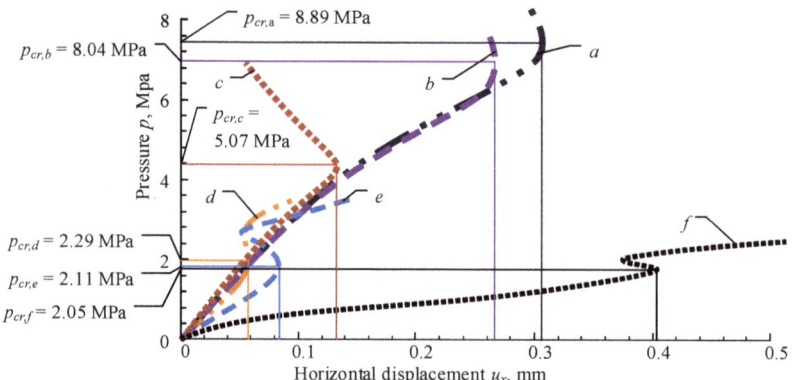

Figure 12. Load dependency graph. Displacement in horizontal direction at point A (Figure 11).

3.5. Discussion on Model Limitations

Creep. The deformations of bone under the load are time dependent not only due to osteoporosis but also due to creep [42–44]. Therefore, the long-term critical force or long-term strength of the bone is less than the short-term critical force or short-term strength. In case of the long-term deformation, long term deformation of the bone subject to long-term loading can be modelled properly using well-developed viscoelasticity or creep theories developed in the mechanics of materials provided that the characteristics of the bone is known, for example, modulus of elasticity, compliance function, or creep function. However, in the case of osteoporosis, the common viscoelasticity theories are not suitable due to fact that, in the classic viscoelasticity theories, the derivatives of the modulus of elasticity and the creep functions with respect to the time are nonnegative. In other words, the modulus of elasticity is a non-decreasing function with respect to time. However, in the case of osteoporosis, these conditions are violated and the long term analysis of the bone deformations when the osteoporosis simultaneously takes place is a much more complicated problem that also demands profound theoretical reconsiderations of the existing creep or viscoelasticity theories. The raised issue demands separate profound investigations which is not possible in the present study.

Anisotropy. Trabeculae bone tissues are strongly anisotropic materials with individual mechanical and topological properties for each patient. Good known representative volume elements (RVE) and homogenization-based methods [45] require topology of trabeculae, which needs micro-CT or micro-MRI scans. In the case of lumbar vertebra, they are impossible or very expansive. Therefore, modelling of mechanical behaviour of patient-specific lumbar vertebra is the challenge and we needs some indirect methods for evaluating mechanical properties of patient-specific lumbar veretbra trabeculae. Wolf's law [46] helps to understand the anisotropy of mechanical properties of bone, and from theoretical point of view, we can still investigate simplified trabecular structures arranged in the direction of external stresses as a suitable mechanical model if we want to understand mechanical behaviour of trabeculae inside a vertebral body. On the other hand, it is experimentally observed fact that, in vertebra L1, trabeculae arrangement is remodelled to withstand maximal compression loads. So, choosing of numerical compression tests is logical too.

Yield criteria. In general, lumbar vertebrae are strongly anisotropic plastic biological tissue. Therefore, failure criteria should be based on yield surface, which can be expressed as a Taylor expansion [47]

$$\left(\sum_{ik} a_{ik}\sigma_{ik}\right)^{\alpha} + \left(\sum_{pqmn} a_{pqmn}\sigma_{pq}\sigma_{mn}\right)^{\beta} + \left(\sum_{rstlmn} a_{rstlmn}\sigma_{rs}\sigma_{tl}\sigma_{mn}\right)^{\gamma} \leq 1 \qquad (15)$$

where $a_{ik}, a_{pqmn}, a_{rstlmn}$ are strength tensors of different order. von Mises [48] proposed yield criterion for isotropic materials. Hill [49] extended the von Mises yield criterion of isotropic materials to anisotropic materials. Later Tsai [50] extended this criterion for anisotropic materials to a unidirectional lamina. It is easy to show that von Mises or Tsai–Hill failure criteria can be derived form Goldenblar–Kopnov failure criteria. Two-dimensional failure propagation simulations by Korenczuk et al. [51] showed that the von Mises failure criterion did not capture the failure type, location, or propagation direction nearly as well as the Tsai–Hill criterion. Both the von Mises and Tsai–Hill failure criteria severely underpredicted the amount of displacement needed to produce initial failure in the porcine abdominal aortas. Therefore, using of von Mises or Tsai–Hill failure criteria would overestimate lumbar vertebra fracture risk.

Remodelling. One-time resonant destruction of vertebra is a very rare clinical dysfunction, which was not investigated in our model. On the other hand, according to Wolf's low, long range loads enable the increase of bone strength in the greatest load direction and opposite decrease strength in lowest load direction. Therefore, we would take into account additionally bone remodelling or its fatigue property, but this article does not include an investigation of vertebra remodelling.

3.6. Validation of Mechanical Model

Extracting physical and micro-geometrical properties of vertebrae is very complicated. If we want to know micro-geometry of human bones, quantitative computational tomography (QCT) can be used on leg or hand bones but not on whole human spine or one of vertebra. Therefore, an alternating methodology of investigation of vertebrae mechanical properties can be 3-D printing. As is stated in Reference [52], today, 3-D printing is practical, useful technology in surgical planing or spine implantation. Obviously, knowing mechanical characteristics, 3-D printed vertebrae is the basic step in successful applications of such kind of structures.

The validation of numerical modelling was aided in our case by a physical test of the printed polylactide (PLA) vertebrae geometrical model (Figure 13a). The whole procedure took the following the steps:

1. The printing of the vertebrae model;
2. The printing of the cylindrical PLA sample for mechanical properties of PLA to define;
3. The compression test of the printed PLA sample;
4. The compression test of the printed PLA vertebrae;
5. The determination of the mechanical properties of PLA by verifying the obtained load-displacement curve of the cylindrical sample;
6. The implementation of the defined stress-strain curve of PLA onto the numerical calculation;
7. The comparison of the results of the experimental and numerical studies.

The printing process was realized by using self-made 3-D printer, based on Prusa-i3 model (Figure 13b). The selection of this device was justified by its parameters: printer type FDM, build volume, $25 \times 21 \times 20$ cm^3, minimal layer height 50 µm, and nozzle diameter 0.2 mm. The printing process took about 20 h, while the printing was completed. The properties of the osteoporotic sample of vertebrae was as follow: thickness of cortical shell, 0.5 mm, 0.1 BV/TV ratio, and 1.2 TBS.

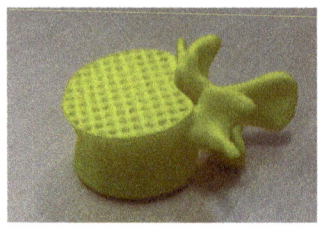
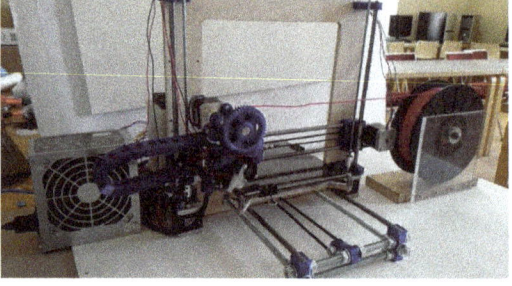

(a) Printed polylactide (PLA) vertebrae.

(b) The 3-D printer based on the Prusa-i3 model.

Figure 13. The 3-D printer and printed vertebra.

The physical experiment was performed by using a MultiTest 2.5-i compression machine (Figure 14). The selection of this device was based on suitable range of load 0–2500 N and relatively high precision ($\pm 0.1\%$ of full scale). The sample vertebra was tested under the constant loading speed (10 mm/min), and the displacement values were obtained: They are presented in Figure 15a. The same test was accomplished for the printed cylindrical sample too.

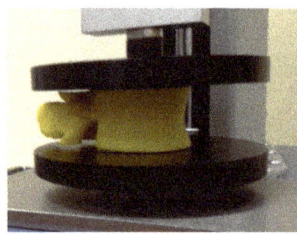

Figure 14. Testing of printed vertebrae by the compression machine.

As Figure 15a shows, the nonlinear behaviour of the printed PLA was revealed. The mechanical properties of PLA were determined by processing the load-displacement curve of the cylindrical sample (20 mm length, 15 mm diameter), and the stress–strain relation of PLA was defined.

The defined stress–strain curve of PLA (Figure 15a) was integrated into the numerical model of the vertebrae, and the finite element study was compared to the results of the physical experiment (Figure 15b).

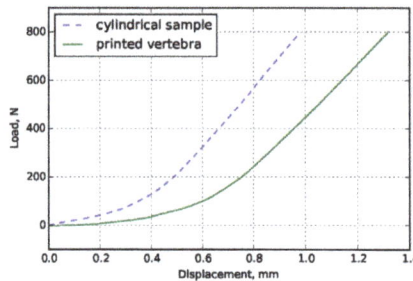
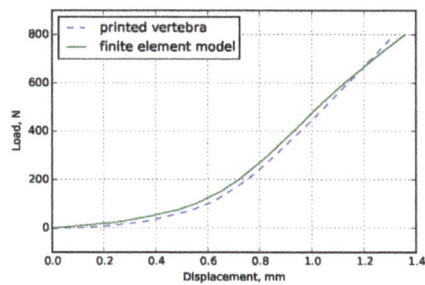

(a) Compression test of cylindrical PLA sample and printed model of the vertebrae.

(b) Compression test of 3-D printed and FEM models of lumbar vertebrae.

Figure 15. The load-displacement curves.

As Figure 15b shows, the curves present corresponding characters, and the biggest difference between the results is constant (about 4%) until the value of load becomes 700 N. Then, the curves demonstrate similar magnitudes of displacement values, which does not exceed 5%. These results approve the adequacy of finite element model and shows that the method offered for osteoporotic bone validation is reliable.

4. Conclusions

The proposed method based on the cancellous bone and cortical shell in silico finite element modelling includes basic principles of evaluating fracture risk of the mechanical system and can be used after clinical researches to estimate the quantiles of the load-bearing capacity of a lumbar vertebra as well as the fracture risk of individual patients by applying the peculiar anatomical properties of the lumbar vertebra.

The results show that the fracture risk is substantially higher at relatively low levels of apparent BV/TV ratios and critical due to thinner cortical shells, suggesting high risk levels even during daily activities of typical external loads.

Author Contributions: Conceptualization, A.M., V.A., M.T., and R.K.; data curation, A.M., O.A., and O.C.; formal analysis, A.M. and D.Z.; funding acquisition, A.M.; investigation, A.M., O.A., O.C., and D.Z.; methodology, A.M., D.Z., and R.K.; project administration, A.M.; resources, A.M.; software, A.M. and D.Z.; supervision, A.M.; validation, A.M., O.A., O.C., and D.Z.; visualization, O.A., O.C., and D.Z.; writing—original draft, A.M., V.A., D.Z., and M.T.; writing—review and editing, A.M., V.A., D.Z., and M.T.

Funding: This research received no external funding.

Conflicts of Interest: The authors declare no conflict of interest.

Abbreviations

The following abbreviations are used in this manuscript:

FEM	Finite element method
FE	Finite element
IVD	intervetebral disk
BV/TV	Bone volume vs total volume
QCT	Quantitative computational tomography
BMD	Bone mineral density
DXA	Dual-energy X-ray absorptiometry

References

1. Agrawal, A.; Kalia, R. Osteoporosis: Current Review. *J. Orthop. Traumatol. Rehabil.* **2014**, *7*, 101. [CrossRef]
2. Lin, J.T.; Lane, J.M. Osteoporosis: A review. *Clin. Orthop. Relat. Res.* **2004**, *425*, 126–134. [CrossRef]
3. Cooper, C.; Cole, Z.A.; Holroyd, C.R.; Earl, S.C.; Harvey, N.C.; Dennison, E.M.; Melton, L.J.; Cummings, S.R.; Kanis, J.A.; The IOF CSA Working Group on Fracture Epidemiology. Secular trends in the incidence of hip and other osteoporotic fractures. *Osteoporos. Int.* **2011**, *22*, 1277–88. [CrossRef]
4. Cummings, S.R.; Melton, L.J., III. Epidemiology and outcomes of osteoporotic fractures. *Lancet* **2002**, *359*, 1761–1767. [CrossRef]
5. Doblaré, M.; García, J.M.; Gómez, M.J. Modelling bone tissue fracture and healing: A review. *Eng. Fract. Mech.* **2004**, *71*, 1809–1840. [CrossRef]
6. Łodygowski, T.; Kakol, W.; Wierszycki, M. Ogurkowska, B.M. Three-dimensional nonlinear finite element model of the human lumbar spine segment. *Acta Bioeng. Biomech.* **2005**, *7*, 17–28.
7. Su, J.; Cao, L.; Li, Z.; Yu, B.; Zhang, C.; Li, M. Three-dimensional finite element analysis of lumbar vertebra loaded by static stress and its biomechanical significance. *Chin. J. Traumatol.* **2009**, *12*, 153–156.

8. Jones, A.C.; Wilcox, R.K. Finite element analysis of the spine: Towards a framework of verification, validation and sensitivity analysis. *Med. Eng. Phys.* **2008**, *30*, 1287–1304. [CrossRef]
9. Crawford, R.P.; Cann, C.E.; Keaveny, T.M. Finite element models predict in vitro vertebral body compressive strength better than quantitative computed tomography. *Bone* **2003**, *33*, 744–750. [CrossRef]
10. Maquer, G.; Schwiedrzik, J.; Huber, G.; Morlock, M.M.; Zysset, P.K. Compressive strength of elderly vertebrae is reduced by disc degeneration and additional flexion. *J. Mech. Behav. Biomed. Mater.* **2015**, *42*, 54–66. [CrossRef]
11. Provatidis, C.; Vossou, C.; Koukoulis, I.; Balanika, A.; Baltas, C.; Lyritis, G. A pilot finite element study of an osteoporotic L1-vertebra compared to one with normal T-score. *Comput. Methods Biomech. Biomed. Eng.* **2010**, *13*, 185–95. [CrossRef]
12. McDonald, K.; Little, J.; Pearcy, M.; Adam, C. Development of a multi-scale finite element model of the osteoporotic lumbar vertebral body for the investigation of apparent level vertebra mechanics and micro-level trabecular mechanics. *Med. Eng. Phys.* **2010**, *32*, 653–661. [CrossRef]
13. Garo, A.; Arnoux, P.J.; Wagnac, E.; Aubin, C.E. Calibration of the mechanical properties in a finite element model of a lumbar vertebra under dynamic compression up to failure. *Med. Biol. Eng. Comput.* **2011**, *49*, 1371–1379. [CrossRef]
14. Kim, Y.H.; Wu, M.; Kim, K. Stress Analysis of Osteoporotic Lumbar Vertebra Using Finite Element Model with Microscaled Beam-Shell Trabecular-Cortical Structure. *J. Appl. Math.* **2013**, *2013*, 285165. [CrossRef]
15. Wierszycki, M.; Szajek, K.; Łodygowski, T.; Nowak, M. A two-scale approach for trabecular bone microstructure modeling based on computational homogenization procedure. *Comput. Mech.* **2014**, *54*, 287–298. [CrossRef]
16. Wolfram, U.; Gross, T.; Pahr, D.H.; Schwiedrzik, J.; Wilke, H.J.; Zysset, P.K. Fabric-based Tsai-Wu yield criteria for vertebral trabecular bone in stress and strain space. *J. Mech. Behav. Biomed. Mater.* **2012**, *15*, 218–228. [CrossRef]
17. El-Rich, M.; Arnoux, P.J.; Wagnac, E.; Brunet, C.; Aubin, C.E. Finite element investigation of the loading rate effect on the spinal load-sharing changes under impact conditions. *J. Biomech.* **2009**, *42*, 1252–1262. [CrossRef]
18. Pothuaud, L.; Carceller, P.; Hans, D. Correlations between grey-level variations in 2D projection images (TBS) and 3D microarchitecture: Applications in the study of human trabecular bone microarchitecture. *Bone* **2008**, *42*, 775–778. [CrossRef]
19. Hans, D.; Barthe, N.; Boutroy, S.; Pothuaud, L.; Winzenrieth, R.; Krieg, M.-A. Correlations Between Trabecular Bone Score, Measured Using Anteroposterior Dual-Energy X-Ray Absorptiometry Acquisition, and 3-Dimensional Parameters of Bone Microarchitecture: An Experimental Study on Human Cadaver Vertebrae. *J. Clin. Densitom.* **2011**, *14*, 302–312. [CrossRef]
20. Kanis, J.A.; Oden, V.; Johnell, O.; Johansson, H.; De Laet, C.; Brown J.; Burckhardt, P.; Cooper, C.; Christiansen, C.; Cummings, S.; et al. The use of clinical risk factors enhances the performance of BMD in the prediction of hip and osteoporotic fractures in men and women. *Osteoporos. Int.* **2007**, *18*, 1033–1046. [CrossRef]
21. Marshall, D.; Johnell O.; Wedel, H. Meta-analysis of how well measures of bone mineral density predict occurrence of osteoporotic fractures. *BMJ* **1996**, *312*, 1254–1259. [CrossRef]
22. Taylor, B.C.; Schreiner, P.J.; Stone K.L.; Fink, H.A.; Cummings, S.R.; Nevitt, M.C.; Bowman, P.J.; Ensrud, K.E. Long-term prediction of incident hip fracture risk in elderly white women: Study of osteoporotic fractures. *J. Am. Geriatr. Soc.* **2004**, *52*, 1479–1486. [CrossRef]
23. Kanis, J.A.; Oden, A.; Johansson, H.; Borgstrom, F.; Strom O.; McCloskey, E. FRAX and its applications to clinical practice. *Bone* **2009**, *44*, 734–743. [CrossRef]
24. Kanis, J.A.; Johnell, O.; Oden, A.; Johansson H.; McCloskey, E. FRAX and the assessment of fracture probability in men and women from the UK. *Osteoporos. Int.* **2008**, *19*, 385–397. [CrossRef]
25. Timothy, H.K.; Brandeau, J.F. Mathematical modeling of the stress strain-strain rate behavior of bone using the Ramberg-Osgood equation. *J. Biomech.* **1983**, *16*, 445–450.
26. Nazarian, A.; von Stechow, D.; Zurakowski, D.; Muller, R.; Snyder, B.D. Bone Volume Fraction Explains the Variation in Strength and Stiffness of Cancellous Bone Affected by Metastatic Cancer and Osteoporosis. *Calcif. Tissue Int.* **2008**, *83*, 368–379. [CrossRef]

27. Abaqus FEA, SIMULIA Web Site. Dassault Systèmes, Retrieved 2017. Available online: https://www.3ds.com/ (accessed on 25 July 2019).
28. Linthorne, N.P. Analysis of standing vertical jumps using a force platform. *J. Sports Sci. Med.* **2010**, *9*, 282–287. [CrossRef]
29. Dodson, B.; Noland, D. *Reliability Engineering Handbook*; CRC Press LLC Main Office: Boca Raton, FL, USA, 1999; p. 592.
30. Melton, L.J., III; Achenbach, S.J.; Atkinson, E.J.; Therneau, T.M.; Amin, S. Long-term mortality following fractures at different skeletai sites: A population-based cohort study. *Osteoporos. Int.* **2013**, *24*, 1689–1696. [CrossRef]
31. R Core Team. *R: A Language and Environment for Statistical Computing*; R Foundation for Statistical Computing: Vienna, Austria, 2017. Available online: https://www.R-project.org/ (accessed on 25 July 2019).
32. Pinheiro, J.; Bates, D.; DebRoy, S.; Sarkar, D.; R Core Team (2017). Nlme: Linear and Nonlinear Mixed Effects Models. R Package Version 3.1-131. 2017. Available online: https://CRAN.R-project.org/package=nlme (accessed on 25 July 2019).
33. Fields, A.J.; Eswaran, S.K.; Jekir, M.G.; Keaveny, T.M. Role of trabecular microarchitecture in whole-vertebral body biomechanical behavior. *J. Bone Miner. Res.* **2009**, *24*, 1523–1530. [CrossRef]
34. Roux, J.P.; Wegrzyn, J.; Arlot, M.E.; Guyen, O.; Delmas, P.D.; Chapurlat, R.; Bouxsein, M.L. Contribution of trabecular and cortical components to biomechanical behavior of human vertebrae: An ex vivo study. *J. Bone Miner. Res.* **2010**, *25*, 356–361. [CrossRef]
35. Jaumard, N.V.; Bauman, J.A.; Weisshaar, C.L.; Guarino, B.B.; Welch, W.C.; Winkelstein, B.A. Contact pressure in the facet joint during sagittal bending of the cadaveric cervical spine. *J. Biomech. Eng.* **2011**, *133*, 071004. [CrossRef]
36. Venables, W.N.; Ripley, B.D. *Modern Applied Statistics with S*, 4th ed.; Springer: New York, NY, USA, 2002; ISBN 0-387-95457-0.
37. Mann K.A.; Miller, M.A. Fluid-structure interactions in micro-interlocked regions of the cement-bone interface. *Comput. Methods Biomech. Biomed. Eng.* **2014**, *17*, 1809–1820. [CrossRef]
38. Souzanchi, M.F.; Palacio-Mancheno, P.; Borisov, Y.A.; Cardoso, L.; Cowin, S.C. Microarchitecture and bone quality in the human calcaneus: Local variations of fabric anisotropy. *J. Bone Min. Res.* **2012**, *27*, 2562–2572. [CrossRef]
39. Polikeit, A.; Nolte, L.P.; Ferguson, S.J. Simulated influence of osteoporosis and disc degeneration on the load transfer in a lumbar functional spinal unit. *J. Biomech.* **2004**, *37*, 1061–1069. [CrossRef]
40. Helgason, B.; Perilli, E.; Schileo, E.; Taddei, F.; Brynjólfsson, S.S.; Viceconti, M. Mathematical relationships between bone density and mechanical properties: A literature review. *Clin. Biomech.* **2008**, *23*, 135–146. [CrossRef]
41. Genant, H.K.; Wu, C.Y.; van Kuijk, C.; Nevitt, M.C. Vertebral fracture assessment using a semiquantitative technique. *J. Bone Min. Res.* **1993**, *8*, 1137–1148. [CrossRef]
42. Lakes, R.S.; Katz, J.L.; Sternstein, S.S. Viscoelastic properties of wet cortical bone: Part I, torsional and biaxial studies. *J. Biomech.* **1979**, *12*, 657–678. [CrossRef]
43. Lakes, R.S.; Katz, J.L. Viscoelastic properties of wet cortical bone: Part II, relaxation mechanisms. *J. Biomech.* **1979**, *12*, 679–687. [CrossRef]
44. Lakes, R.S.; Katz, J.L. Viscoelastic properties of wet cortical bone: Part III, A non-linear constitutive equation. *J. Biomech.* **1979**, *12*, 689–698. [CrossRef]
45. Burczinski, T. Multiscale Modelling of Osseous Tissues. *J. Theor. Appl. Mech.* **2010**, *48*, 855–870.
46. Wolf, J. *Das Gesetz der Transformation der Knochen*; Hirschwald: Berlin, Germany, 1892.
47. Goldenblar, I.I.; Kopnov, A. Strength of Glass Reinforced Plastics in the Complex Stress State. *Polym. Mech.* **1966**, *1*, 54–60. [CrossRef]
48. von Mises, R. Mechanik der festen Körper im plastisch deformablen Zustand Göttin. *Nachr. Math. Phys.* **1913**, *1*, 582–592.
49. Hill, R. *The Mathematical Theory of Plasticity*; Oxford, U.P.: Oxford, UK, 1950.
50. Tsai, S.W. Strength Theories of Filamentary Structures. In *Fundamental Aspects of Fibre Reinforced Plastic Composites*; Schwartz, R.T., Schwartz, H.S., Eds.; Interscience: New York, NY, USA, 1968; Chapter 1.

51. Korenczuk, C.E.; Votava, L.E.; Dhume, R.Y.; Kizilski, S.B.; Brown, G.E.; Narain, R.; Barocas, V.H. Isotropic Failure Criteria Are Not Appropriate for Anisotropic Fibrous Biological Tissues. *J. Biomech. Eng.* **2017**, *139*, 071008. [CrossRef]
52. Wilcox, B.; Mobbs, R.J.; Wu, A.M.; Phan, K. Systematic review of 3D printing in spinal surgery: The current state of play. *J. Spine Surg.* **2017**, *3*, 433–443. [CrossRef]

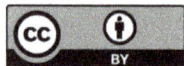

© 2019 by the authors. Licensee MDPI, Basel, Switzerland. This article is an open access article distributed under the terms and conditions of the Creative Commons Attribution (CC BY) license (http://creativecommons.org/licenses/by/4.0/).

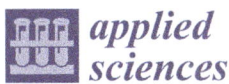

Article

A Comparative Study of Continuum and Structural Modelling Approaches to Simulate Bone Adaptation in the Pelvic Construct

Dan T. Zaharie [1,2,*] and Andrew T.M. Phillips [1,2]

1   The Royal British Legion Centre for Blast Injury Studies, Imperial College London, London SW7 2AZ, UK
2   Department of Civil and Environmental Engineering, Structural Biomechanics, Imperial College London, London SW7 2AZ, UK
*   Correspondence: dan.zaharie10@imperial.ac.uk

Received: 27 June 2019; Accepted: 7 August 2019; Published: 13 August 2019

Abstract: This study presents the development of a number of finite element (FE) models of the pelvis using different continuum and structural modelling approaches. Four FE models were developed using different modelling approaches: continuum isotropic, continuum orthotropic, hybrid isotropic and hybrid orthotropic. The models were subjected to an iterative adaptation process based on the Mechanostat principle. Each model was adapted to a number of common daily living activities (walking, stair ascent, stair descent, sit-to-stand and stand-to-sit) by applying onto it joint and muscle loads derived using a musculoskeletal modelling framework. The resulting models, along with a structural model previously developed by the authors, were compared visually in terms of bone architecture, and their response to a single load case was compared to a continuum FE model derived from computed tomography (CT) imaging data. The main findings of this study were that the continuum orthotropic model was the closest to the CT derived model in terms of load response albeit having less total bone volume, suggesting that the role of material directionality in influencing the maximum orthotropic Young's modulus should be included in continuum bone adaptation models. In addition, the hybrid models, where trabecular and cortical bone were distinguished, had similar outcomes, suggesting that the approach to modelling trabecular bone is less influential when the cortex is modelled separately.

Keywords: biomechanics; finite element modelling; pelvis; bone adaptation; musculoskeletal modelling

1. Introduction

The pelvic construct is the region of load transition between the upper body and lower limbs and plays a number of roles, such as protecting the organs and vessels in the lower abdomen. It also facilitates the transfer of forces between the lower limbs and the upper body during physical activities such as walking and stair climbing, withstanding loads at the hip joints of up to around six times body weight [1–3].

Continuous adaptation of bone tissue in response to the mechanical environment surrounding it provides an explanation for the different architecture of bones in the skeletal system [4]. Long bones, such as the femur and tibia, develop thick cortical shafts with trabecular bone concentrated at the joints to transfer contact forces [5,6], whereas the pelvis is viewed as a sandwich structure where a thin layer of cortical bone surrounds a structure of trabecular bone [7–9].

Finite element (FE) modelling is a very common approach to investigate the biomechanics of the pelvic ring due to its versatility and low cost compared to clinical investigations, with the added characteristic of enabling the design of bone scaffolds or implants. Computational modelling of bone adaptation to the mechanical environment surrounding it has emerged into an important component in aiding the interpretation of experimental findings and exploring further issues [10,11]. Bone adaptation models have been previously developed using both continuum elements [12–15] or structural elements [6,16–18]. Early FE models either used simplified geometries [19–22], were axisymmetric [23,24] or reduced the three-dimensional pelvis to a two-dimensional slice [25–29].

The first FE model of the bony pelvis based on subject specific geometry and material properties from medical imaging data was developed by Dalstra et al. [30] using continuum solid elements, validating it against experimentally obtained data from a cadaveric pelvis loaded at the hip joint. Anderson et al. [9] developed an FE model of the pelvic innominate by distinguishing between cortical and trabecular bone using different element types. Cortical bone was modelled using structural shell elements with location dependent thickness derived from medical imaging data. Trabecular bone was modelled using continuum isotropic elements and the model was validated against experimental data by comparing cortical bone strains. The majority of recent FE models representing the pelvic construct were developed from CT imaging data with a tendency of using an isotropic material model to represent bone and distinguishing between trabecular and cortical bone by adding a layer of shell elements [9,31,32]. Notably, Anderson et al. [9] also developed a purely continuum model in which the surface nodes were assigned the highest Young's modulus they found for cancellous bone (approximately 3.8 GPa) which performed similarly to the model with a shell element layer. Although modelling bone using isotropic material properties has the benefit of reducing computational time, it is insufficient to provide information on directionality of the bone microstructure [33]. Orthotropy has been found to offer a good approximation of bone's anisotropy at the continuum level [34].

The aim of this study was to develop a number of computational models of the pelvic construct using different continuum and structural FE bone adaptation modelling approaches with the purpose of investigating their effects on bone adaptation and predicted mechanical behaviour of the pelvis in comparison to a CT scan derived FE model. The modelling approaches were divided into isotropic and orthotropic material models, followed by a continuum or hybrid approach, where cortical and trabecular bone were distinguished. The motivation behind developing a number of different models was to assess their sensitivity to the approach used. Each model was subjected to an iterative adaptation algorithm based on the Mechanostat principle [4] and tailored for the type of elements used [6,14]. Bone adaptation was driven by the strains generated by a loading environment derived from five daily living activities (walking, stair ascent, stair descent, sit-to-stand and stand-to-sit).

2. Methods

2.1. Musculoskeletal Modelling

To obtain a physiologically relevant morphological representation of the pelvic construct, the base FE models were subjected to a loading environment derived from musculoskeletal simulations of the five most frequent daily living activities [35]: walking, stair ascent, stair descent, sit-to-stand and stand-to-sit. The simulations were performed using a bilateral musculoskeletal model of the lower limbs. The model was based on an ipsilateral model developed by Modenese et al. [36] based on an anatomical dataset published by Horsman et al. [37] and implemented in OpenSim [38]. The model was validated at the hip joint. The bilateral model had a total of 76 muscles and 326 actuators. Further details can be found in Zaharie and Phillips [39].

Gait data for the selected physical activities were collected from a male volunteer (age: 23 years, weight: 93 kg, height: 188 cm) at the Human Biodynamics Lab in the Imperial College Research Labs at Charing Cross Hospital and processed using Vicon Nexus and the Biomechanical ToolKit [40]. A total of 59 reflective markers were positioned on bony landmarks and tracked using a Vicon system (Oxford Metrics, Oxford, UK) equipped with 10 infrared cameras. Ground reaction forces (GRFs) were measured using three force plates (Type 9286BA, sampling rate 1000 Hz, Kistler Instruments Ltd, Hook, UK). For walking, the force plates were placed to form a walkway (speed: 1.34 m/s, stride length:

0.64 m, cadence: 115.54 steps/min). A staircase was instrumented with the force plates to record stair ascent and stair descent GRFs (step height 15 cm and step depth 25 cm). Three force plates were set, one under each foot and another on a stool with a height of 52.5 cm from the floor to measure ground and seat reaction forces during sit-to-stand and stand-to-sit.

The body segments of the model were scaled to the anatomical dimensions of the volunteer by calculating the ratios between the lengths given by experimental and virtual markers. The inertial properties of each segment were updated using the regression equations of Dumas et al. [41]. The joint angles for each recorded activity were derived using an inverse kinematic approach [42]. Static optimization with a cost function minimising the sum of muscle activations squared was performed to estimate the muscle forces throughout each activity's cycle. The muscle insertion points on the pelvis along with the direction and magnitude of each muscle force were extracted using the MuscleForceDirection (v1.0) plugin [6,43]. The hip joint contact forces were calculated using the JointReaction tool available in OpenSim [44]. The musculoskeletal modelling was performed using OpenSim (Version 3.3) [38]. The loads applied on the pelvis throughout the duration of each activity cycle (hip joint reaction forces, muscle forces and inertial forces) were determined and subsampled to maintain computational efficiency, resulting in a total of 39 load cases representing the five physical activities.

2.2. Finite Element Modelling

2.2.1. Base Model

The base FE model used in this study was generated from a tetrahedral mesh previously developed by the authors [39]. The volumetric mesh of the pelvis was generated in Mimics (Materialise, Leuven, Belgium) from a CT scan (399 × 3 mm thick slices, 512 × 512 pixels, 0.91 mm/pixel) of a cadaveric pelvis and lower limbs (Male, age: 55, weight: 94.3 kg, height: 188 cm) provided by the Royal British Legion Centre for Blast Injury Studies at Imperial College London, to which the volunteer was height and weight matched. The base FE model consisted of 377,362 tetrahedral elements with an average edge length of 3.76 mm [39]. In the present study, four predictive models of the pelvic construct were developed: two purely continuum models with orthotropic and isotropic material properties, and two hybrid models where trabecular and cortical bone were differentiated using continuum and shell elements respectively, while assigning orthotropic and isotropic material properties to elements representing trabecular bone (Table 1). In addition, a structural model previously developed by the authors [39] was included for comparison.

Table 1. Element type used to model cortical and trabecular bone for each model developed.

Model	Cortical Bone	Trabecular Bone
Orthotropic		Tetrahedral elements
Isotropic		Tetrahedral elements
Hybrid orthotropic	Shell elements	Tetrahedral elements
Hybrid isotropic	Shell elements	Tetrahedral elements
Structural	Shell elements	Truss elements

2.2.2. Ligaments

To realistically model the load transfer between the three pelvic bones, the ligaments associated with the pelvic ring (sacro-iliac, pubic, sacrospinous, sacrotuberous and inguinal) were included in the model. The anatomical attachment areas of each ligament were visually defined on the model based on descriptions in the literature [45–48].

Each ligament was modelled using truss elements between each pair of closest nodes from the two surfaces corresponding to the insertions areas. All truss elements representing ligaments were assigned linear elastic material properties and zero stiffness in compression. A set of truss elements with a low compressive Young's modulus was overlaid with the initial truss elements for each ligament to ensure numerical stability. For the joints containing cartilage, truss elements were included to allow the transfer of compressive forces. The tensile and compressive material properties assigned to the ligaments and cartilage were taken from a previous study [39].

2.2.3. Loading and Boundary Conditions

The 39 load cases resulting from the musculoskeletal simulations were applied on the model in successive analysis steps. The muscle forces obtained from the musculoskeletal model were applied as point loads on the closest three nodes to each muscle insertion point [39,49]. The hip joint contact forces and the inertial loads were applied at the joint centres and the centre of mass of the pelvic segment, respectively. In addition, for sit to stand and stand to sit, the reaction load from the seat was applied at the inferior ischium for the duration of contact. To spread the hip joint contact forces over the corresponding bone surface, they were applied using 'load applicators' comprising of four layers of continuum wedge elements, each with a thickness of 2 mm, as they allow for a reduction in CPU time in comparison to modeling contact at each joint. The two first layers were assigned material properties akin to cartilage (E = 10 MPa, ν = 0.49), with the furthest two being assigned stiffnesses of 10 MPa (ν = 0.3) and 500 MPa (ν = 0.3), respectively [6,39]. In addition, an 'inertial applicator' was designed to spread the inertial load of the pelvis over the whole construct by linking its centre of mass to every node of the model with truss elements with a radius of 0.1 mm and low stiffness (E = 0.1 MPa, ν = 0.3) to avoid artificially stiffening the model. The L5S1 interface between the lumbar spine and the sacrum was constrained in the three translational degrees of freedom via four layers of wedge elements to avoid fixing nodes directly on the bone surface resulting in artificial stress concentrations. The layers were respectively assigned the same thickness and material properties as the load applicators.

The load cases obtained from the musculoskeletal model were applied in consecutive analysis steps to the FE model.

2.3. Bone Adaptation

The base FE models were subjected iteratively to the aforementioned load cases using an adaptation algorithm based on the Mechanostat principle [4] proposed by Geraldes and Phillips [14] for the continuum orthotropic and isotropic elements used in the continuum and hybrid models. After each iteration, the material properties of each orthotropic element were adjusted depending on the stresses and strains occuring due to the applied loading regime. A guiding step was selected for each element based on the absolute maximum principal strain value from all analysis steps. The stress tensor associated with that step was then used to extract the principal stresses and their orientation by performing an eigenanalysis.

The axes representing the orthotropic orientations of each element were aligned to the vectors defining the principal stress directions for the guiding frame (Figure 1).

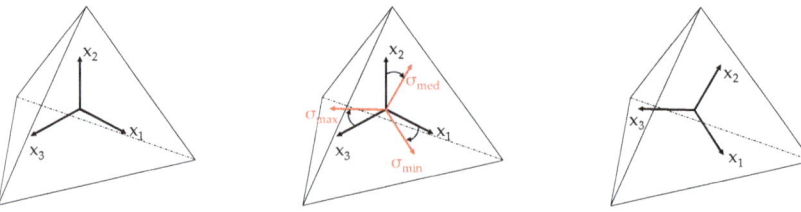

Figure 1. Orientation of element updated based on the principal stress directions of guiding frame.

Young's moduli and shear moduli were updated proportional to the absolute maximum normal and shear strains for the orientation obtained from the guiding step across all analysis steps, compared to the normal strain target and shear strain target, respectively. Poisson's ratios for each element were altered to satisfy the thermodynamic restrictions on the elastic constant of bone and maintain the compliance matrix as positive definite [15].

For the isotropic elements, the Young's modulus of each element was updated proportionally to the absolute maximum principal strain taken across all loading frames, while Poisson's ratio was kept constant. Concerning the hybrid models, shell elements representing cortical bone were adjusted in a similar fashion by modifying their thickness according to the in-plane absolute maximum strain as implemented in previous work from the research group [6,39,50].

To satisfy the Mechanostat principle [4], material and geometric properties of the elements were adjusted to bring the local normal strains towards a target strain, assigned a value of 1250 $\mu\varepsilon$. The lazy zone interval was defined between 1000 $\mu\varepsilon$ and 1500 $\mu\varepsilon$. In the case of models with orthotropic elements, the shear target strain was assigned a value of 1443 $\mu\varepsilon$ with a lazy zone of 1154 $\mu\varepsilon$ and 1732 $\mu\varepsilon$, in concordance with previous studies from the research group [6,14,15]. In addition, normal strains lower than 250 $\mu\varepsilon$ were associated with the dead zone.

The elements of the continuum models were assigned an initial Young's modulus value of 3000 MPa and a Poisson's ratio of 0.3. In addition, for the continuum orthotropic model, the initial values of shear modulus were set at 1500 MPa. The Young's modulus values were limited between 10 and 18,000 MPa [30]. The limits of shear modulus values for continuum orthotropic model were set between 5 and 15000 MPa. Elements with strains in the dead zone were assigned the minimum allowable Young's modulus and were not re-adjusted in subsequent iterations of the the adaptation process. The convergence criterion was defined as when the average change in Young's moduli of elements with absolute normal strain values above 250 $\mu\varepsilon$ and Young's moduli above the minimum was less than 2% between successive iterations [13].

In the case of the hybrid models, a distinction was made between cortical and trabecular bone. Continuum elements, representing trabecular bone, were assigned initial Young's modulus values of 300 MPa, limited between 10 and 2000 MPa and Possion's ratio values of 0.3 [30]. For the hybrid orthotropic model, elements were assigned initial shear modulus values of 150 MPa, limited between 5 and 1500 MPa. Each shell element, representative of cortical bone, was assigned a Young's modulus of 18,000 MPa, a Poisson's ratio of 0.3 and an initial thickness of 0.1 mm [6]. Cortical thickness was limited between 0.1 mm and 5 mm [39]. The thickness of cortical elements was updated proportional to the largest value of maximum principal strain across all load cases and the target normal strain. The convergence criterion for shell elements adaptation was defined as when less than 1% of shell elements changed their thickness between successive iterations [6]. Convergence of the hybrid models was achieved only when both structural and continuum convergence criteria were met simultaneously.

A structural model of the pelvis developed previously [39] was included in the comparison. Briefly, the structural model was developed using a network of truss elements to represent trabecular bone and shell elements to represent cortical bone. The thickness of shells and cross-sectional area of trusses were updated proportional to absolute maximum principal strains resulting from the same set of load cases used in this study and the same target normal strain. Similarly, convergence was achieved when less than 2% of elements changed their thickness or cross-sectional area between successive iterations.

2.4. Comparison with CT Scan Derived Model

The tetrahedral mesh of the right hemipelvis was assigned varying material properties derived from the CT scan data (Figure 2) using Bonemat [51]. Assuming a linear relationship between the Hounsfield units (HU) values in the scans and bone ash density [52], bone ash density distribution was derived from the medical images. Young's moduli (GPa) for each element were derived from the ash density (g/cm^3) using a power relationship [53]. This model was not used in the adaptation and was developed to provide an independent comparison for the adaptive models. The response of the resulting CT derived FE model and the corresponding adapted models to a vertical load of

2 kN applied at the acetabulum representing a standing stance were compared. The hemipelvis was constrained at the pubic and sacroiliac joint surfaces.

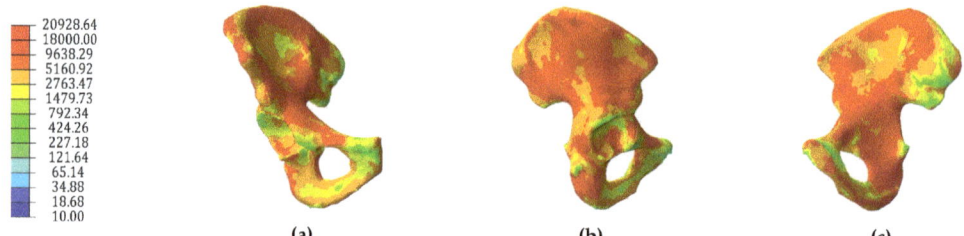

Figure 2. Distribution of Young's modulus (MPa) across the CT scan derived model - shown for (**a**) frontal, (**b**) lateral, and (**c**) medial views.

3. Results

3.1. Continuum Models

The continuum isotropic model converged to an adapted solution after 25 iterations. The Young's modulus distribution of the converged isotropic model is shown in Figure 3a–c. Regions with high stiffness were found along the arcuate line, anterior superior sacrum, superior pubis ramus, acetabulum and near the greater sciatic notch. Conversely, large parts of the ilium, inferior pubis ramus and inferior sacrum were found to have a low stiffness.

The continuum orthotropic model of the pelvis was found to converge after 60 iterations. The distributions of the mean and dominant Young's moduli across the model are shown in Figure 3d–i. The mean Young's modulus for each element was calculated as the average of the three directional Young's moduli, whereas the dominant Young's modulus was selected as the maximum value of the three directional moduli. Regions with high mean stiffness were found around the sacroiliac joint, along the arcuate line, around the top of the sacrum, along the superior pubis ramus, in the acetabulum and between the posterior inferior iliac spine and greater sciatic notch. Low mean stiffnesses were found at the iliac fossa, ischial tuberosity and inferior sacrum. Both models produced trabecular distributions which were broadly consistent with previous findings [9].

Visually, the distributions of isotropic Young's modulus and orthotropic dominant Young's modulus share more similarities than with the distribution of mean orthotropic Young's modulus. Although the CT scan derived model has generally a higher stiffness across the whole surface compared to the adaptive continuum models, an interesting aspect to note is a region at the top of the ilium medially where the dominant Young's modulus values of the orthotropic model were similar to the same region in the CT scan derived model. In addition, the same region appeared to have a lower stiffness in the case of the isotropic model.

A frequency distribution of Young's modulus values for the orthotropic model, isotropic model and CT scan derived model suggests that both predictive models have similar distributions of elastic moduli, with over 75% of elements having a stiffness lower than 2 GPa. On the other hand, the CT derived model had less than 50% of elements with a stiffness lower than 2 GPa (Table 2).

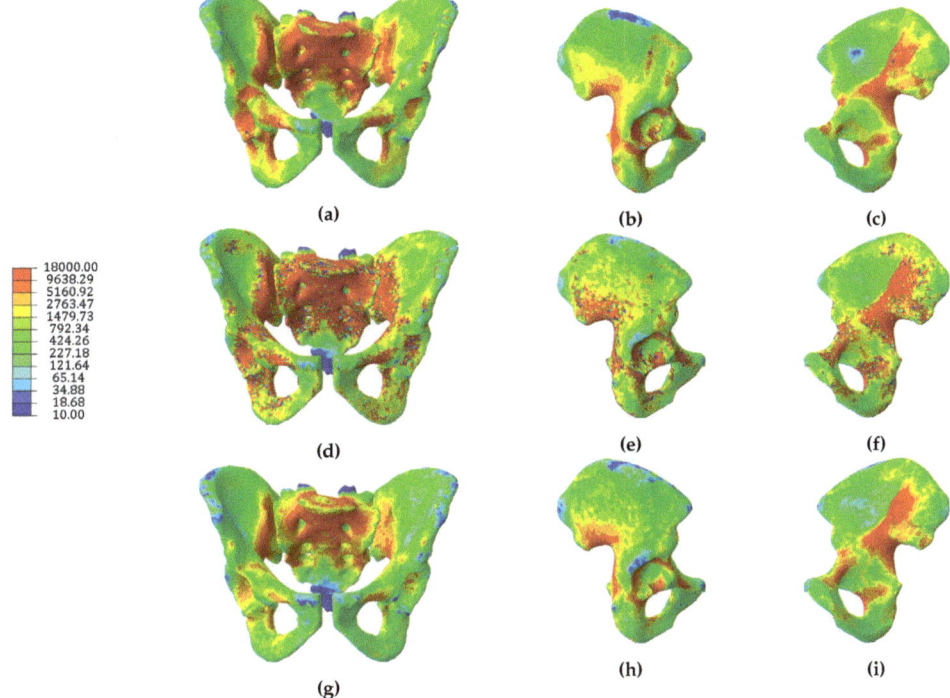

Figure 3. Distributions of Young's modulus (MPa) for the isotropic model (**a**–**c**), dominant Young's modulus (**d**–**f**) and mean Young's modulus (**g**–**i**) for the orthotropic model.

Table 2. Cumulative distribution (%) of elastic moduli of the three continuum models: CT scan derived, isotropic and orthotropic.

	CT Scan Model	Isotropic Model	Orthotropic Model E_1	Orthotropic Model E_2	Orthotropic Model E_3	Orthotropic Model E_{dom}	Orthotropic Model E_{mean}
10–1000 MPa	26.32	63.83	86.33	91.45	89.37	71.89	81.79
10–2000 MPa	47.37	77.88	89.64	93.89	92.27	78.85	87.56
10–3000 MPa	59.48	84.23	91.44	95.10	93.74	82.57	90.43
10–5000 MPa	73.74	91.01	93.53	96.39	95.38	86.82	93.57
10–10,000 MPa	90.43	96.78	95.93	97.81	97.14	91.63	99.42
10–15,000 MPa	98.51	98.27	97.14	98.50	98.01	94.06	99.97
10–18,000 MPa	99.91	100.00	100.00	100.00	100.00	100.00	100.00
Mean (MPa)	3727.6	1688.7	1059.4	616.4	781.9	2161.3	819.2
Std. dev. (MPa)	3817.5	3076.9	3411.5	2559.7	2898.7	4646.9	1841.8

3.2. Hybrid Continuum Models

The hybrid isotropic model reached a state of convergence after 24 iterations. The cortical thickness distribution is shown in Figure 4a–c. Shell elements were the thickest at the superior sacrum, along the arcuate line, around the sacroiliac joint, along the superior pubic ramus and in the region of the greater sciatic notch. Areas with thin shell elements were found on the superior ilium, inferior pubic ramus, ischial tuberosity, pubic tubercle and supraacetabular region.

The Young's modulus distribution of the continuum elements in the hybrid isotropic model are shown in Figure 5a–c. Regions with high stiffness were found along the arcuate line, anterior superior sacrum, superior pubis ramus, acetabulum and near the greater sciatic notch. Conversely, large parts of the ilium, inferior pubis ramus and inferior sacrum were found to have a low stiffness.

The hybrid orthotropic model of the pelvis was found to converge after 44 iterations. The cortical thickness distribution is illustrated in Figure 4d–f. Thick shell elements appeared at the superior sacrum, around the sacroiliac joint, along the superior pubic ramus and in the region of the greater sciatic notch. Areas with thin shell elements were found on the superior ilium, inferior pubic ramus, ischial tuberosity and supraacetabular region.

The distribution of mean and dominant Young's moduli of the continuum elements of the hybrid orthotropic model is shown in Figure 5d–i. Regions with high Young's moduli were found around the sacroiliac joint, on the arcuate line close to the sacrum, around the top of the sacrum, along the superior pubis ramus, around the superior acetabulum and between the posterior inferior iliac spine and greater sciatic notch. Low Young's moduli were found at the iliac fossa, ischial tuberosity, inferior sacrum and superior ilium, similar to the hybrid isotropic model. Similar to the distributions of the continuum models, distributions of dominant Young's moduli of the hybrid orthotropic model were visually more similar to the distributions of isotropic Young's moduli than the distributions of orthotropic mean Young's moduli.

A structural model previously developed by the authors [39] was included in this comparison. Cortical thickness was highest at the superior sacrum, along the gluteal surface, around the sacroiliac joint, superior pubic ramus, posterior iliac crest and greater sciatic notch. Cortical bone had a thickness between 0.1 mm and 0.5 mm at the ischium, acetabulum, pubic tubercle, iliac fossa and posterior superior iliac spine (Figure 4g–i). The main differences between the structural model and the hybrid continuum models in terms of cortical thickness distribution were found on the ilium superior to the acetabular region, where the structural model predicted an increase in cortical thickness with respect to the hybrid continuum models, and in the area of the sacroiliac joint, where both hybrid continuum models predicted cortical thickness close to the upper limit, whereas the structural model predicted lower thicknesses, with a few elements 5 mm thick.

Clusters of elements with large radii were found at the superior sacrum, supra acetabular region, pubic tubercle and greater sciatic notch. Regions with a small number of active elements were found at the iliac fossa, ischial tuberosity and inferior sacrum (Figure 6). The trabecular architecture predicted by the structural model was visually similar to the trabecular stiffness distributions predicted by the hybrid continuum models, particularly at the top of the sacrum, iliac crest, above the sciatic notch and in the acetabular region.

Frequency distributions of the trabecular Young's moduli for the hybrid orthotropic and hybrid isotropic models are shown in Table 3. Over 80% of elements in the hybrid orthotropic model had at least one directional elastic modulus lower than 200 MPa, whereas the Young's modulus values of the hybrid isotropic model were more distributed, with consistently more elements than the hybrid orthotropic model for values ranging from 200 MPa to 2000 MPa.

The frequency distribution of the cortical shell thickness across the hybrid models is shown in Table 4, along with the cortical thickness distribution of the structural model. The thickness distributions of the hybrid models were largely similar, whereas the structural model had a greater number of thicker shell elements. This difference can be attributed to the hybrid models having continuum elements in contact with the shell, taking a larger proportion of the surface loading as opposed to the truss elements of the structural model.

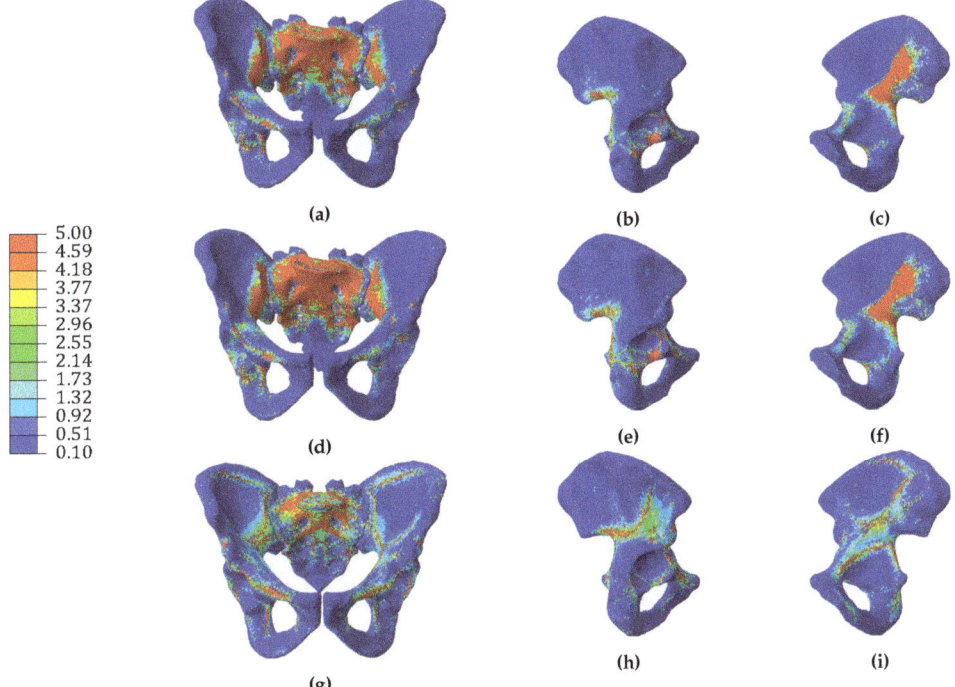

Figure 4. Distributions of cortical thickness (mm) for the hybrid isotropic model (**a**–**c**), hybrid orthotropic model (**d**–**f**) and structural model (**g**–**i**).

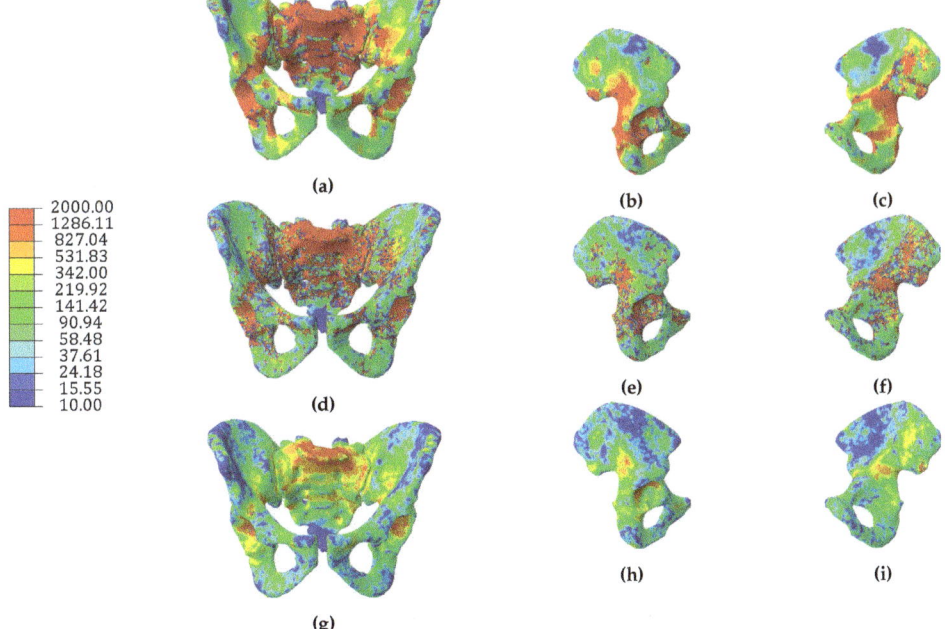

Figure 5. Distributions of trabecular Young's modulus (MPa) for the hybrid isotropic model (**a**–**c**), dominant Young's modulus (**d**–**f**) and mean Young's modulus (**g**–**i**) for the hybrid orthotropic model.

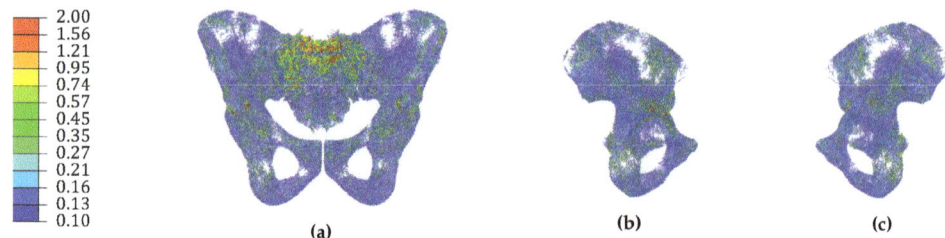

Figure 6. Trabecular elements' radii distribution (mm) of the structural model - shown for (**a**) frontal, (**b**) lateral, and (**c**) medial views. Trabecular elements with a radius <0.1 mm were excluded for clarity.

Table 3. Cumulative distribution (%) of trabecular elastic moduli for the hybrid isotropic and hybrid orthotropic models.

	Isotropic Model	Orthotropic Model E_1	Orthotropic Model E_2	Orthotropic Model E_3	Orthotropic Model E_{dom}	Orthotropic Model E_{mean}
10–100 MPa	33.87	80.06	87.98	83.05	59.76	69.44
10–200 MPa	45.01	83.56	90.62	86.42	66.88	76.33
10–300 MPa	52.78	85.56	91.99	88.24	70.84	80.16
10–500 MPa	63.33	88.00	93.58	90.41	75.71	84.84
10–1000 MPa	76.30	91.22	95.45	93.28	82.13	98.02
10–1500 MPa	83.79	93.04	96.42	94.80	85.75	99.86
10–2000 MPa	100.00	100.00	100.00	100.00	100.00	100.00
Mean (MPa)	585.5	213.3	121.0	171.0	422.8	168.5
Std. dev. (MPa)	689.1	522.4	389.1	461.9	685.9	281.4

Table 4. Cumulative distribution of the cortical thickness for the hybrid isotropic, hybrid orthotropic and structural models.

	Isotropic Model (%)	Orthotropic Model (%)	Structural Model (%)
0.1–0.3 mm	47.33	45.51	37.46
0.1–0.5 mm	62.21	58.99	56.30
0.1–1 mm	75.60	72.27	76.61
0.1–2 mm	83.68	81.06	88.72
0.1–3 mm	86.91	85.00	93.38
0.1–4 mm	88.81	87.10	95.66
0.1–5 mm	100.00	100.00	100.00
Mean (mm)	1.1	1.2	0.9
Std. dev. (mm)	1.5	1.6	1.1

3.3. Comparison to CT Scan Derived Model

The minimum and maximum principal strains on the surface of each model as a result of a loading scenario associated with upright standing (described in Zaharie and Phillips [39]) were compared to the homologous strains for the CT scan derived model subjected to the same loading scenario (Figures 7 and 8). The plots indicate that the continuum isotropic model had the worst match with the CT scan derived model, whereas the continuum orthotropic model had the best match. Both hybrid continuum models compared similarly to the CT scan derived model. Finally, the structural model was found to have the second best match in terms of fit, with a clustering of elements more similar to the hybrid models than the continuum models, indicating that the inclusion of a shell has a considerable effect on the overall stiffness of the models.

The determination coefficients and gradients of lines of best fit between each adaptive model and the CT scan derived model are shown in Table 5. Values of gradient below 1 indicate that the adapted model is less stiff than the CT scan derived model. In addition, determination coefficients and gradients of lines of best fit between each pair of adaptive models are shown in Tables 6 and 7.

Bone volumes of each model were calculated and, where applicable, were divided into cortical and trabecular volumes (Table 8). For the continuum models, relative density and volume were calculated for each element, with their product giving a bone volume value. The relative density of each element was derived from the Young's modulus using an approach developed by Geraldes et al. [15], described in the electronic supplementary material of that study. Total bone volume was obtained by summing bone volumes of all elements. The volumes of structural elements were calculated without having to take into account relative density. The CT scan derived model had a much higher volume of bone compared to any of the adapted models.

Table 5. Coefficients of determination and slopes of the line of best fit for each adaptive model compared to the CT scan derived model. A slope value of 1 means a perfect match between models.

Model	$\varepsilon_{min}(R^2)$	$\varepsilon_{max}(R^2)$	ε_{min} (Slope)	ε_{max} (Slope)
Isotropic	0.64	0.63	0.33	0.33
Orthotropic	0.78	0.79	0.87	0.84
Hybrid isotropic	0.71	0.72	0.60	0.59
Hybrid orthotropic	0.70	0.69	0.60	0.59
Structural	0.66	0.65	0.69	0.70

Table 6. Coefficients of determination between each pair of adaptive models for maximum principal strains (above table diagonal) and minimum principal strains (below table diagonal).

Model	Isotropic	Orthotropic	Hybrid Isotropic	Hybrid Orthotropic	Structural
Isotropic	N/A	0.35	0.81	0.63	0.62
Orthotropic	0.49	N/A	0.49	0.53	0.53
Hybrid isotropic	0.84	0.57	N/A	0.83	0.85
Hybrid orthotropic	0.63	0.61	0.81	N/A	0.99
Structural	0.61	0.61	0.84	0.99	N/A

Table 7. Gradients of lines of best fit between each pair of adaptive models for maximum principal strains (above table diagonal) and minimum principal strains (below table diagonal).

Model	Isotropic	Orthotropic	Hybrid Isotropic	Hybrid Orthotropic	Structural
Isotropic	N/A	1.49	0.59	0.36	0.36
Orthotropic	1.85	N/A	0.97	0.69	0.7
Hybrid isotropic	0.53	1.07	N/A	1.06	0.71
Hybrid orthotropic	0.33	0.74	1.1	N/A	0.98
Structural	0.33	0.74	0.71	0.98	N/A

Table 8. Predicted bone volumes for the adapted models and the CT scan derived model.

Model	Cortical Bone Volume (mm^3)	Trabecular Bone Volume (mm^3)	E < 2 GPa (mm^3)	E > 2 GPa (mm^3)	Total Bone Volume (mm^3)
CT scan	N/A	N/A	23269.04	163487.15	186756.20
Isotropic	N/A	N/A	25041.63	30499.45	55541.09
Orthotropic	N/A	N/A	26810.03	34241.34	61051.37
Hybrid isotropic	14941.68	25750.14	N/A	N/A	40691.82
Hybrid orthotropic	16465.59	17396.64	N/A	N/A	33862.23
Structural	17969.76	42321.05	N/A	N/A	60290.81

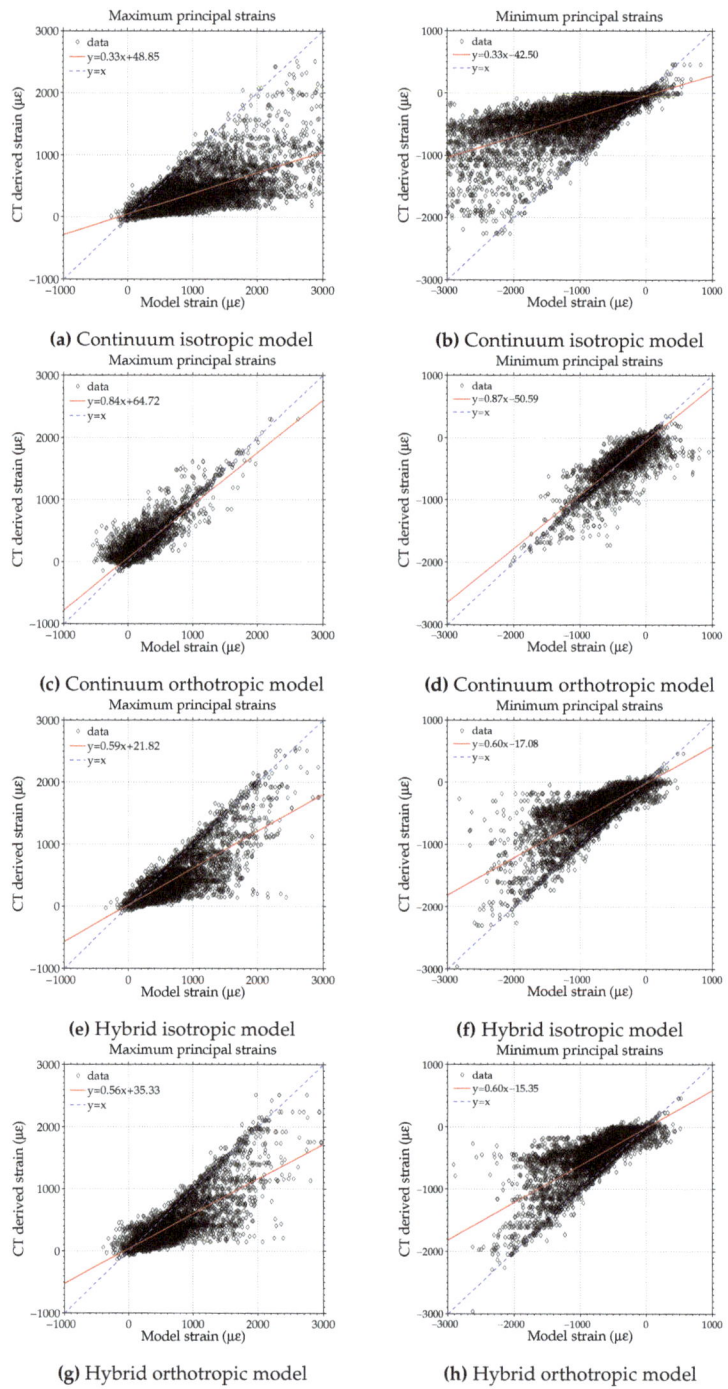

Figure 7. Comparison between the maximum (**a**,**c**,**e**,**g**) and minimum (**b**,**d**,**f**,**h**) principal strains across the surface of the continuum and hybrid models (x-axis) and CT derived model (y-axis). Lines of best fit are shown in red for each case, with the $y = x$ line shown in dashed blue.

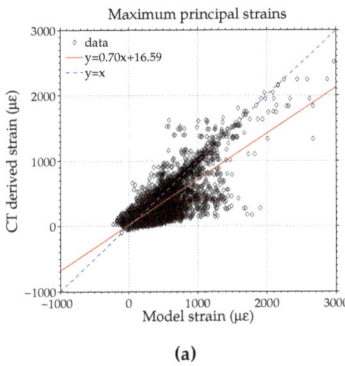 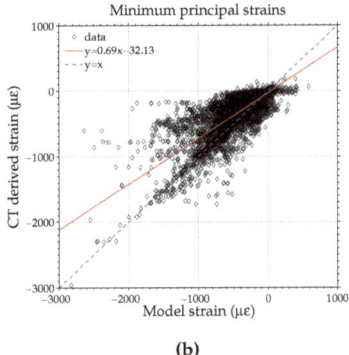

Figure 8. Comparison between the maximum (a) and minimum (b) principal strains across the surface of the structural model (x-axis) and CT derived model (y-axis). Lines of best fit are shown in red for each case, with the $y = x$ line shown in dashed blue.

4. Discussion

The current study sought to compare different FE modelling approaches to simulate bone adaptation in the pelvic construct. A number of computational models were developed and subjected to an iterative adaptation in response to a loading environment associated with physical activities of daily life. The converged models were compared in terms of the predicted bone architecture and response to an upright standing load case along with a CT scan derived continuum model and a previously developed structural model [39]. The converged models and the CT scan derived model are freely available in the Supplementary Materials.

Both continuum models had a much greater number of low stiffness elements present compared to CT data (Table 2). Although the average stiffness of the orthotropic model (819.2 MPa) was lower than both the isotropic and CT derived models' average stiffnesses (1689 MPa and 3728 MPa, respectively), its behaviour under loading was more similar to the CT derived model than the isotropic model (Table 5). This can be attributed to the directional material properties of the orthotropic model, which allows regions of bone to have different stiffnesses in different directions. This approach enables the use of less bone material while maintaining a higher overall directional stiffness, compared to an isotropic approach, similar to the findings of Geraldes and Phillips [14]. In addition, dominant Young's modulus values in the elements of the orthotropic model increase their stiffness (average 2161 MPa) compared to the isotropic model, whereas the mean Young's modulus values of the orthotropic model are lower than the corresponding values in the isotropic model. An important aspect to consider regarding the stiffness of the adaptive models is the target strain used to drive bone adaptation, as a lower target strain value would result in stiffer models.

The two hybrid models presented in this study were developed with the objective of differentiating between cortical and trabecular bone by using different element types. Interestingly, both hybrid models fared similarly when compared to the CT derived model (Table 5), meaning that the addition of a layer of shell elements to represent the cortex reduced the effect of considering the orthotropy of cancellous bone. An explanation can be provided by the change in the elastic modulus distributions for the continuum isotropic models, where more elements had a Young's modulus closer to the upper limit for the hybrid isotropic model than the continuum isotropic model. Conversely, the distribution of Young's moduli for the continuum and hybrid orthotropic models were largely similar. In addition, there were few discrepancies in the cortical thickness distributions of the two hybrid models (Table 4). The inclusion of shell elements to represent cortical bone seemed to reduce the importance of deciding between isotropic and orthotropic properties assigned to trabecular bone when comparing resulting bone architectures and overall stiffness of models.

A structural model previously developed by the authors [39] was included in this study to assess how a structural approach compared against continuum and hybrid approaches. The structural model compared well to the CT scan derived model, with only the continuum orthotropic model predicting a closer response (Table 5). Although the coefficients of determination for the structural model were lower than for both hybrid models, the gradient of the line of best fit was higher, indicating a better stiffness match with the CT scan derived model. Interestingly, the hybrid orthotropic model and structural model were found to be very similar (Tables 6 and 7), suggesting that both approaches result in similar directionality dependent behaviour and both can be used in the design of bone scaffold structures. In addition, a structural representation of the trabecular bone provides a clear image of bone architecture, suggesting that this approach is capable of picking up trabecular motifs present in bone.

The total bone volume of the CT scan derived model was much greater than any of the adapted models (Table 8). A reason for this discrepancy could be attributed to the adaptation algorithm being set up to generate the minimum amount of bone required to sustain the load cases tested. In addition, the selected load cases do not capture the full loading environment that a pelvis is subjected to and develops in throughout its lifetime, including strenuous activities such as running, which would result in higher muscle and joint contact forces. The disappearance of bone in the dead zone was modelled as instantaneous in the algorithm, whereas, in reality, this process is time dependent.

In addition, the grayscale values defining the material distribution of the CT scan model might overestimate the true stiffness of local regions. At the scale of clinical CT imaging, directional stiffnesses are not clearly defined which can lead to inaccuracies when quantifying the stiffness using a single isotropic value.

The modelling framework presented in this study has a number of limitations that must be acknowledged. In the musculoskeletal model used to derive the loading environment applied on the pelvis, muscle actuators did not take into account contraction dynamics and force-length-velocity relationships [49]. Furthermore, the muscle actuators were not spread over bone attachment areas and compressive forces of muscles applied on bone were not taken into account. This limitation was partially overcome by having a large number of muscle actuators in the musculoskeletal model. The FE model was developed to contain only bone, ligaments and cartilage. The lack of internal organs and soft tissue associated with the pelvic region could have an impact on the resulting bone architecture in some regions. A potential limitation of the FE models is the scale at which they were developed. The average edge length of the continuum elements was 3.76 mm, closer to the macroscale rather than the microscale, as discussed in the supplementary material in Zaharie and Phillips [39]. In addition, this scale would not allow for bone voids to be modelled. However, the adapted models could potentially allow for assessment of bone voids and bone microarchitecture using macro-to-micro conversion relationships [54].

The lack of separate cortical and trabecular bone representations in the continuum models can be a hindrance in the cases when bone architecture needs to be assessed locally. Similarly, the resolution of the clinical CT scan was not suitable to allow cortical bone to be distinguished from trabecular bone throughout the pelvis. Although the hybrid continuum models overcome this limitation, they do not provide sufficient information on bone architecture. The hybrid orthotropic model provides trabecular bone directionality in addition to the hybrid isotropic model, but it does not allow for an assessment of trabecular bone architecture locally. This capability is provided by the structural model. On the other hand, the high stiffness of the shell elements in the hybrid and structural models followed immediately by elements with lower stiffness can pose a limitation as moments that may be present in the cortex might not be transferred to the trabecular bone in its vicinity.

All models were found to have run times of approximately three minutes for a single loadcase on a workstation PC with one Intel Xeon E5-2630 v2 2.60 GHz (Dell Computer Corporation, Round Rock, TX, USA) and 64 GB of RAM. The overall run times for adapting the models to the full loading regime were approximately 24 h for the isotropic model, 40 h for the orthotropic model, 25 h for the hybrid isotropic model and 38 h for the hybrid orthotropic model. The continuum and hybrid isotropic models reported similar runtimes to the structural model. The main factor in slowing down the adaptation of the orthotropic and hybrid orthotropic models was post-processing. Adapting a model with a much finer mesh to the same loading regime would result in a longer runtime. Thus, although the scale poses a limitation, the models are considered to present a reasonable balance between accuracy and computational efficiency.

The computational models presented in this study were developed with the purpose of simulating bone adaptation in the pelvic construct using different modelling approaches and material models and comparing the effect that different modelling approaches have on bone adaptation. A distinct advantage of using predictive modelling is the potential of gaining insight into the role of different activities and corresponding muscle loading patterns on driving bone adaptation without requiring information from CT data.

Considering that the CT derived model is isotropic, it is unexpected that those models which include directionality either through the use of structural elements or material directionality all compare more favourably with the CT derived model than the predicted isotropic continuum model. A potential explanation for this is that the conversion going from HU values in the CT images to the Young's modulus values in the FE model picks up the dominant rather than the mean Young's modulus. To assess this, a combined model was generated in which the material directionalities and ratios between the Young's moduli found for the converged adapted orthotropic continuum model were imposed on the CT derived model, while setting the dominant Young's modulus value to that given by the CT scan, resulting in an overall average stiffness of 2403 MPa. If the conversion process finds the dominant Young's modulus value, then this combination of the predicted continuum orthotropic and CT derived model would be expected to have a similar response to the unaltered CT derived model for the single leg stance load case. The slopes of the lines of best fit for the hybrid model compared to the CT derived model are 0.96 and 0.99 for the maximum and minimum principal strains, respectively, indicating that the conversion from HU to Young's modulus does find the dominant rather than the mean Young's modulus.

5. Conclusions

The findings of this study suggest that material directionality plays an important factor in the balance between overall stiffness and total volume of material used in the case of the continuum and structural models. On the other hand, distinguishing between cortical and trabecular bone leads to a reduction in the effect of material directionality on overall stiffness, potentially due to the directionality imposed through the use of shell elements to represent cortical bone. In cases where distinguishing between trabecular and cortical bone is important, both hybrid approaches and the structural approach seem appropriate with the caveat that a structural approach could potentially have a further advantage of directly providing architecture that can be additively manufactured. In addition, despite using two different approaches, the orthotropic, hybrid and structural models predicted similar outcomes while the isotropic predictive model compared least favourably with the CT derived model, indicating that using an isotropic approach to model bone adaptation might not be a suitable solution.

In addition to providing information on the particularities of orthotropic and isotropic material modelling or the use of structural shell elements to model cortical bone, the adaptive models can be used to simulate the mechanical behaviour of bone seeded scaffolds designed to fill bone defects or to aid tissue regeneration. Furthermore, as the models are strain driven, they can be used with different materials to design scaffolds or implants that will be supporting the bone architecture surrounding them, as well as stimulating bone growth. The models can also be used in applications such as rehabilitation programs, informing the user on what type of physical activity is required to stimulate a specific region, or to predict the evolution of skeletal diseases, such as osteoporosis, by modifying the target strain, remodelling rate or set of activities within the adaptation process.

Supplementary Materials: The following are available at http://www.mdpi.com/2076-3417/9/16/3320/s1.

Author Contributions: Conceptualization, D.Z. and A.P.; methodology, D.Z. and A.P.; formal analysis, D.Z.; investigation, D.Z.; writing—original draft preparation, D.Z.; writing—review and editing, A.P.; supervision, D.Z.; project administration, A.P.; funding acquisition, A.P.

Funding: This work was conducted under the auspices of the Royal British Legion Centre for Blast Injury Studies at Imperial College London. The authors would like to acknowledge the financial support of the Royal British Legion.

Conflicts of Interest: The authors declare no conflict of interest. The funders had no role in the design of the study; in the collection, analyses, or interpretation of data; in the writing of the manuscript, or in the decision to publish the results.

References

1. Michaeli, D.A.; Murphy, S.B.; Hipp, J.A. Comparison of predicted and measured contact pressures in normal and dysplastic hips. *Med. Eng. Phys.* **1997**, *19*, 180–186. [CrossRef]
2. van den Bogert, A.J.; Read, L.; Nigg, B.M. An analysis of hip joint loading during walking, running, and skiing. *Med. Sci. Sports Exerc.* **1999**, *31*, 131–142. [CrossRef] [PubMed]
3. Bergmann, G.; Deuretzabacher, G.; Heller, M.; Graichen, F.; Rohlmann, A.; Strauss, J.; Duda, G.N. Hip forces and gait patterns from routine activities. *J. Biomech.* **2001**, *34*, 859–871. [CrossRef]
4. Frost, H.M. Bone's mechanostat: A 2003 update. *Anat. Rec. Part A Discov. Mol. Cell. Evolut. Biol.* **2003**, *275*, 1081–1101. [CrossRef] [PubMed]
5. Treece, G.M.; Gee, A.H.; Mayhew, P.M.; Poole, K.E.S. High resolution cortical bone thickness measurement from clinical CT data. *Med. Image Anal.* **2010**, *14*, 276–290. [CrossRef]
6. Phillips, A.T.M.; Villette, C.C.; Modenese, L. Femoral bone mesoscale structural architecture prediction using musculoskeletal and finite element modelling. *Int. Biomech.* **2015**, *2*, 43–61. [CrossRef]
7. Jacob, H.A.C.; Huggler, A.H.; Dietschi, C.; Schreiber, A. Mechanical function of subchondral bone as experimentally determined on the acetabulum of the human pelvis. *J. Biomech.* **1976**, *9*, 625–627. [CrossRef]
8. Dalstra, M.; Huiskes, R.; Odgaard, A.; van Erning, L. Mechanical and textural properties of pelvic trabecular bone. *J. Biomech.* **1993**, *26*, 523–535. [CrossRef]
9. Anderson, A.E.; Peters, C.L.; Tuttle, B.D.; Weiss, J.A. Subject-Specific Finite Element Model of the Pelvis: Development, Validation and Sensitivity Studies. *J. Biomech. Eng.* **2005**, *127*, 364. [CrossRef]
10. Giorgi, M.; Verbruggen, S.W.; Lacroix, D. In silico bone mechanobiology: Modeling a multifaceted biological system. *Wiley Interdiscip. Rev. Syst. Biol. Med.* **2016**, *8*, 485–505. [CrossRef]
11. Wang, L.; Dong, J.; Xian, C.J. Computational modeling of bone cells and their biomechanical behaviors in responses to mechanical stimuli. *Crit. Rev. Eukaryot. Gene Expr.* **2019**, *29*, 51–67. [CrossRef] [PubMed]
12. Tsubota, K.I.; Suzuki, Y.; Yamada, T.; Hojo, M.; Makinouchi, A.; Adachi, T. Computer simulation of trabecular remodeling in human proximal femur using large-scale voxel FE models: Approach to understanding Wolff's law. *J. Biomech.* **2009**, *42*, 1088–1094. [CrossRef] [PubMed]
13. Geraldes, D.; Phillips, A. A novel 3d strain-adaptive continuum orthotropic bone remodelling algorithm: prediction of bone architecture in the femur. In Proceedings of the 6th World Congress of Biomechanics (WCB 2010), Singapore, 1–6 August 2010; Springer: Berlin, Germany, 2010; pp. 772–775.
14. Geraldes, D.M.; Phillips, A. A comparative study of orthotropic and isotropic bone adaptation in the femur. *Int. J. Numer. Methods Biomed. Eng.* **2014**, *30*, 873–889. [CrossRef] [PubMed]
15. Geraldes, D.M.; Modenese, L.; Phillips, A.T. Consideration of multiple load cases is critical in modelling orthotropic bone adaptation in the femur. *Biomech. Model. Mechanobiol.* **2016**, *15*, 1029–1042. [CrossRef] [PubMed]
16. Marzban, A.; Nayeb-Hashemi, H.; Vaziri, A. Numerical simulation of load-induced bone structural remodelling using stress-limit criterion. *Comput. Methods Biomech. Biomed. Eng.* **2015**, *18*, 259–268. [CrossRef] [PubMed]
17. Villette, C.C.; Phillips, A.T. Informing phenomenological structural bone remodelling with a mechanistic poroelastic model. *Biomech. Model. Mechanobiol.* **2016**, *15*, 69–82. [CrossRef] [PubMed]
18. Villette, C.; Phillips, A. Microscale poroelastic metamodel for efficient mesoscale bone remodelling simulations. *Biomech. Model. Mechanobiol.* **2017**, *16*, 2077–2091. [CrossRef]

19. Goel, V.K.; Valliappan, S.; Svensson, N.L. Stresses in the normal pelvis. *Comput. Biol. Med.* **1978**, *8*, 91–104. [CrossRef]
20. Oonishi, H.; Isha, H.; Hasegawa, T. Mechanical analysis of the human pelvis and its application to the artificial hip joint–by means of the three-dimensional, finite element method. *J. Biomech.* **1983**, *16*, 427–444. [CrossRef]
21. Landjerit, B.; Jacquard-Simon, N.; Thourot, M.; Massin, P. Physiological loadings on human pelvis: A comparison between numerical and experimental simulations. *Proc. ESB* **1992**, *8*, 195.
22. Schuller, H.; Dalstra, M.; Huiskes, R.; Marti, R. Total hip reconstruction in acetabular dysplasia. A finite element study. *J. Bone Joint Surg. Br.* **1993**, *75B*, 468–474. [CrossRef]
23. Pedersen, D.R.; Crowninshield, R.D.; Brand, R.A.; Johnston, R.C. An axisymmetric model of acetabular components in total hip arthroplasty. *J. Biomech.* **1982**, *15*, 305–315. [CrossRef]
24. Huiskes, R. Finite element analysis of acetabular reconstruction. Noncemented threaded cups. *Acta Orthop. Scand.* **1987**, *58*, 620–625. [CrossRef] [PubMed]
25. Vasu, R.; Carter, D.R.; Harris, W.H. Stress distributions in the acetabular region-I. Before and after total joint replacement. *J. Biomech.* **1982**, *15*, 155–157. [CrossRef]
26. Carter, D.R.; Vasu, R.; Harris, W.H. Stress distributions in the acetabular region-II. Effects of cement thickness and metal backing of the total hip acetabular component. *J. Biomech.* **1982**, *15*, 165–170. [CrossRef]
27. Rapperport, D.; Carter, D.; Schurman, D. Contact finite element stress analysis of the hip joint. *J. Orthop. Res.* **1985**, *3*, 435–446. [CrossRef] [PubMed]
28. Oonishi, H.; Tatsumi, M.; Kawaguchi, A. Biomechanical studies on fixations of an artificial hip joint acetabular socket by means of 2D-FEM. In *Biological and Biomechanical Performance of Biomaterials*; Christel, P., Meunier, A., Lee, A.J.C., Eds.; Elsevier: Amsterdam, The Netherlands, 1986; pp. 513–518.
29. Phillips, A.T.M.; Pankaj, P.; Usmani, A.S.; Howie, C.R. Numerical modelling of the acetabular construct following impaction grafting. In Proceedings of the International Symposium on Computer Methods in Biomechanics and Biomedical Engineering, Madrid, Spain, 25–28 February 2004.
30. Dalstra, M.; Huiskes, R.; van Erning, L. Development and validation of a three-dimensional finite element model of the pelvic bone. *J. Biomech. Eng.* **1995**, *117*, 272–278. [CrossRef]
31. Li, Z.; Kim, J.E.; Davidson, J.S.; Etheridge, B.S.; Alonso, J.E.; Eberhardt, A.W. Biomechanical response of the pubic symphysis in lateral pelvic impacts: a finite element study. *J. Biomech.* **2007**, *40*, 2758–2766. [CrossRef] [PubMed]
32. Zhang, Q.H.; Wang, J.Y.; Lupton, C.; Heaton-Adegbile, P.; Guo, Z.X.; Liu, Q.; Tong, J. A subject-specific pelvic bone model and its application to cemented acetabular replacements. *J. Biomech.* **2010**, *43*, 2722–2727. [CrossRef]
33. Pankaj, P. Patient-specific modelling of bone and bone-implant systems: the challenges. *Int. J. Numer. Methods Biomed. Eng.* **2013**, *29*, 233–249. [CrossRef]
34. Ashman, R.; Cowin, S.; Van Buskirk, W.; Rice, J. A continuous wave technique for the measurement of the elastic properties of cortical bone. *J. Biomech.* **1984**, *17*, 349–361. [CrossRef]
35. Morlock, M.; Schneider, E.; Bluhm, A.; Vollmer, M.; Bergmann, G.; Müller, V.; Honl, M. Duration and frequency of every day activities in total hip patients. *J. Biomech.* **2001**, *34*, 873–881. [CrossRef]
36. Modenese, L.; Gopalakrishnan, A.; Phillips, A. Application of a falsification strategy to a musculoskeletal model of the lower limb and accuracy of the predicted hip contact force vector. *J. Biomech.* **2013**, *46*, 1193–1200. [CrossRef] [PubMed]
37. Horsman, M.D.K.; Koopman, H.; der Helm, F.C.T.; Prosé, L.P.; Veeger, H.E.J. Morphological muscle and joint parameters for musculoskeletal modelling of the lower extremity. *Clin. Biomech.* **2007**, *22*, 239–247. [CrossRef] [PubMed]
38. Delp, S.; Anderson, F.; Arnold, A.; Loan, P.; Habib, A.; John, C.; Guendelman, E.; Thelen, D. OpenSim: Open source to create and analyze dynamic simulations of movement. *IEEE Trans. Biomed. Eng.* **2007**, *54*, 1940–1950. [CrossRef]
39. Zaharie, D.T.; Phillips, A.T. Pelvic construct prediction of trabecular and cortical bone structural architecture. *J. Biomech. Eng.* **2018**, *140*, 091001. [CrossRef] [PubMed]
40. Barre, A.; Armand, S. Biomechanical ToolKit: Open-source framework to visualize and process biomechanical data. *Comput. Methods Programs Biomed.* **2014**, *114*, 80–87. [CrossRef]

41. Dumas, R.; Chèze, L.; Verriest, J.P. Adjustments to McConville et al. and Young et al. body segment inertial parameters. *J. Biomech.* **2007**, *40*, 543–553. [CrossRef]
42. Lu, T.W.; O'Connor, J.J. Bone position estimation from skin marker co-ordinates using global optimisation with joint constraints. *J. Biomech.* **1999**, *32*, 129–134. [CrossRef]
43. van Arkel, R.J.; Modenese, L.; Phillips, A.T.; Jeffers, J.R. Hip abduction can prevent posterior edge loading of hip replacements. *J. Orthop. Res.* **2013**, *31*, 1172–1179. [CrossRef]
44. Steele, K.M.; DeMers, M.S.; Schwartz, M.H.; Delp, S.L. Compressive tibiofemoral force during crouch gait. *Gait Posture* **2012**, *35*, 556–560. [CrossRef]
45. Phillips, A.; Pankaj, P.; Howie, C.; Usmani, A.; Simpson, A. Finite element modelling of the pelvis: Inclusion of muscular and ligamentous boundary conditions. *Med. Eng. Phys.* **2007**, *29*, 739–748. [CrossRef]
46. Hammer, N.; Steinke, H.; Slowik, V.; Josten, C.; Stadler, J.; Böhme, J.; Spanel-Borowski, K. The sacrotuberous and the sacrospinous ligament—A virtual reconstruction. *Ann. Anat. Anat. Anz.* **2009**, *191*, 417–425. [CrossRef]
47. Hammer, N.; Steinke, H.; Böhme, J.; Stadler, J.; Josten, C.; Spanel-Borowski, K. Description of the iliolumbar ligament for computer-assisted reconstruction. *Ann. Anat. Anat. Anz.* **2010**, *192*, 162–167. [CrossRef]
48. Moore, K.L.; Agur, A.M.R.; Dalley, A.F.; Moore, K.L. *Essential Clinical Anatomy*; Wolters Kluwer Health: Alphen aan den Rijn, The Netherlands, 2015.
49. Modenese, L.; Phillips, A.T.M.; Bull, A.M.J. An open source lower limb model: Hip joint validation. *J. Biomech.* **2011**, *44*, 2185–2193. [CrossRef]
50. Phillips, A.T.M. Structural optimisation: Biomechanics of the femur. *Proc. ICE Eng. Comput. Mech.* **2012**, *165*, 147–154. [CrossRef]
51. Taddei, F.; Schileo, E.; Helgason, B.; Cristofolini, L.; Viceconti, M. The material mapping strategy influences the accuracy of CT-based finite element models of bones: An evaluation against experimental measurements. *Med. Eng. Phys.* **2007**, *29*, 973–979. [CrossRef]
52. Les, C.; Keyak, J.; Stover, S.; Taylor, K.; Kaneps, A. Estimation of material properties in the equine metacarpus with use of quantitative computed tomography. *J. Orthop. Res.* **1994**, *12*, 822–833. [CrossRef]
53. Keller, T.S. Predicting the compressive mechanical behavior of bone. *J. Biomech.* **1994**, *27*, 1159–1168. [CrossRef]
54. Teo, J.C.; Si-Hoe, K.M.; Keh, J.E.; Teoh, S.H. Relationship between CT intensity, micro-architecture and mechanical properties of porcine vertebral cancellous bone. *Clin. Biomech.* **2006**, *21*, 235–244. [CrossRef]

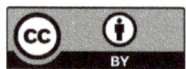

© 2019 by the authors. Licensee MDPI, Basel, Switzerland. This article is an open access article distributed under the terms and conditions of the Creative Commons Attribution (CC BY) license (http://creativecommons.org/licenses/by/4.0/).

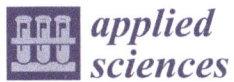

Review

Continuum Modeling and Simulation in Bone Tissue Engineering

Jose A. Sanz-Herrera * and Esther Reina-Romo

Escuela Técnica Superior de Ingeniería, Universidad de Sevilla, 41092 Sevilla, Spain
* Correspondence: jsanz@us.es; Tel.: +34-95-448-7293

Received: 30 July 2019; Accepted: 23 August 2019; Published: 5 September 2019

Featured Application: Bone tissue engineering (BTE) can be investigated by means of mathematical modeling and numerical tools complementary to the experimental methods. In particular, the design process of a bone tissue engineering product or protocol can be enhanced by computer simulation as evidenced in a number of papers in the last decades. In this work, we review the most relevant contributions of continuum models and simulations applied to different stages and problems of interest found in the field of BTE.

Abstract: Bone tissue engineering is currently a mature methodology from a research perspective. Moreover, modeling and simulation of involved processes and phenomena in BTE have been proved in a number of papers to be an excellent assessment tool in the stages of design and proof of concept through in-vivo or in-vitro experimentation. In this paper, a review of the most relevant contributions in modeling and simulation, in silico, in BTE applications is conducted. The most popular in silico simulations in BTE are classified into: (i) Mechanics modeling and scaffold design, (ii) transport and flow modeling, and (iii) modeling of physical phenomena. The paper is restricted to the review of the numerical implementation and simulation of continuum theories applied to different processes in BTE, such that molecular dynamics or discrete approaches are out of the scope of the paper. Two main conclusions are drawn at the end of the paper: First, the great potential and advantages that in silico simulation offers in BTE, and second, the need for interdisciplinary collaboration to further validate numerical models developed in BTE.

Keywords: bone tissue engineering; biomaterials; computational mechanobiology; numerical methods in bioengineering

1. Introduction

Bone tissue engineering (BTE) aims to persuade bone tissue to regenerate and/or heal under diverse circumstances. These circumstances include the repair of long bone defects where the body has limited regeneration capability, treatment of bone diseases such as osteoporosis, or to accelerate the process of bone fracture healing [1]. The bone healing process can be summarized in the following steps [2]: (i) A hematoma is formed from injury in the periosteum; (ii) osteocytes near the fracture site die due to blood disruption following a demand for repair; (iii) macrophages and fibroblasts are recruited to the site to remove tissue debris and to express extracellular matrix, then growth factors and cytokines released by these inflammatory cells, mesenchymal stem cells are recruited from the bone marrow and periosteum, which then proliferate and differentiate into progenitor cells; (iv) those osteoprogenitor cells differentiate into osteoblasts and form osteoid which is rapidly calcified into bone. Finally, (v) the uncalcified material is resorbed and new bone is deposited. The woven bone is then remodeled into lamellar bone and the process is completed by the return of normal bone marrow within trabecular regions, while in repairing cortical bone the spaces between trabeculae are gradually filled in with successive layers of bone thus forming new Haversian canals.

In order to mimic the process of natural bone healing described above, BTE methodology involves the use of porous biomaterials as a structure support, i.e., scaffolds, which serve to temporally cover the bone defect, as well as providing room for bone cells to invade, proliferate, and develop their specific functions to segregate new bone matrix. Ideally, the structural support (scaffold) should degrade over time resulting in the formation of a new bony structure [1].

The base scaffold biomaterial should mimic the natural bone matrix; therefore, ceramics and polymers are extensively used in BTE applications. On the one hand, bioceramics including hydroxyapatite (HA) and calcium phosphate are used. They show excellent ability to bond to bone, good biocompatibility behavior, and reasonably good mechanical properties [3–10].

On the other hand, polymeric biomaterials are used since they are biodegradable, either natural polymer matrices: Polysaccharides (starch, alginate, chitin/chitosan, hyaluronic acid derivates) or proteins (soy, collagen, fibrin gels, silk). Moreover, synthetic biodegradable polymers for BTE include saturated aliphatic polyesters: Poly(lactic acid) (PLA), poly(glycolic acid) (PGA), poly(lactic-co-glycolide) (PLGA) copolymers, and poly(e-caprolactone); unsaturated linear polyesters: Polypropylene fumarate (PPF); and aliphatic polyesters: Polyhydroxyalkanoates and derived products (PHB, PHBV, P4HB, PHBHHx, PHO). Due to the limited mechanical strength of polymeric biomaterials, a variety of biofibers such as lignocellulosic natural fibers are used as a reinforcement [11].

Bioactive glasses are a class of inorganic biomaterials discovered by Hench in 1969 [12]. Bioactive glass materials have the ability to bond new bone tissue enhanced by a reaction that takes place once the biomaterial is inserted in the body environment. A number of commercial scaffolds have been developed such as Bioglass® in bone defects, PerioGlas™ for periodontal disease, and NovaBone™ as a bone filler [13]. Some drawbacks of bioactive glasses are their low fracture toughness and mechanical strength, especially in a porous form. These drawbacks are enhanced by a HA particulate reinforcement [14].

In order to promote new bone tissue regeneration, following the natural process of bone healing, the BTE methodology usually combines a seeding strategy along the biomaterial surface of the scaffold prior to implantation. Usually bone marrow stromal cells (BMSC), mesenchymal stem cells (MSC), or preosteoblasts are combined with bone morphogenetic proteins (BMP) or growth factors such as transforming growth factor-β (TGF-β), within porous scaffolds with the use of a bioreactor. In particular, BMSC-seeded ceramics were implanted in a large tibial defect in ewes [15]. Mechanical stability at the defect site was obtained either by an internal plate or by external fixation. Results show around 10% of bone volume to total volume regeneration. Mastrogiacomo et al. [16] also presented the same tissue engineering strategy for segmental tibial defect in sheep, resulting in a progressive scaffold resorption coincident with new bone deposition [16]. A comparison of bone regeneration in rabbits among BMSC-harvested poly(lactide-co-glycolide) scaffolds, non-harvested ones, and without scaffolds was presented in [17]. The defect consisted of a unilateral femoral osteotomy gap created surgically under general anesthetic and stabilized by a mandibular reconstruction plate fixated with three screws on either side of the osteotomy site. The obtained results showed that there were no significant differences between the use of the scaffold alone and the cell-seeded scaffold although faster in this case. On the contrary, the non-scaffold strategy presented less regenerated tissue. Using biodegradable scaffolds as well, Holy et al. [18] performed a trabecular-like, three-dimensional structure to repair bone. BMCS-preseeded scaffolds were implanted in a non-healing rabbit segmental bone defect achieving bony union within eight weeks. Biodegradable scaffolds medical-grade polycaprolactone–calcium phosphate (mPCL–CaP) seeded with BMSC were implanted under the skin of nude rats. It presented neo cortical and well-vascularized cancellous bone up to 40% of bone volume [19]. Savarino et al. [20] presented a study involving the use of poly-e-caprolactone scaffolds (PCL) loaded with BMSC and BMP-4. PCL without cells showed scarce bone formation and scaffold resorption, whereas PCL seeded with BMSC stimulated new tissue formation. In conclusion, the combination of BMSC with BMP-4 strongly favored osteoinductivity of cellular constructs.

Bone tissue undergoes a piezoelectric effect such that bone cells are stimulated to remodel by means of an electrical filed, induced by a strain field, which recruits and aggregates macromolecules and ions in the extracellular matrix [21]. This feature has been exploited in bone tissue regeneration using piezoelectric scaffolds which mimic the natural collagen matrix, such as piezopolymers. The reader is referred to [22] for a review of piezoelectric scaffolds.

Mathematical modeling and computer simulation have been demonstrated to be a powerful tool both in the design and evaluation stages of scaffolds in BTE applications. In the design phase, the mechanical properties (elasticity modulus, strength, toughness) and fluidic properties (diffusivity and permeability) are essential for the overall success of the scaffold. Moreover, the degradation properties and characteristics are also of interest for a certain BTE experiment. The overall behavior during implantation of BTE processes has also been simulated through the incorporation of biomechanical and mechanobiological theories. In the next sections, the state-of-the-art of continuum approaches and simulation of the referred BTE phenomena are reviewed. The new challenges, perspectives, and some conclusions are drawn at the end of the paper.

2. Mechanics Modeling

2.1. Constitutive Behavior Modeling and Scaffold Design

According to the evidences, the optimal scaffold design, i.e., microarchitecture, should include high porosity, proper pore structure interconnection, and enough specific surface to attach cells to segregate new matrix and proliferate [1]. In particular, porosity values in the range 60–80% are recommended for load-bearing BTE applications [1,11]. These features can be controlled via a computer aided design (CAD) technique of the scaffold in the design step. On the other hand, permeability is an important parameter in tissue engineering applications, linked to pore structure and porosity, and related to the flow of nutrients and waste removal which are essential processes during cell activity. Moreover, the overall constitutive mechanical behavior is a design variable of the scaffold microstructure for load bearing in BTE, as well as the distribution of the mechanical stimuli to activate bone cell functions [23].

Both permeability and overall mechanical properties are macroscopic quantities which describe the fluid and solid mechanical behavior of the scaffold. They can be tailored by getting control over some scaffold parameters microscopically, e.g., mean pore size, porosity, and virgin biomaterial mechanical properties. Hollister and co-workers have focused on the design of bone scaffolds as an optimization problem to get a microstructure as similar as possible (mechanical properties, porosity, pore size, etc.) to that of the implanted region. For this purpose, the homogenization theory was extensively applied during design [24–26]. In the same context, the asymptotic homogenization theory was applied to validate the experimental Darcian permeability and mechanical properties of a specific scaffold, Sponceram®, available for BTE applications [27]. On the one hand, the homogenization theory computes the overall macroscopic stiffness tensor $\mathbb{C}^0$ as follows,

$$\mathbb{C}^0 = \frac{1}{V} \int_V \mathbb{C}^{\varphi}(\mathbf{I}_{kh} + \varepsilon^{\varphi}(\chi_{kh})) dV, \qquad (1)$$

where $\varepsilon^{\varphi}(\chi_{kh})$ are elementary unit strain solutions with associated displacement field χ_{kh}. $\mathbf{I}_{kh}$ is the identity fourth order tensor, $\mathbb{C}^{\varphi}$ the stiffness tensor of the base (bulk) material, and V the volume of the microscopic cell.

On the other hand, the permeability tensor $\mathbf{K}$ is obtained following the homogenization theory as,

$$\mathbf{K} = \frac{1}{V} \int_V \kappa_j^i dV, \qquad (2)$$

with κ_j^i the characteristic fluid velocities associated with unit pressure gradients.

The homogenization theory has been further developed in connection with topology optimization in the scaffold design [28]. Coelho et al. [29] used again the homogenization theory and topological optimization connected to the fabrication and testing of the optimal scaffold. Moreover, the mechanical properties of a multiphasic scaffold composed of poly(propylene fumarate) reinforced with silicon particles were obtained in terms of elasticity and shear moduli by means of theoretical developments based on the Eshelby theory [30]. The overall mechanical properties of porous and multiphasic scaffolds have been also obtained by means of theoretical (analytical) methods [31–33]. A review of these methods can be seen in [34].

As seen in the cited papers above, the design of the scaffold microstructure can be posed as an optimization problem to achieve the optimal overall constitutive behavior. The same optimization design procedure was followed to achieve a uniform shear stress as an objective function [35]. This criterion was established to get an optimal erosion along the microstructure. In the same context, Boccaccio et al. [36] determined the optimal loading for a number of 3D printed scaffold microarchitectures to enhance new bone tissue growth. This study may be used in patient-specific BTE applications.

The design of the scaffold microstructure has been recently linked to advanced manufacturing techniques mainly based on 3D printing. Egan et al. [37] analyzed lattice-based scaffold microstructural parameters of different families (Figure 1). Results concluded that each family may find an application depending on its specific characteristics. The mechanical performance of 3D printed scaffolds was evaluated as well with a focus on the distribution of the mechanical stimuli along the scaffold microstructure [38].

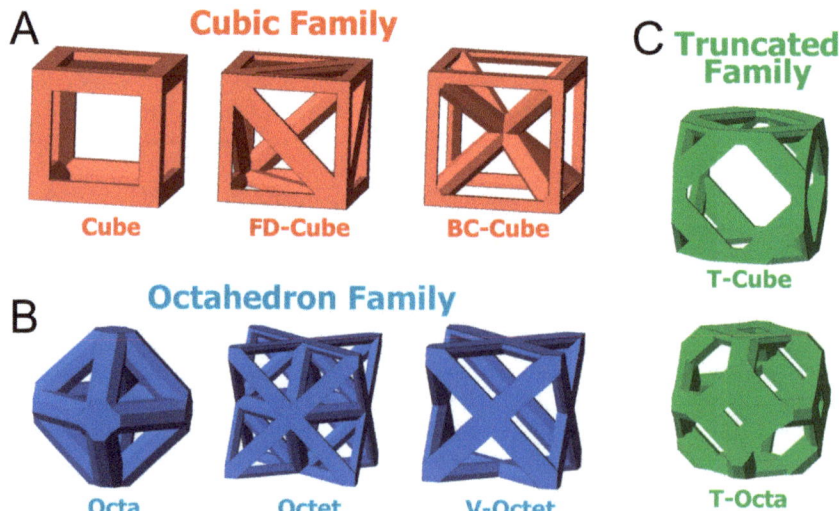

Figure 1. Potential lattice-based scaffold microstructures analyzed for bone tissue engineering (BTE) applications. Reprinted with permission from [37].

2.2. Simulation of Applications of Interest

In silico modeling in BTE is becoming a predictive tool for bone regeneration simulation within the scaffold reducing the number of in vivo/in vitro experiments that need to be performed.

Bone tissue regeneration in vivo using scaffolds inherently attends to two well-differentiated spatial and temporal scales. One is the tissue level or macroscopic scale, with the other one being named as pore level or micro/mesoscopic scale. Therefore, the mathematical and in silico modeling of tissue growth within scaffolds has been usually restricted to one of these scales.

At the macroscopic scale, finite element analyses (FEA) has been used to analyze the solid mechanical behavior of the scaffold. Two different modeling approaches can be found in the literature at this scale: FEA models, that simulate the fluid flow with poroelastic materials (in which the flow is defined according to Darcy's law) and computational fluid dynamics (CFD) models, which solve the governing equations of fluid flow dynamics.

On the one hand, FEA have tried to investigate the effect of scaffold architecture on the neotissue formed within the scaffold. The mathematical model of cell/tissue differentiation proposed by Prendergast et al. [39] has been widely used in bone tissue engineering applications [40–47]. In these studies, cell proliferation is modeled as a diffusion problem and macroscopic variables, such as the shear strain and fluid flow, are considered as stimuli for cell differentiation. Osteochondral defect repair using scaffolds has been simulated in [40]. Khayyeri et al. [42] predicted tissue differentiation with FEA by means of a lattice modeling approach in a bone chamber and compared the numerical results with in vivo bone formation. Olivares et al. [41] used a CAD-based model to analyze the effects of scaffold pore morphology on cell differentiation stimulus values. These models are either based on computer aided design (CAD) [42] or on micro-computed tomography (μCT) [43,44,47]. However, CAD models are not able to capture the strain distributions seen in the μCT [48].

On the other hand, CFD characterizes the hydrodynamic field imposed on cells within different types of scaffolds [48–53]. They allow numerical prediction of the shear stresses induced at the internal walls in relation with the scaffold geometry and, thus, they qualitatively relate the flow of culture medium with the macroscopic 3D shear stresses [54,55]. It is well known that flow-induced shear stress produces a significant stimulatory effect and plays a critical role in the physiological responses [56–59]. More recent studies have predicted the new tissue formed and have related the wall shear stresses (WSS) with cellular processes such as proliferation, differentiation, or mineralization of the extracellular matrix by means of CFD analyses. In particular, Sonnaert et al. [60] investigated the influence of fluid-flow-induced shear stress on the proliferation, differentiation, and matrix deposition of human periosteal-derived cells in 3D Ti6Al4V scaffolds. Nava et al. [61] numerically described the growth of a neotissue in a perfusion bioreactor where the growth was coupled to oxygen concentration and shear stress. Zhao et al. [62] calculated the optimal fluid flow rate to be applied to the bioreactor for BTE experiments by means of CFD for different scaffold pore shapes, pore diameters, and porosities. They employed a combination of CFD with mechano-regulation theories to optimize the external flow rate for a perfusion bioreactor. Such flow rate would maximize the scaffold surface fraction, whose WSS was in the range required for mineralization.

In the microscopic scale, Byrne et al. [63] have presented a mechanobiological model applied to a periodic unit cell of the scaffold microstructure. In this model, the influence of several factors such as permeability, mechanical properties, and others have been analyzed in tissue regeneration. In the same scale, bone tissue regeneration within a scaffold unit cell has been numerically reproduced [64] using concepts and hypothesis previously established for a remodeling theory [65]. At a nanoscale level, the mechanisms of cell adhesion to the walls has also been studied [66,67].

Finally, the use of multiscale methods and homogenization has allowed the analysis of different phenomena of bone regeneration within scaffolds [68–73]. Sanz-Herrera et al. [68,69] proposed for the first time a coupled micro–macro mathematical approach for bone tissue regeneration in tissue engineering applications, see Figure 2. In these works, at the tissue level, the macroscopic mechanical, diffusive, and flow properties are derived by means of the asymptotic homogenization theory. At the microscopic scale, bone tissue regeneration at the scaffold microsurface is simulated using a bone growth model based on a bone remodeling theory [23], whereas scaffold degradation is implemented following a previous model [64]. This multiscale model was later used to analyze the effect of scaffold microarchitecture in new bone tissue growth [72]. Nguyen et al. [74] performed a multiscale approach based on a CFD analysis on two scales to predict cell growth inside a given macroporous scaffold put in a perfusion bioreactor. Their objective was to determine the optimal flow rate in order to enhance cell proliferation and to improve an upcoming bone reconstruction.

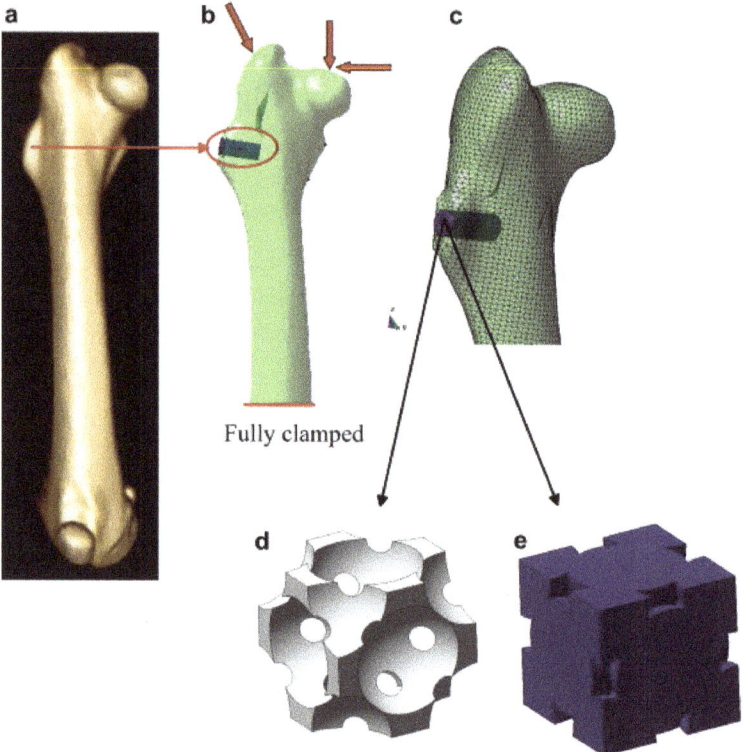

Figure 2. Multiscale computer simulation in BTE to predict new bone tissue growth in a unit cell of a predefined scaffold microstructure. (**a**) CT reconstruction of a rabbit femur, (**b**) model of the femur, scaffold implantation, loads and boundary conditions, (**c**) detailed mesh of the model, (**d**) unit cell microstructure of the scaffold solid domain, and (**e**) unit cell microstructure of the scaffold fluid domain. Reprinted with permission from [69].

3. Transport and Flow Modeling

Fluid circulation, transport of nutrients, and waste removal are essential processes that must take place inside the scaffold microstructure in a successful BTE product. In fact, vascularization, i.e., invasion of blood vessel and formation of new vasculature, is one of the main drawbacks in tissue engineering [75]. Moreover, fluid percolation and circulation is important as well in vitro in BTE assisted by bioreactors. Therefore, flow mechanics and diffusion mechanisms have been theoretically modeled and simulated during design of BTE scaffolds.

Permeability is an overall parameter that (macroscopically) condenses the information about how a fluid penetrates in a porous medium. It is a clear design parameter in BTE scaffolds. Scaffold permeability has been measured experimentally in several papers using pumped water [76,77], with a gravity-induced pressure using water [78–80] or using compressed air [81], to cite a few. Indeed, permeability was numerically validated using the homogenization theory versus an experimental gravity-induced pressure setup, for a specific commercial scaffold for BTE applications [27]. In the same context, Truscello et al. [82] validated the permeability values of Ti6Al4V scaffolds using CFD simulations. An interesting study [83] obtained the permeability of simulated cancellous bone structure by means of CFD analyses over a unit cell of the scaffold. Results concluded which wasthe best-suited scaffold microarchitecture for BTE in terms of blood circulation inside the microstructure.

The study presented in [84], see Figure 3, shows a CFD analysis over a complex non regular microstructure of a poly(L-lactic acid) scaffold. The microstructural geometry was obtained by microCT and results analyzed both the permeability parameter as well as the wall shear stress, which is an important mechanobiological output as a mechanical stimulus [39], as seen before. The experimental results validated the simulations in the referred work. Similar studies were conducted for irregular pore geometries and regular ones [41,46]. Homogeneous fluid flow distribution was found for irregular microstructures, in contrast to regular ones, due to irregular interconnection between the pores [85].

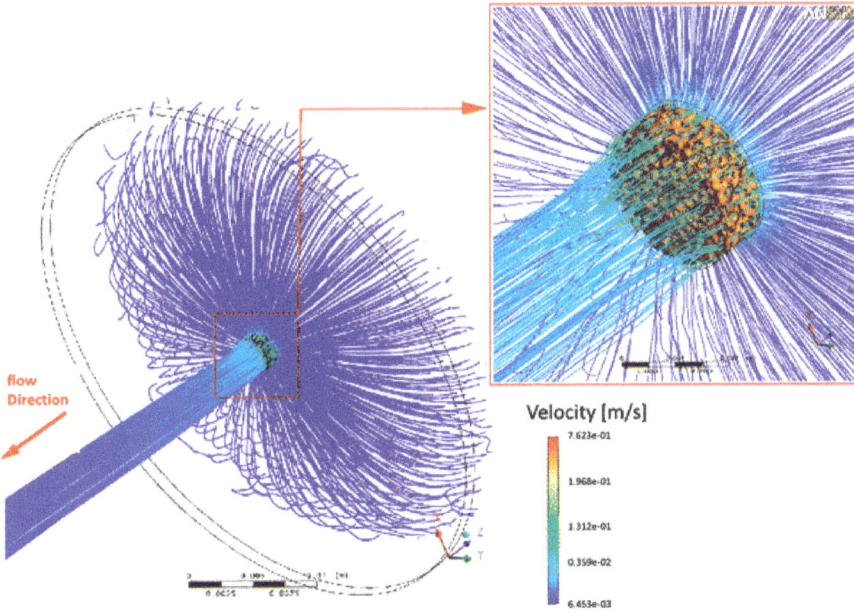

Figure 3. Fluid velocity streamlines along poly(L-lactic acid) non regular scaffold computed by means of computational fluid dynamics (CFD) analysis. Reprinted with permission from [84].

On the other hand, diffusion and transport of nutrients have been simulated in the design of scaffold microstructure. The macroscopic diffusivity of porous scaffolds, as an analogy to Darcian permeability, was analyzed as a function of the pore microarchitecture [68]. These results were used in a full multiscale model accounting for microstructural growth and resorption, and subsequent macroscopic evolution. Li et al. [86] showed finite element simulations of the diffusion and evolution of oxygen concentration along the interior of regular scaffold microstructures.

The evolution of tissue growth coupled with nutrient supply and also including mechanistic effects has been mathematically modeled mostly for in vitro (bioreactor) conditions. In particular, Lemon et al. [87] proposed a continuum and multiphasic model including scaffold, cells, and water (medium) as the main phases. The model was applied to the study of the mobility and aggregation of a population of cells seeded into an artificial polymeric scaffold. This model was extended in [88]. A similar approach, which includes coupling between tissue growth and nutrients consumption, was proposed in [89]. The model was numerically elaborated, implemented, and solved in a hollow-fiber membrane bioreactor as an application, validating existing results available in the literature.

4. Modeling of Physical Phenomena

In this section, we review the modeling and simulation of the most relevant physical phenomena that take place in biomaterials in BTE applications, such as biodegradation. Most BTE products exploit the ability of biomaterials to dissolve over time, finally resulting in the removal of the scaffold implant. This class of biomaterials are synthetic polymers: Lactide polymer (trimethylene carbonate D,L-lactide (TMCDLLA)) [90], poly-e-caprolactone (PCL) [91,92], polylactic acid (PLA) [93], and polyglycolic acid (PGA) [94,95], to cite a few. Even though the degradation products are naturally evacuated from the human body, some secondary problems have been reported in the reaction of these residuals with the living tissues [96].

Modeling and simulation of biodegradation of polymeric biomaterials were mainly developed after the theory proposed by Gopferich [97]. This modeling was the basis for the development of a number of applications in BTE using polymeric scaffolds and it considers water diffusion within the bulk polymeric biomaterial according to a Fickean law as follows,

$$\dot{d} = \alpha \Delta d \text{ in } \Omega + \text{boundary and initial conditions,} \tag{3}$$

where d is the water (aqueous) concentration, α the diffusion coefficient, and Δ the Laplacian operator. The dot on d denotes time derivative and Ω the biomaterial domain. Water concentration, W, within the polymer is then related to the change rate of the molecular weight of the biomaterial due to hydrolysis and assumed to depend on the local water content,

$$W = -\beta d \text{ in } \Omega. \tag{4}$$

where β is a constant property of the material.

The model introduced above was applied to the study of the degradation of a unit cell of the scaffold microstructure [66] and coupled with a bone growth multiscale model [68,69,73]. Other researchers [98,99] presented a similar but extended model to analyze degradation of biopolymers, which takes into consideration crystallization. Further studies [100,101] introduced a mathematical continuum formulation based on the mixture theory to model degradation, transport of molecules across the extracellular matrix, and swelling in a hydrogel scaffold. The model was useful to investigate hydrolytic and enzymatic degradation. Moreover, a similar model for the simulation of the hydrolysis phenomena in polymeric biomaterials was presented in [102]. In this approach, the hydrolysis reaction was modeled by a fundamental stochastic process and an additional autocatalytic effect. Results were shown over different polymeric matrices providing a good agreement with experimental data in the literature.

Inorganic bioactive materials, such as bioglasses, are widely used in BTE due to their ability to react with the body fluid and dissolve, finally resulting in the formation of a hydroxyapatite surface layer. This layer can form stable bonds with the adjacent living tissue, which is specially well suited to bone implants and BTE [11,103–107].

Dissolution of bioactive glasses was macroscopically modeled using a physical–chemical model which turned into a reaction–diffusion continuum model [108]. Dissolution was represented using the Voxel-FEM approach. Additionally, a reaction–diffusion modeling approach was proposed for the simulation of degradation of calcium phosphate scaffolds [109]. Recently, a generic mathematical framework for the simulation and design of dissolution of biomaterials for tissue engineering and drug delivery applications has been introduced [110]. The model was experimentally validated by means of a straightforward ad hoc setup that considered the dissolution of bicarbonate pellets.

Even though magnesium implants have been used since several decades ago, they have gained an increasing interest in the last years. The main motivations are the great advantages they offer versus traditional metallic, bioceramic, or polymeric implants. On one hand, the absence of a second surgery for removal due to their biodegradability characteristic [111]. Moreover, magnesium implants show similar mechanical properties to bone tissue, avoiding bone resorption due to stress shielding in the neighborhood of the implant and hence minimizing osseointegration problems. Finally, magnesium implants can be used as a load-bearing scaffold being then an ideal candidate for BTE applications [111–113]. As a main drawback, magnesium biomaterials release hydrogen gas as a consequence of biodegradation which may prove dangerous under uncontrolled fast dissolution reaction rates [114]. Modeling and simulation of magnesium biodegradation is therefore identified as a useful assessment tool in the design phase of magnesium implants and BTE applications both to understand and control the dissolution process of such biomaterials. In this context, Grogan et al. [115,116] presented physically based continuum models, based on reaction–diffusion equations, available to analyze the corrosion of magnesium metal stents. A similar mathematical modeling was shown in [117] but using the level-set strategy to simulate the dissolution of the biomaterial. Sanz-Herrera et al. [118] developed a continuum model for the biodegradation of magnesium accounting for the dynamics and evolution of secondary species, such as pH or corrosion products. The model was qualitatively validated with previous results found in the literature (Figure 4).

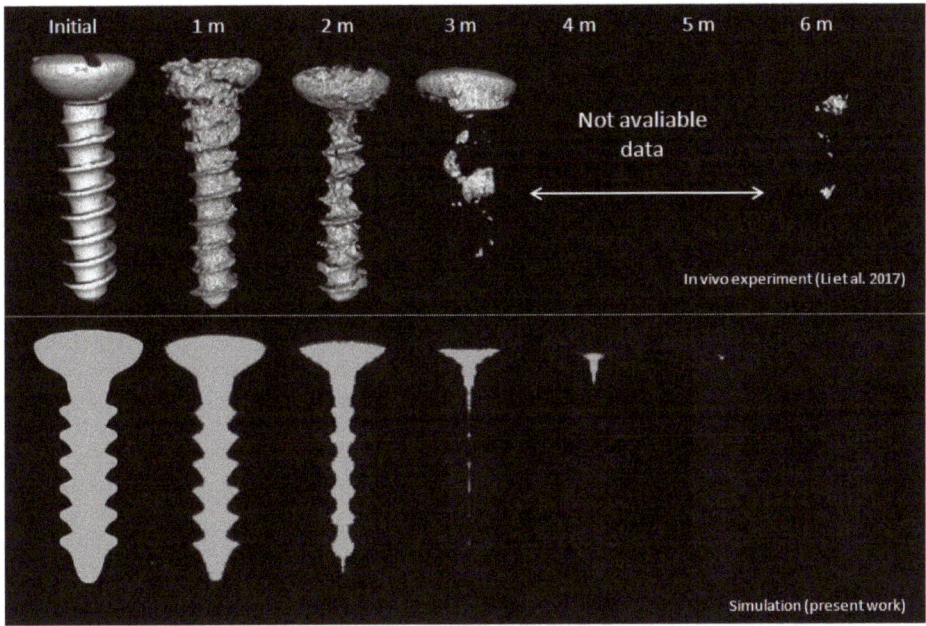

Figure 4. Validation of the simulation of magnesium screw degradation obtained by the mathematical modeling presented by Sanz-Herrera et al. [118] (**bottom**), compared with the experimental setup by Li et al. [119] (**top**). Reprinted with permission from [118].

The general continuum modeling framework proposed above based on reaction–diffusion equations, numerical implementation, and simulation has been applied to drug delivery systems [120]. Additional mathematical models have been proposed in this field in the last decades. Since this is not the focus of this paper, the reader is addressed to [121] for a review of models in drug delivery.

5. Perspectives

Continuum modeling and simulation in BTE has been proved to be a useful tool at several stages of the methodology according to the revised literature. On one hand, the design of the scaffold in terms of its desired characteristics, such as porosity, pore connectivity, permeability, or overall mechanical behavior, according to a specific application, has been a niche of research using numerical methods. The literature is nowadays vast regarding computer-aided scaffold design, and, traditionally, researchers involved in this part have not always been connected with the fabrication process, which has been performed in collaboration with biomaterial scientists. Currently, 3D printing has brought both fields together, and now computer design of scaffolds is usually complemented by 3D printing of prototypes and mechanical testing of the specimens in the lab [122]. In addition, bioprinting techniques, i.e., 3D printing technology using biological materials, are being explored as an alternative to traditional BTE [123–127]. Numerical methods can be particularly useful in this context for the design of the printing strategy and simulation of the biofabrication technique [128–133].

Other physical phenomena that are relevant to analyze in the design phase of a BTE product have not been treated and investigated in detail by computer simulation. These phenomena include biomaterial dissolution and biodegradation since a limited number of mathematical models have been presented in the literature, despite the clear advantages that introduce simulation-based design of degradable materials as concluded in the referred examples. This is a clear line for future research in the modeling of BTE.

On the other hand, the evolution of the scaffold in terms of tissue growth, tissue differentiation, and tissue–scaffold interaction has been extensively modeled and simulated in BTE applications in the last decades. Some elaborated models including multiscale, multiphasic, and multiphysics elements have been presented in several examples of interest, showing a great potential. First, the models predict in silico the performance of a certain in vivo applications by means of a virtual assay conducted in the computer. The simulation can be patient-specific accounting for the specific characteristics in hands. Second, in silico simulations reduce time and cost of the assays, as well as reducing animal experimentation with its subsequent ethical implications. However, the main drawback of the computer simulation of clinical BTE applications is the fact that the models are based on empirical laws of tissue growth and evolution. These theories have not been sufficiently validated although some of them were proposed several decades ago. It is therefore necessary to advance the validation of the models in connection with a multidisciplinary team of clinicians, veterinarians and biologists, by no means a trivial task. Model validation is then identified as another research line in BTE collateral to in silico BTE. Moreover, multiscale and multiphasic analyses have been limited by the computational cost of this kind of modeling. In particular, multiphasic models traditionally consider both the solid and fluid domains of the scaffold in a simplified way, either using diffusive or poroelastic approaches. A coupled CFD (fluid phase) and mechanical (solid phase) approach, including solid–fluid interaction, can be useful to account in a detailed fashion both the mechanobiological stimulus, as well as degradation phenomena that take place in the biomaterial.

Finally, even a model available for BTE simulation that has been validated at some conditions, may not be predictive in a different scenario. This fact is due to the highly phenomenological nature of this kind of continuum model. Usually, models for BTE include an average of 10–15 model parameters to be calibrated by experimental setups. It is therefore needed to establish a magnified and more fundamental observation scale in the continuum models, even lower than the pore scaffold scale; which allows to consider in a detailed fashion cell–biomaterial sensing and interaction, as well as specific functions of the cell such as proliferation, migration, or apoptosis. These models, posed at the cell scale, may violate the continuum assumption and other discrete models, such as agent-based models, including lattice or particle methods can be of application at this scale. Nonetheless, the discrete models defined at the cell scale may be useful at meso- or macroscopic continuum scale models by fitting complex correlations at this scale a priori or feeding with information at higher scales using a multiscale coupling approach.

6. Conclusions

Through this review, the usefulness and potential of continuum models and computer simulation, both in the in silico design of scaffolds for BTE and in the prediction of the evolution of bone tissue growth in BTE, have been demonstrated. Even though some issues regarding in silico design of scaffolds can be explored in more detail, these simulations are usually calibrated and contrasted with experimental results. On the other hand, the predictive capability of in silico models of applications of interest in BTE needs to be enhanced. The empirical mechanobiological rules underlying those models need further validation via interdisciplinary collaboration among the different involved researchers. In the improvement of the predictive capability of continuum approaches in BTE, it may help to pose the problem in a higher and magnified observation scale, and hence less phenomenological scale, using discrete numerical approaches such as agent-based modeling or molecular dynamics simulations. All these efforts may contribute to make BTE a clinical viable reality in the next years.

Author Contributions: J.A.S.-H. and E.R.-R. analyzed the state of the art in the field, discussed the previous work and perspectives, and wrote the review paper.

Funding: This research was funded by the Ministerio de Economía y Competitividad del Gobierno España, grant number DPI2017-82501-P.

Conflicts of Interest: The authors declare no conflict of interest.

References

1. Hutmacher, D.W. Scaffolds in tissue engineering bone and cartilage. *Biomaterials* **2000**, *21*, 2529–2543. [CrossRef]
2. Hing, K.A. Bone repair in the twenty-first century: Biology, chemistry or engineering? *Philos. Trans. R. Soc. A* **2004**, *362*, 2821–2850. [CrossRef] [PubMed]
3. Kato, A.; Aoki, H.; Tabata, T.; Ogiso, M. Biocompatibility of apatite ceramics mandibles. *Biomater. Med. Devices. Artif. Organs* **1979**, *7*, 291–297. [CrossRef] [PubMed]
4. Jarcho, M. Calcium phosphate ceramics as hard tissue prosthetics. *Clin. Ortho.* **1981**, *157*, 259–278. [CrossRef]
5. Eggli, P.S.; Muller, W.; Schenk, P.K. Porous hydroxyapatite and tricalcium phosphate cylinders with two different pore size ranges implanted in the cancellous bone of rabbits. A comparative histomorphometric and histology study of bony in-growth and implant substitution. *Clin. Ortho.* **1988**, *232*, 127–138. [CrossRef]
6. LeGeros, R.Z. Calcium phosphate materials in restorative dentistry. *Adv. Dent. Res.* **1988**, *2*, 164–180. [CrossRef] [PubMed]
7. Ohgushi, H.; Goldberg, V.M.; Caplan, A.I. Heterotopic osteogenesis in porous ceramics induced by marrow cells. *J. Ortho. Res.* **1989**, *7*, 568–578. [CrossRef]
8. Ohgushi, H.; Okumura, M.M.; Tamai, S.; Shors, E.C.; Caplan, A.I. Marrow cell induced osteogenesis in porous hydroxyapatite and tricalcium phosphate. *J. Biomed. Mat. Res.* **1990**, *24*, 1563–1570. [CrossRef]
9. Okumura, M.; Ohgushi, H.; Tamai, S. Bonding osteogenesis in coralline hydroxyapatite combined with bone marrow cells. *Biomaterials* **1991**, *12*, 411–416. [CrossRef]
10. Ohgushi, H.; Dohi, Y.; Yoshikawa, T.; Tamai, S.; Tabata, S.; Okunaga, K.; Shibuya, T. Osteogenic differentiation of cultured marrow stromal stem cells on the surface of bioactive glass ceramic. *J. Biomed. Mater. Res.* **1996**, *32*, 341–348. [CrossRef]
11. Rezwan, K.; Chen, Q.Z.; Blaker, J.J.; Boccaccini, A.R. Biodegradable and bioactive porous polymer/inorganic composite scaffolds for bone tissue engineering. *Biomaterials* **2006**, *27*, 3413–3431. [CrossRef] [PubMed]
12. Hench, L.L.; Splinter, R.J.; Allen, W.C. Bonding mechanisms at the interface of ceramic prosthetic materials. *J. Biomed. Mater. Res. Symp.* **1971**, *2*, 117–141. [CrossRef]
13. Hench, L.L. Bioceramics. *J. Am. Ceram. Soc.* **1998**, *81*, 1705–1728. [CrossRef]
14. Chen, Q.Z.; Boccaccini, A.R. Poly(D,L-lactic acid) coated 45S5 Bioglass®-based R-based scaffolds: Processing and characterization. *J. Biomed. Mat. Res. A* **2006**, *77*, 445–457. [CrossRef] [PubMed]
15. Mastrogiacomo, M.; Muraglia, A.; Komlev, V.; Peyrin, F.; Rustichelli, F.; Crovace, A.; Cancedda, R. Tissue engineering of bone: Search for a better scaffold. *Orthod. Craniofac. Res.* **2005**, *8*, 277–284. [CrossRef]
16. Mastrogiacomo, M.; Papadimitropoulos, A.; Cedola, A.; Peyrin, F.; Giannoni, P.; Pearce, S.G.; Alini, M.; Giannini, C.; Guagliardi, A.; Cancedda, R. Engineering of bone using bone marrow stromal cells and a silicon-stabilized tricalcium phosphate bioceramic: Evidence for a coupling between bone formation and scaffold resorption. *Biomaterials* **2007**, *28*, 1376–1384. [CrossRef] [PubMed]
17. Fialkov, J.A.; Holy, C.E.; Shoichet, M.S.; Davies, J.E. In vivo bone engineering in a rabbit femur. *J. Craniofac. Surg.* **2003**, *14*, 324–332. [CrossRef]
18. Holy, C.E.; Fialkov, J.A.; Davies, J.E.; Shoichet, M.S. Use of a biomimetic strategy to engineer bone. *J. Biomed. Mater. Res. A* **2003**, *65*, 447–453. [CrossRef]
19. Zhou, Y.; Chen, F.; Ho, S.T.; Woodruff, M.A.; Lim, T.M.; Hutmacher, D.W. Combined marrow stromal cell-sheet techniques and high-strength biodegradable composite scaffolds for engineered functional bone grafts. *Biomaterials* **2007**, *28*, 814–824. [CrossRef]

20. Savarino, L.; Baldini, N.; Greco, M.; Capitani, O.; Pinna, S.; Valentini, S.; Lombardo, B.; Esposito, M.T.; Pastore, L.; Ambrosio, L.; et al. The performance of poly-e-caprolactone scaffolds in a rabbit femur model with and without autologous stromal cells and BMP4. *Biomaterials* **2007**, *28*, 3101–3109. [CrossRef]
21. Bassett, C.A.L. Biologic significance of piezoelectricity. *Calcif. Tissue Int.* **1967**, *1*, 252–272. [CrossRef]
22. Rajabi, A.H.; Jaffe, M.; Arinzeh, T.L. Piezoelectric materials for tissue regeneration: A review. *Acta Biomater.* **2015**, *24*, 12–23. [CrossRef] [PubMed]
23. Beaupre, G.S.; Orr, T.E.; Carter, D.R. An approach for time-dependent bone modelling and remodelling: Theoretical development. *J. Orthop. Res.* **1990**, *8*, 651–661. [CrossRef] [PubMed]
24. Hollister, S.J.; Maddox, R.D.; Taboas, J.M. Optimal design and fabrication of scaffolds to mimic tissue properties and satisfy biological constraints. *Biomaterials* **2002**, *23*, 4095–4103. [CrossRef]
25. Lin, C.Y.; Kikuchi, N.; Hollister, S.J. A novel method for biomaterial scaffold internal architecture design to match bone elastic properties with desired porosity. *J. Biomech.* **2004**, *37*, 623–636. [CrossRef]
26. Taboas, J.M.; Maddox, R.D.; Krebsbach, P.H.; Hollister, S.J. Indirect solid free form fabrication of local and global porous, biomimetic and composite 3D polymer-ceramic scaffolds. *Biomaterials* **2003**, *24*, 181–194. [CrossRef]
27. Sanz-Herrera, J.A.; Kasper, C.; van Griensven, M.; Garcia-Aznar, J.M.; Ochoa, I.; Doblare, M. Mechanical and flow characterization of Sponceram® carriers: Evaluation by homogenization theory and experimental validation. *J. Biomed. Mater. Res. B* **2008**, *87*, 42–48. [CrossRef]
28. Sturm, S.; Zhou, S.; Mai, Y.W.; Li, Q. On stiffness of scaffolds for bone tissue engineering-a numerical study. *J. Biomech.* **2010**, *43*, 1738–1744. [CrossRef]
29. Coelho, P.G.; Hollister, S.J.; Flanagan, C.L.; Fernandes, P.R. Bioresorbable scaffolds for bone tiss engineering: Optimal design, fabrication, mechanicaltesting and scale-size effects analysis. *Med. Eng. Phys.* **2015**, *37*, 287–296. [CrossRef]
30. Ranganathan, S.I.; Yoon, D.M.; Henslee, A.M.; Nair, M.B.; Smid, C.; Kasper, F.K.; Tasciotti, E.; Mikos, A.G.; Decuzzi, P.; Ferrari, M. Shaping the micromechanical behavior of multi-phase composites for bone tissue engineering. *Acta Biomater.* **2010**, *6*, 3448–3456. [CrossRef]
31. Scheiner, S.; Sinibaldi, R.; Pichler, B.; Komlev, V.; Renghini, C.; Vitale-Brovarone, C.; Rustichelli, F.; Hellmich, C. Micromechanics of bone tissue-engineering scaffolds, based on resolution error-cleared computer tomography. *Biomaterials* **2009**, *30*, 2411–2419. [CrossRef] [PubMed]
32. Fritsch, A.; Dormieux, L.; Hellmich, C.; Sanahuja, J. Mechanical behavior of hydroxyapatite biomaterials: An experimentally validated micromechanical model for elasticity and strength. *J. Biomed. Mater. Res. A* **2009**, *88*, 149–161. [CrossRef] [PubMed]
33. Kariem, H.; Pastrama, M.I.; Roohani-Esfahani, S.I.; Pivonka, P.; Zreiqat, H.; Hellmich, C. Micro-poro-elasticity of baghdadite-based bone tissue engineering scaffolds: A unifying approach based on ultrasonics, nanoindentation, and homogenization theory. *Mater. Sci. Eng. C Mater. Biol. Appl.* **2015**, *46*, 553–564. [CrossRef] [PubMed]
34. Scheiner, S.; Komlev, V.S.; Hellmich, C. Computational methods for the predictive design of bone tissue engineering scaffolds. In *3D Printing and Biofabrication*; Springer: Berlin/Heidelberg, Germany, 2018.
35. Chen, Y.; Schellekens, M.; Zhou, S.; Cadman, J.; Li, W.; Appleyard, R.; Li, Q. Design optimization of scaffold microstructures using shear stress criterion towards regulated flow-induced erosion. *J. Biomech. Eng.* **2011**, *133*, 081008. [CrossRef] [PubMed]
36. Boccaccio, A.; Uva, A.E.; Fiorentino, M.; Monno, G.; Ballini, A.; Desiate, A. Optimal load for bone tissue scaffolds with an assigned geometry. *Int. J. Med. Sci.* **2018**, *15*, 16–22. [CrossRef] [PubMed]
37. Egan, P.F.; Gonella, V.C.; Engensperger, M.; Ferguson, S.J.; Shea, K. Computationally designed lattices with tuned properties for tissue engineering using 3D printing. *PLoS ONE* **2017**, *12*, e0182902. [CrossRef] [PubMed]
38. Castro, A.P.G.; Lacroix, D. Micromechanical study of the load transfer in a polycaprolactone-collagen hybrid scaffold when subjected to unconfined and confined compression. *Biomech. Model. Mechanobiol.* **2018**, *17*, 531–541. [CrossRef] [PubMed]
39. Prendergast, P.J.; Huiskes, R.; Søballe, K. Biophysical stimuli on cells during tissue ifferentiation at implant interfaces. *J. Biomech.* **1997**, *30*, 539–548. [CrossRef]
40. Kelly, D.J.; Prendergast, P.J. Prediction of the optimal mechanical properties for a scaffold used in osteochondral defect repair. *Tissue Eng.* **2006**, *12*, 2509–2519. [CrossRef]

41. Olivares, A.L.; Marsal, E.; Planell, J.A.; Lacroix, D. Finite element study of scaffold architecture design and culture conditions for tissue engineering. *Biomaterials* **2009**, *30*, 6142–6149. [CrossRef] [PubMed]
42. Khayyeri, H.; Checa, S.; Tägil, M.; Prendergast, P.J. Corroboration of mechanobiological simulations of tissue differentiation in an in vivo bone chamber using a lattice-modeling approach. *J. Orthop. Res.* **2009**, *27*, 1659–1666. [CrossRef] [PubMed]
43. Sandino, C.; Lacroix, D. A dynamical study of the mechanical stimuli and tissue differentiation within a CaP scaffold based on micro-CT finite element models. *Biomech. Model. Mechanobiol.* **2011**, *10*, 565–576. [CrossRef] [PubMed]
44. Sandino, C.; Checa, S.; Prendergast, P.J.; Lacroix, D. Simulation of angiogenesis and cell differentiation in a CaP scaffold subjected to compressive strains using a lattice modeling approach. *Biomaterials* **2010**, *31*, 2446–2452. [CrossRef] [PubMed]
45. Checa, S.; Prendergast, P.J. Effect of cell seeding and mechanical loading on vascularization and tissue formation inside a scaffold: A mechanobiological model using a lattice approach to simulate cell activity. *J. Biomech.* **2010**, *43*, 961–968. [CrossRef] [PubMed]
46. Milan, J.L.; Planell, J.A.; Lacroix, D. Computational modelling of the mechanical environment of osteogenesis within a polylactic acid–calcium phosphate glass scaffold. *Biomaterials* **2009**, *30*, 4219–4226. [CrossRef] [PubMed]
47. Milan, J.L.; Planell, J.A.; Lacroix, D. Simulation of bone tissue formation within a porous scaffold under dynamic compression. *Biomech. Model Mechanobiol.* **2010**, *9*, 583–596. [CrossRef]
48. Hendrikson, W.J.; van Blitterswijk, C.A.; Verdonschot, N.; Moroni, L.; Rouwkema, J. Modeling mechanical signals on the surface of microCT and CAD based rapid prototype scaffold models to predict (early stage) tissue development. *Biotechnol. Bioeng.* **2014**, *111*, 1864–1875. [CrossRef] [PubMed]
49. Hutmacher, D.W.; Singh, H. Computational fluid dynamics for improved bioreactor design and 3D culture. *Trends Biotechnol.* **2008**, *26*, 166–172. [CrossRef]
50. Hossain, M.S.; Chen, X.B.; Bergstrom, D.J. Investigation of the in vitro culture process for skeletal-tissue-engineered constructs using computational fluid dynamics and experimental methods. *J. Biomech. Eng.* **2012**, *134*, 121003. [CrossRef]
51. Patrachari, A.R.; Podichetty, J.T.; Madihally, S.V. Application of computational fluid dynamics in tissue engineering. *J. Biosci. Bioeng.* **2012**, *114*, 123–132. [CrossRef]
52. Voronov, R.; VanGordon, S.; Sikavitsas, V.I.; Papavassiliou, D.V. Computational modeling of flow-induced shear stresses within 3D salt-leached porous scaffolds imaged via micro-CT. *J. Biomech.* **2010**, *43*, 1279–1286. [CrossRef] [PubMed]
53. Hendrikson, W.J.; Deegan, A.J.; Yang, Y.; van Blitterswijk, C.A.; Verdonschot, N.; Moroni, L.; Rouwkema, J. Influence of additive manufactured scaffold architecture on the distribution of surface strains and fluid flow shear stresses and expected osteochondral cell differentiation. *Front. Bioeng. Biotechnol.* **2017**, *5*, 6. [CrossRef] [PubMed]
54. Raimondi, M.T.; Bridgen, D.T.; Laganà, M.; Cioffi, M.; Boschetti, F. Integration of experimental and computational microfluidics in 3D tissue engineering. In *Methods in Bioengineering: 3D Tissue Engineering*. Boston: Artech House; Berthiaume, F., Morgan, J., Eds.; Artech House: Norwood, MA, USA, 2010; pp. 237–252.
55. Sadir, S.; Kadir, M.R.A.; Harun, M.N. Simulation of direct perfusión through 3D cellular scaffolds with different porosity. *Bioinformatics* **2011**, *5*, 123–126.
56. Sikavitsas, V.I.; Bancroft, G.N.; Holtorf, H.L.; Jansen, J.A.; Mikos, A.G. Mineralized matrix deposition by marrow stromal osteoblasts in 3D perfusion culture increases with increasing fluid shear forces. *Proc. Natl. Acad. Sci. USA* **2003**, *100*, 14683–14688. [CrossRef] [PubMed]
57. Holtorf, H.L.; Jansen, J.A.; Mikos, A.G. Flow perfusion culture induces the osteoblastic differentiation of marrow stromal cell-scaffold constructs in the absence of dexamethasone. *J. Biomed. Mater. Res. A* **2005**, *72*, 326–334. [CrossRef] [PubMed]
58. Stolberg, S.; McCloskey, K.E. Can shear stress direct stem cell fate? *Biotechnol. Prog.* **2009**, *25*, 10–19. [CrossRef] [PubMed]
59. Kreke, M.R.; Sharp, L.A.; Lee, Y.W.; Goldstein, A.S. Effect of intermittent shear stress on mechanotransductive signaling and osteoblastic differentiation of bone marrow stromal cells. *Tissue Eng. Part. A* **2008**, *14*, 529–537. [CrossRef] [PubMed]

60. Sonnaert, M.; Papantoniou, I.; Bloemen, V.; Kerckhofs, G.; Luyten, F.P.; Schrooten, J. Human periosteal-derived cell expansion in a perfusion bioreactor system: Proliferation, differentiation and extracellular matrix formation. *J. Tissue Eng. Regen. Med.* **2017**, *11*, 519–530. [CrossRef]
61. Nava, M.M.; Raimondi, M.T.; Pietrabissa, R. A multiphysics 3D model of tissue growth under interstitial perfusion in a tissue-engineering bioreactor. *Biomech. Model. Mechanobiol.* **2013**, *12*, 1169–1179. [CrossRef]
62. Zhao, F.; van Rietbergen, B.; Ito, K.; Hofmann, S. Flow rates in perfusion bioreactors to maximise mineralisation in bone tissue engineering in vitro. *J. Biomech.* **2018**, *79*, 232–237. [CrossRef]
63. Byrne, D.P.; Lacroix, D.; Planell, J.A.; Kelly, D.J.; Prendergast, P.J. Simulation of tissue differentiation in a scaffold as a function of porosity, Young's modulus and dissolution rate: Application of mechanobiological models in tissue engineering. *Biomaterials* **2007**, *28*, 5544–5554. [CrossRef] [PubMed]
64. Adachi, T.; Osako, Y.; Tanaka, M.; Hojo, M.; Hollister, S.J. Framework for optimal design of porous scaffold microstructure by computational simulation of bone regeneration. *Biomaterials* **2006**, *27*, 3964–3972. [CrossRef] [PubMed]
65. Adachi, T.; Tsubota, K.I.; Tomita, Y.; Hollister, S.J. Trabecular surface remodeling simulation for cancellous bone using microstructural voxel finite element models. *J. Biomech. Eng. T ASME* **2001**, *123*, 403–409. [CrossRef] [PubMed]
66. Comisar, W.A.; Kazmers, N.H.; Mooney, D.J.; Linderman, J.J. Engineering RGD nanopatterned hydrogels to control preosteoblast behavior: A combined computational and experimental approach. *Biomaterials* **2007**, *28*, 4409–4417. [CrossRef] [PubMed]
67. Chen, V.J.; Smith, L.A.; Ma, P.X. Bone regeneration on computer-designed nano-fibrous scaffolds. *Biomaterials* **2006**, *27*, 3973–3979. [CrossRef] [PubMed]
68. Sanz-Herrera, J.A.; García-Aznar, J.M.; Doblaré, M. Micro–macro numerical modelling of bone regeneration in tissue engineering. *Comput. Methods Appl. Mech. Eng.* **2008**, *197*, 3092–3107. [CrossRef]
69. Sanz-Herrera, J.A.; García-Aznar, J.M.; Doblaré, M. On scaffold designing for bone regeneration: A computational multiscale approach. *Acta Biomater.* **2009**, *5*, 219–229. [CrossRef] [PubMed]
70. Shipley, R.J.; Jones, G.W.; Dyson, R.J.; Sengers, B.G.; Bailey, C.L.; Catt, C.J.; Please, C.P.; Malda, J. Design criteria for a printed tissue engineering construct: A mathematical homogenization approach. *J. Theor. Biol.* **2009**, *259*, 489–502. [CrossRef]
71. Chan, K.S.; Liang, W.; Francis, W.L.; Nicolella, D.P. A multiscale modeling approach to scaffold design and property prediction. *J. Mech. Behav. Biomed. Mat.* **2010**, *3*, 584–593. [CrossRef]
72. Sanz-Herrera, J.A.; García-Aznar, J.M.; Doblaré, M. Scaffold microarchitecture determines internal bone directional growth structure: A numerical study. *J. Biomech.* **2010**, *43*, 2480–2486. [CrossRef]
73. Sanz-Herrera, J.A.; García-Aznar, J.M.; Doblaré, M. A mathematical approach to bone tissue engineering. *Proc. R. Soc. A* **2009**, *367*, 2055–2078. [CrossRef] [PubMed]
74. Nguyen, T.K.; Carpentier, O.; Monchau, F.; Chai, F.; Hornez, J.C.; Hivart, P. Numerical optimization of cell colonization modelling inside scaffold for perfusion bioreactor: A multiscale model. *Med. Eng. Phys.* **2018**, *57*, 40–50. [CrossRef] [PubMed]
75. Liu, Y.; Chan, J.K.; Teoh, S.H. Review of vascularised bone tissue-engineering strategies with a focus on co-culture systems. *J. Tissue Eng. Regen. Med.* **2015**, *9*, 85–105. [CrossRef] [PubMed]
76. Shimko, D.A.; Nauman, E.A. Development and characterization of a porous poly(methyl methracrylate) scaffold with controllable modulus and permeability. *J. Biomed. Mater. Res.* **2007**, *80*, 360–369. [CrossRef] [PubMed]
77. Swider, P.; Conroy, M.; Pedrono, A.; Ambard, D.; Mantell, S.; Søballe, K.; Bechtold, J.E. Use of high-resolution MRI for investigation of fluid flow and global permeability in a material with interconnected porosity. *J. Biomech.* **2007**, *40*, 2112–2118. [CrossRef] [PubMed]
78. Li, S.; de Wijn, J.R.; Li, J.; Layrolle, P.; de Groot, K. Macroporous biphasic calcium phosphate scaffold with high permeability/porosity ratio. *Tissue Eng.* **2003**, *9*, 535–548. [CrossRef]
79. Shimko, D.A.; Shimko, V.F.; Sander, E.A.; Dickson, K.F.; Nauman, E.A. Effect of porosity on the fluid flow characteristics and mechanical properties of tantalum scaffolds. *J. Biomed. Mater. Res.* **2005**, *73*, 315–324. [CrossRef]
80. Ochoa, I.; Sanz-Herrera, J.A.; García-Aznar, J.M.; Doblaré, M.; Yunos, D.M.; Boccaccini, A.R. Permeability evaluation of 45S5 Bioglass®-based scaffolds for bone tissue engineering. *J. Biomech.* **2009**, *42*, 257–260. [CrossRef]

81. Chor, M.V.; Li, W. A permeability measurement system for tissue engineering scaffolds. *Meas. Sci. Technol.* **2007**, *18*, 208–216. [CrossRef]
82. Truscello, S.; Kerckhofs, G.; Van Bael, S.; Pyka, G.; Schrooten, J.; Van Oosterwyck, H. Prediction of permeability of regular scaffolds for skeletal tissue engineering: A combined computational and experimental study. *Acta Biomater.* **2012**, *8*, 1648–1658. [CrossRef]
83. Syahrom, A.; Abdul Kadir, M.R.; Abdullah, J.; Öchsner, A. Permeability studies of artificial and natural cancellous bone structures. *Med. Eng. Phys.* **2013**, *35*, 792–799. [CrossRef] [PubMed]
84. Acosta Santamaría, V.A.; Malvè, M.; Duizabo, A.; Mena Tobar, A.; Gallego Ferrer, G.; García Aznar, J.M.; Doblaré, M.; Ochoa, I. Computational methodology to determine fluid related parameters of non regular three-dimensional scaffolds. *Ann. Biomed. Eng.* **2013**, *41*, 2367–2380. [CrossRef] [PubMed]
85. Olivares, A.L.; Lacroix, D. Computational methods in the modeling of scaffolds for tissue engineering. In *Computational Modeling in Tissue Engineering. Studies in Mechanobiology, Tissue Engineering and Biomaterials*; Geris, L., Ed.; Springer: Berlin/Heidelberg, Germany, 2012; Volume 10.
86. Li, E.; Chang, C.C.; Zhang, Z.; Li, Q. Characterization of tissue scaffolds for time dependent biotransport criteria—A novel computational procedure. *Comput. Methods Biomech. Biomed. Eng.* **2016**, *19*, 210–224. [CrossRef] [PubMed]
87. Lemon, G.; King, J.R.; Byrne, M.H.; Jensen, O.E.; Shakesheff, K.M. Mathematical modelling of engineered tissue growth using a multiphase porous flow mixture theory. *J. Math. Biol.* **2006**, *52*, 571–594. [CrossRef] [PubMed]
88. Lemon, G.; King, J.R. Multiphase modelling of cell behaviour on artificial scaffolds: Effects of nutrient depletion and spatially nonuniform porosity. *Math. Med. Biol.* **2007**, *24*, 57–83. [CrossRef] [PubMed]
89. Mohebbi-Kalhori, D.; Behzadmehr, A.; Doillon, C.J.; Hadjizadeh, A. Computational modeling of adherent cell growth in a hollow-fiber membrane bioreactor for large-scale 3-D bone tissue engineering. *J. Artif. Organs* **2012**, *15*, 250–265. [CrossRef] [PubMed]
90. Pego, A.P.; Siebum, B.; Van Luyn, M.J.; Gallego Van Seijen, X.J.; Poot, A.A.; Grijpma, D.W.; Feijen, J. Preparation of degradable porous structures based on 1,3-trimethylene carbonate and D,L-lactide (co)polymers for heart tissue engineering. *Tissue Eng.* **2003**, *9*, 981–994. [CrossRef]
91. Shin, M.; Ishii, O.; Sueda, T.; Vacanti, J.P. Contractile cardiac grafts using a novel nanofibrous mesh. *Biomaterials* **2004**, *25*, 3717–3723. [CrossRef] [PubMed]
92. Ishii, O.; Shin, M.; Sueda, T.; Vacanti, J.P. In vitro tissue engineering of a cardiac graft using a degradable scaffold with an extracellular matrix-like topography. *J. Thorac. Cardiovasc. Surg.* **2005**, *130*, 1358–1363. [CrossRef]
93. Zong, X.; Bien, H.; Chung, C.Y.; Yin, L.; Fang, D.; Hsiao, B.S.; Chu, B.; Entcheva, E. Electrospun fine-textured scaffolds for heart tissue constructs. *Biomaterials* **2005**, *26*, 5330–5338. [CrossRef]
94. Carrier, R.L.; Rupnick, M.; Langer, R.; Schoen, F.J.; Freed, L.E.; Vunjak Novakovic, G. Perfusion improves tissue architecture of engineered cardiac muscle. *Tissue Eng.* **2002**, *8*, 175–188. [CrossRef] [PubMed]
95. Carrier, R.L.; Rupnick, M.; Langer, R.; Schoen, F.J.; Freed, L.E.; Vunjak Novakovic, G. Effects of oxygen on engineered cardiac muscle. *Biotechnol. Bioeng.* **2002**, *78*, 617–625. [CrossRef] [PubMed]
96. Schrumpf, M.A.; Lee, A.T.; Weiland, A.J. Foreign-body reaction and osteolysis induced by an intraosseous poly-L-lactic Acid suture anchor in the wrist: Case report. *J. Hand Surg. Am.* **2011**, *36*, 1769–1773. [CrossRef]
97. Gopferich, A. Polymer bulk erosion. *Macromolecules* **1997**, *30*, 2598–2604. [CrossRef]
98. Wang, Y.; Pan, J.; Han, X.; Sinka, C.; Ding, L. A phenomenological model for the degradation of biodegradable polymers. *Biomaterials* **2009**, *29*, 3393–3401. [CrossRef]
99. Han, X.; Pan, J. A model for simultaneous crystallisation and biodegradation of biodegradable polymers. *Biomaterials* **2009**, *30*, 423–430. [CrossRef]
100. Dhote, V.; Vernerey, F.J. Mathematical model of the role of degradation on matrix development in hydrogel scaffold. *Biomech. Model. Mechanobiol.* **2004**, *13*, 167–183. [CrossRef]
101. Akalp, U.; Bryant, S.J.; Vernerey, F.J. Tuning tissue growth with scaffold degradation in enzyme-sensitive hydrogels: A mathematical model. *Soft Matter* **2016**, *12*, 7505–7520. [CrossRef]
102. Chen, Y.; Zhou, S.; Li, Q. Mathematical modeling of degradation for bulk-erosive polymers: Applications in tissue engineering scaffolds and drug delivery systems. *Acta Biomater.* **2011**, *7*, 1140–1149. [CrossRef]
103. Hench, L.L.; Paschall, H.A. Direct chemical bond of bioactive glass ceramic materials to bone and muscle. *J. Biomed. Mater. Res. Symp.* **1973**, *4*, 25–42. [CrossRef]

104. Wilson, J.; Low, S.B. Bioactive ceramics for periodontal treatment: Comparative studies in the Patus monkey. *J. Appl. Biomater.* **1992**, *3*, 123–169. [CrossRef] [PubMed]
105. Hench, L.L.; West, J.K. Biological applications of bioactive glasses. *Life Chem. Rep.* **1996**, *13*, 187–241.
106. Roether, J.A.; Boccaccini, A.R.; Hench, L.L.; Maquet, V.; Gautier, S.; Jerome, R. Development and in vitro characterisation of novel bioresorbable and bioactive composite materials based on polylactide foams and bioglasss for tissue engineering applications. *Biomaterials* **2002**, *23*, 3871–3878. [CrossRef]
107. Chen, Q.Z.; Thompson, I.D.; Boccaccini, A.R. 45S5 Bioglass derived glass-ceramic scaffolds for bone tissue engineering. *Biomaterials* **2006**, *27*, 2414–2425. [CrossRef] [PubMed]
108. Sanz-Herrera, J.A.; Boccaccini, A.R. Modelling bioactivity and degradation of bioactive glass based tissue engineering scaffolds. *Int. J. Solids Struct.* **2011**, *48*, 257–268. [CrossRef]
109. Manhas, V.; Guyot, Y.; Kerckhofs, G.; Chai, Y.C.; Geris, L. Computational modelling of local calcium ions release from calcium phosphate-based scaffolds. *Biomech. Model. Mechanobiol.* **2017**, *16*, 425–438. [CrossRef] [PubMed]
110. Sanz-Herrera, J.A.; Soria, L.; Reina-Romo, E.; Torres, Y.; Boccaccini, A.R. Model of dissolution in the framework of tissue engineering and drug delivery. *Biomech. Model. Mechanobiol.* **2018**, *17*, 1331–1341. [CrossRef]
111. Kraus, T.; Fischerauer, S.F.; Hänzi, A.C.; Uggowitzer, P.J.; Löffler, J.F.; Weinberg, A.M. Magnesium alloys for temporary implants in osteosynthesis: In vivo studies of their degradation and interaction with bone. *Acta Biomater.* **2012**, *8*, 1230–1238. [CrossRef]
112. Brar, H.S.; Platt, M.O.; Sarntinoranont, M.; Martin, P.I.; Manuel, M.V. Magnesium as a biodegradable and bioabsorbable material for medical implants. *JOM* **2009**, *61*, 31–34. [CrossRef]
113. Castellani, C.; Lindtner, R.A.; Hausbrandt, P.; Tschegg, E.; Stanzl-Tschegg, S.E.; Zanoni, G.; Beck, S.; Weinberg, A.M. Bone-implant interface strength and osseointegration: Biodegradable magnesium alloy versus standard titanium control. *Acta Biomater.* **2011**, *7*, 432–440. [CrossRef]
114. Staiger, M.P.; Pietak, A.M.; Huadmai, J.; Dias, G. Magnesium and its alloys as orthopedic biomaterials: A review. *Biomaterials* **2006**, *27*, 1728–1734. [CrossRef] [PubMed]
115. Grogan, J.A.; Brien, B.J.O.; Leen, S.B.; McHugh, P.E. A corrosion model for bioabsorbable metallic stents. *Acta Biomater.* **2011**, *7*, 3523–3533. [CrossRef] [PubMed]
116. Grogan, J.A.; Leen, S.B.; McHugh, P.E. A physical corrosion model for bioabsorbable metal stents. *Acta Biomater.* **2014**, *10*, 2313–2322. [CrossRef] [PubMed]
117. Bajger, P.; Ashbourn, J.M.A.; Manhas, V.; Guyot, Y.; Lietaert, K.; Geris, L. Mathematical modelling of the degradation behaviour of biodegradable metals. *Biomech. Model. Mechanobiol.* **2017**, *16*, 227–238. [CrossRef] [PubMed]
118. Sanz-Herrera, J.A.; Reina-Romo, E.; Boccaccini, A.R. In silico design of magnesium implants: Macroscopic modeling. *J. Mech. Behav. Biomed. Mater.* **2018**, *79*, 181–188. [CrossRef] [PubMed]
119. Li, Z.; Sun, S.; Chen, M.; Fahlman, B.D.; Liu, D.; Bi, H. In vitro and in vivo corrosion, mechanical properties and biocompatibility evaluation of MgF_2-coated MgZn-Zr alloy as cancellous screws. *Mater. Sci. Eng. C* **2017**, *75*, 1268–1280. [CrossRef] [PubMed]
120. Frenning, G.; Brohede, U.; Stromme, M. Finite element analysis of the release of slowly dissolving drugs from cylindrical matrix systems. *J. Control. Release* **2005**, *107*, 320–329. [CrossRef]
121. Peppas, N.A.; Narasimhan, B. Mathematical models in drug delivery: How modeling has shaped the way we design new drug delivery systems. *J. Control. Release* **2014**, *190*, 75–81. [CrossRef]
122. Mozafari, M.; Sefat, F.; Atala, A. *Handbook of Tissue Engineering Scaffolds*; Elsevier: Amsterdam, The Netherlands, 2019; Volume 1, ISBN 9780081025642.
123. Visconti, R.P.; Kasyanov, V.; Gentile, C.; Zhang, J.; Markwald, R.R.; Mironov, V. Towards organ printing: Engineering an intra-organ branched vascular tree. *Expert. Opin. Biol. Ther.* **2010**, *10*, 409–420. [CrossRef]
124. Derby, B. Printing and prototyping of tissues and scaffolds. *Science* **2012**, *338*, 921–992. [CrossRef] [PubMed]
125. Murphy, S.V.; Atala, A. 3D bioprinting of tissues and organs. *Nat. Biotechnol.* **2014**, *32*, 773–785. [CrossRef] [PubMed]
126. Dababneh, A.B.; Ozbolat, I.T. Bioprinting technology: A current state-of-the-art review. *J. Manuf. Sci. Eng.* **2014**, *136*, 061016. [CrossRef]
127. Mandrycky, C.; Wang, Z.; Kim, K.; Kim, D.H. 3D bioprinting for engineering complex tissues. *Biotechnol. Adv.* **2016**, *34*, 422–434. [CrossRef] [PubMed]

128. Li, M.; Tian, X.; Schreyer, D.J.; Chen, X. Effect of needle geometry on flow rate and cell damage in the dispensing-based biofabrication process. *Biotechnol. Prog.* **2011**, *27*, 1777–1784. [CrossRef]
129. Guyot, Y.; Papantoniou, I.; Chai, Y.C.; Van Bael, S.; Schrooten, J.; Geris, L. A computational model for cell/ECM growth on 3D surfaces using the level set method: A bone tissue engineering case study. *Biomech. Model. Mechanobiol.* **2014**, *13*, 1361–1371. [CrossRef] [PubMed]
130. Guyot, Y.; Luyten, F.P.; Schrooten, J.; Papantoniou, I.; Geris, L. A three dimensional computational fluid dynamics model of shear stress distribution during neotissue growth in a perfusion bioreactor. *Biotechnol. Bioeng.* **2015**, *112*, 2591–2600. [CrossRef]
131. Guyot, Y.; Papantoniou, I.; Luyten, F.P.; Geris, L. Coupling curvature dependent and shear stress-stimulated neotissue growth in dynamic bioreactor cultures: A 3D computational model of a complete scaffold. *Biomech. Model. Mechanobiol.* **2016**, *15*, 169–180. [CrossRef]
132. Billiet, T.; Gevaert, E.; De Schryver, T.; Cornelissen, M.; Dubruel, P. The 3D printing of gelatin methacrylamide cell-laden tissue-engineered constructs with high cell viability. *Biomaterials* **2014**, *35*, 49–62. [CrossRef]
133. Reina-Romo, E.; Papantoniou, I.; Bloemen, V.; Geris, L. Computational design of tissue engineering scaffolds. In *Handbook of Tissue Engineering Scaffolds*; Elsevier: Amsterdam, The Netherlands, 2019.

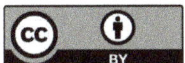

© 2019 by the authors. Licensee MDPI, Basel, Switzerland. This article is an open access article distributed under the terms and conditions of the Creative Commons Attribution (CC BY) license (http://creativecommons.org/licenses/by/4.0/).

MDPI
St. Alban-Anlage 66
4052 Basel
Switzerland
Tel. +41 61 683 77 34
Fax +41 61 302 89 18
www.mdpi.com

Applied Sciences Editorial Office
E-mail: applsci@mdpi.com
www.mdpi.com/journal/applsci

www.ingramcontent.com/pod-product-compliance
Lightning Source LLC
LaVergne TN
LVHW070432100526
838202LV00014B/1584